CONSUMER GUIDE®

The Diet Cookbook

Your Guide to Calorie-Wise Gourmet Cooking

Library of Congress Cataloging in Publication Data

Gibbons, Barbara
    Consumer guide the diet cookbook.

    Includes index.
        1. Cookery. 2. Diet. 3. Consumer education.
I. Consumer guide. II. Title. III. Title: The
diet cookbook.
TX652.G5   641.1   75-11990
ISBN 0-671-22052-7
ISBN 0-671-22053-5 pbk.

Compiled by the Editors of CONSUMER GUIDE
Magazine and published in this edition by New
American Library, New York, NY.

About the Author

Barbara Gibbons is known as "The Slim Gourmet" in a nationally syndicated newspaper column. She also writes the monthly *Family Circle* magazine column, "Creative Low-Calorie Cooking." Mrs. Gibbons weighed over 200 pounds as a teenager. She had to wear a nurse's uniform to her high school graduation because she could not find a white dress in size 20½. She says she lost weight only when she became interested in food and started creating variations of classic gourmet recipes without unnecessary calories. Now, she wears a size 9. Mrs. Gibbons stays slender by following the method of *The Diet Cookbook*: elimination of unneeded calories from favorite recipes.

About the Cover

The "Cheese Pie" on the cover is a perfect example of a classic recipe which has been de-calorized for slim gourmets. The recipe for this mouth-watering dessert can be found in the chapter "Unforbidden Sweets."

Cover design: Frank E. Peiler

Lawrence Teeman
Editor and Publisher

Louis Weber
President

Staff: A.K. Turley, managing editor; Jerold L. Kellman, senior managing editor; Kay Conlon, production editor; Peter Du Pre, editor; Arthur Hammerstrom, editor; Jill Boldt, Joan A. Lepp, Linda Muterspaugh, Helen Parker, assistant editors; Linda Bishop, Gloria Goldberg, Sylvia Greenberg, Sanna Hans, Marian Mirsky, editorial assistants; Frank E. Peiler, art director; Janet Clingerman, Janice Saltz, art assistants; Jack Lynn, production consultant.

Estelle Weber, assistant to the president; Jack Lowell, business manager; Steven Feinberg, public information director.

Contents

CONSUMER GUIDE 7

Turning The Tables On Over~ weight

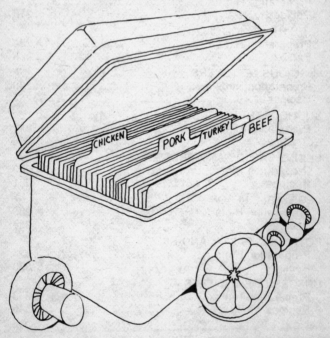

The first step in losing weight is to get back into the kitchen. Declare your independence from gooey frozen pasteries and TV dinners. Take charge of what goes onto your plate, into your mouth, and on your hips. Learn to cook all over again, the low-calorie way.

Most lose-weight prescriptions take just the opposite approach, putting a psychological padlock on the kitchen door by telling the reader to forget about food. How can anybody forget about food? Particularly when we are constantly surrounded by food cues. No-work, no-nutrition, high-calorie snacks scream at us constantly from the TV screen, magazine pages, and supermarket ads. Nobody — least of all a person with a weight problem — can remain immune without alternative satisfactions. However, if you can duplicate the taste and texture of the foods you love — without the unneeded extra calories — you can turn a deaf ear!

Become a low-calorie cook — it needn't be time-consuming. With the variety of foods available today — including many convenience foods which *are* calorie bargains — low-cal cooking is easier than ever. Modern appliances, a well-equipped kitchen, a roomy refrigerator-freezer, and one-stop supermarkets simplify the job.

We recognize that people are busy and that often homemaking is a part-time job fit into a full schedule of community activities or career. So the recipes in this book short-cut preparation time as well as calories.

Why Are You Overweight?

It's your glands or your genes. Or fat cells foisted on you as a helpless infant. You were overfed. Or under-loved. You have a faulty appestat that prevents you from recognizing hunger. It is heredity, environment, or ethnic origin. It is underactivity, over-compensation, or mother's cooking. Even the experts cannot agree on the causes for overweight

Except for one thing.

All concur that overweight is the inevitable outcome of too much energy intake and too little energy outgo. Too many calories, too little exercise.

So let's get it straight at the outset. This book is

about calories — and how to cut them as painlessly and pleasantly as possible. If you can do that — and you can, believe me — you've got the problem licked. No matter what the origin of your overweight, it is impossible to stay fat while consuming fewer calories than your body needs to sustain that fat.

But what about those diets promising magic results? All diets and weight control programs work by causing you to take in fewer calories than you can use up. They work by this method — or they do not work at all. Fat jiggling machines, magic belts, and body wraps are examples of methods that don't work.

Fads, one-food regimens, low-carbohydrate diets, and high-fat diets may work briefly, but not for the reasons their promoters claim — and not in the long run. Your quick "weight" loss at the beginning is simply water — water flushed out of your system which will gradually return. Any true fat loss after that point is due to an automatic reduction in calorie intake — because you have become sick-to-death of eggs, grapefruit, steak, or whatever other limited foods your fad diet permits. Had you consumed the same number of calories on a safer, saner, more satisfying combination of foods, you would have lost the same amount of weight. And more important, you might have stuck with it — whereas the fad diets are doomed to failure. You either tire of them, or are forced to give them up because of failing health.

You Are the Victim of an Epidemic

You are overweight because you take in more calories than you use up . . . but so do millions of other Americans, nearly half the population. The fact that so many others are in the same boat is small comfort. The health costs of carrying around your excess burden are just as high — no matter how many others share your plight.

Nor does the fact that so many people fall beyond the American ideal of slenderness in any way lessen the discrimination overweights are subjected to. Excess pounds cost you money — in terms of lost income and lost opportunity. It has been well documented that fat job applicants lose out to less-qualified slim com-

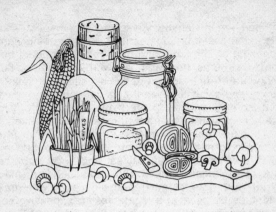

petitors. Fat executives are passed over for promotion. Fat salesmen, waitresses, and taxi drivers lose commissions and tips — often from fat customers. Even fat people don't like fat people!

In no other society has food been so easily attainable for so little physical effort. Yet, despite inflation and soaring prices, despite occasional shortages, Americans still enjoy the "benefits" of a too bountiful breadbasket — with very little "sweat of the brow" in payment. You may hate your job, but sitting down at a desk all day doesn't qualify as "work" not in the physical sense.

It is ironic that a society that makes the accumulation of fat so easy — almost unavoidable — should profess such an intolerance for obesity. The social pressures to avoid overweight are enormous, but they serve a purpose. Our skinny actresses, flat-gutted athletes, society page darlings, and other assorted "beautiful people" do serve a function after all. The standard they set for slimness has made fat unfashionable. And in the long run, vanity is what keeps most of us from eating ourselves into our graves.

Calories: Most Harmful Food Additive

"Three squares a day" . . . "the family dinner hour." These homey concepts have gone the way of parlors and porch swings. Mom's place is no longer in the kitchen — nor is anybody else's for that matter. Family life is increasingly fragmentized, with each individual snacking on the run. Long, late commuter hours from job to suburbs (for Mom as well as Dad), a busy schedule of after-school activities, summers spent at camp, and semesters spent away at college all mean that more Americans of every age are eating outside the home. Even home-cooked meals are less likely to be "cooked" than thawed-and-served. The net result is that Americans have less control than ever before over what goes into the food they eat.

A good Italian cook would make her homemade ravioli with lots of meat and simmer it with fresh tomatoes. But meat and vegetables are expensive, so a food processing firm that packages frozen ravioli is likely to stuff it with yet more starch, flavored with a little meat, and freeze it in a tomato-shy sauce that's thickened with syrups and fillers. The second generation Italian-American wife who serves it to her family concedes wistfully that "it's not quite like Mama used to make." She's probably not aware that the store-bought product is also more fattening and less nourishing — and less filling — because the ravioli is short on appetite-appeasing protein while overly generous with quick-burning carbohydrates. A few hours after their ravioli meal, her family is foraging in the refrigerator for something else to fill their now-empty stomachs. More high-cal snacks fill the void.

This example is multiplied a thousandfold. Just think of all the breaded fish sticks, frozen fried chicken, boiling-bag vegetables, toaster pastries, sugar-coated cereals, stir-and-serve puddings, spray-on-cheese spreads, and can-opener soups and sauces Americans haul home by the tons from supermarkets — in addition to obvious junk foods like candy, soft drinks, chips, dips, and nibbles.

You might think that the American food industry has purposely set out to make us fat. Just when the technological revolution has entrapped an ever-widening circle of Americans of all ages and both sexes into sit-down jobs (or more years of sit-down schooling), just when our national calorie needs are at their lowest, food manufacturers seem to respond with a bulging cornucopia of nutritionally-neutered junk food, food that requires us to eat more and more calories for less and less nutrition.

But food-makers are not intentionally fattening America. It's simply a matter of American business giving the customers what they want. Shoppers want food that's inexpensive, easy-to-serve, and reasonably good-tasting. And the food industry has risen to the challenge — hang nutrition and calories! Today's convenience foods are cooked up by chemists, cost accountants, and advertising copywriters.

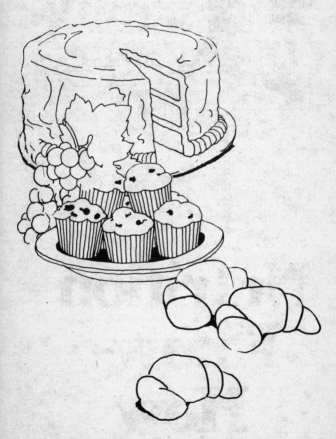

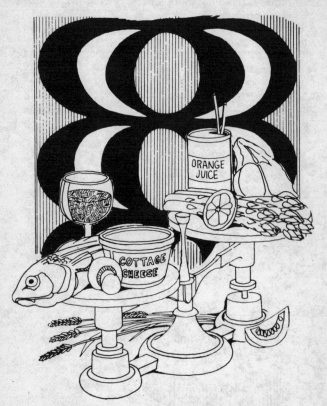

Nutrition Know~ How

Everybody knows that eating lots of food and accumulating extra pounds is no guarantee of adequate nutrition. Many Americans are overfed but undernourished because their tastes run to empty-caloried junk. When a person with a taste for fattening foods attempts to lose weight by simply "cutting down," his or her chances of nutritional deficiency are multiplied. So, before you become a "bookkeeper of calories," it's important to understand that all calories are not alike, and that your calories must come from a variety of food sources to remain healthy.

Spending calories is like managing money. The shrewd manager knows that all bills must be paid before the leftovers can be spent on frills. Some people can live comfortably on little while others spend a great deal and still run into trouble. The undernourished overweight is like a person who buys a car he or she cannot afford, while neglecting to pay the mortgage.

The person who wants to lose weight is in the same situation as somebody who has to live on a reduced income for awhile. Intelligent, imaginative people will find creative ways to do it in reasonable comfort, knowing that the time isn't far off when they can loosen up a little and indulge in a few more luxuries. But the smart dieter knows that the time will *never* come when basic nutritional needs can be ignored.

Protein, Fat, Carbohydrate . . . and Calories

Protein, fat, and carbohydrate are the basic food elements. A balanced diet needs all three. It is nearly impossible to emphasize or eliminate one without causing an unwanted imbalance in another. Therefore, when dieting, it is important to keep each of these elements in a healthy balance and not simply cut out one whole food type.

That's the idea behind the nutritional figures provided with each of the recipes in this book. Once you have computed your daily requirement of calories (see "Computing Your Calorie Needs"), the carbohydrate, protein, and fat figures will help you determine what percentages of your daily intake are being made up of these vital food elements. The last columns tell how much of the fat is saturated fat and how much cholesterol there is. The American Heart Association tells us to keep saturated fats to a minimum because they contain the cholesterol that is believed to be linked with heart disease. Less than 10 percent of the total fat intake should be in the form of saturated fats. And the average daily intake of cholesterol should be approximately 300 milligrams (mg).

Protein is mainly "animal" food — meat, poultry, fish, and eggs. But none is pure protein. Each also contains fat — and the more fat, the less protein. Protein is also found in dairy products like milk and cheese, and in vegetables like beans and nuts (along with fat and carbohydrate).

Protein is vital to life because the body needs it to build and repair itself. Protein is also valuable to dieters because it is slowly digested and helps sustain a feeling of fullness.

Approximately 25 percent of the food you eat should be protein; the minimum is 14 percent. But there is no benefit in having more protein than you need because the excess is stored by the body as fat. Too much protein has been linked with calcium deficiency and kidney disorders.

Fat can be either "animal" — meat fat or butter, for example, or "vegetable" — margarine, salad oil, or the fat found in nuts. Calorically, it does not matter because both animal and vegetable fat have the same calorie count — double the calories of either protein or carbohydrate. It would be both difficult and undesirable to eliminate fat from the diet altogether because a small amount is needed to help the body absorb nutrients properly. But no more than 30-35 percent of the total calories consumed should be in the form of fat. And less than 10 percent of that should be saturated fats.

Carbohydrate is found in the sugars and starches we love so much. A diet plan that attempts to eliminate carbohydrate is a poor idea because fruits and vegetables, which are relatively high in carbohydrate, are the main sources of vital vitamins and minerals, as well as appetite-appeasing roughage. Roughage promotes regularity and guards against overeating.

A DIETER'S DAILY DOZEN

TYPE OF FOOD	SUGGESTIONS
Milk & Dairy Products Skim and low fat milk, plain yogurt, buttermilk, cottage cheese and other low fat cheese	Adults need at least two 8-ounce glasses a day or the equivalent. Can be used as beverage, in cooking, or made into desserts.
Protein Main Courses Lean meat, poultry, seafood, eggs	At least two servings a day (a serving is three ounces, trimmed of all fat and bone).
Other Protein-Rich Foods Cheese and milk products are also complete protein foods. Soybeans and soy products are sources of vegetable protein. Other beans, peas, lentils, and nuts are sources of incomplete protein which can augment the complete protein foods.	These can be used occasionally in place of main course protein foods.
Green or Yellow Fruits and Vegetables Asparagus, broccoli, carrots, collards, escarole, green beans, kale, lettuce, mustard greens, pumpkin, spinach, tomatoes, turnip greens, winter squash, apricots, cantaloupe, mango	At least two half-cup servings every day. Can be cooked, combined with other foods, or served in salads. Raw vegetables make calorie-safe nibbles.

High Vitamin-C Fruits and Vegetables Oranges, grapefruit, lemons, limes, tangerines, strawberries, papayas, tomatoes, broccoli, Brussels sprouts, sweet peppers	At least one serving (6 ounces juice is the equivalent).
Other Fruits and Vegetables Apples, bananas, beets, cauliflower, corn, peaches, pears, potatoes, pineapple, etc.	One potato, apple, banana, peach, or other fresh fruit — or one half-cup serving of canned or frozen vegetable or unsweetened fruit.
Breads, Cereals and Grains Breads, rolls, crackers, breakfast cereals, pasta, rice, flour foods	At least one serving per day. One slice of enriched bread is one serving. Equivalents are 1 cup unsweetened ready-to-eat cereal or 1/2 to 3/4 cup cooked cereal, spaghetti, rice, etc.
Fat Animal fats found in meat, poultry, fish, butter, cheese. Vegetable fats found in shortening, salad oils, margarine, dressings, prepared products	Limit: two tablespoons. Fat is found in so many foods that no additional fat is needed.
Sugar Foods and Sweets White and brown sugar, maple sugar, all syrups, honey	None needed. Limit: one tablespoon. Natural sugar is found in most fruits and vegetables.

Liquids Water, milk, fruit juice, coffee, tea, soft drinks, canned soups, beverages	At least three to four cups liquid a day is needed. Drink cold water before, during, and between meals. Hot bouillon or a fat-skimmed broth before meals is a good idea to curb appetite.
Alcoholic Beverages Beer, wine, scotch, bourbon, gin, vodka, brandy, liqueurs	High in calories, not more than one serving. When used in cooking, the alcohol (and alcohol calories) evaporates.
Non-Nutritive Foods Coffee, tea, sugar substitutes, salt, most spices and seasonings	No calories. Use freely unless you have a special diet problem. (Follow your doctor's advice.)

Approximately 43 percent of a balanced diet should be carbohydrate. A diet that's low in carbohydrate is likely to be too high in fat and protein — with possibly serious consequences. To maintain health, at least 60 grams of carbohydrate must be present in any daily diet. What should be avoided in the carbohydrate category are refined sugars and over-processed starches which have been stripped of everything worthwhile — leaving nothing but calories.

And calories? A calorie is actually a measure of heat — "fuel" to power our bodies. If we consume more "fuel" than we can use up, the excess is stored as unsightly bulges. Calories exist in all foods, otherwise they would not be food. There are roughly four calories in every gram of protein or carbohydrate, and about nine calories in every gram of fat. We need to eat a variety of foods that are high in nutritional value but low in fuel value — calories — so that the body is forced to use up its excess.

Computing Your Calorie Needs

If you are an extremely inactive person who eats 3000 calories a day, your weight will eventually stabilize somewhere over the 200 mark. On the other hand, a young active person forced to live on 1500 calories might eventually become a 98-pound weakling. The right combination for you is somewhere in between those two extremes.

Most diets expect the lifelong overeater to become an undereater overnight. It is unrealistic to believe that a 3000-calorie-a-day person can summon up the willpower to eat like a 98-pound weakling — unrealistic and unnecessary. If those same overweights simply began eating like the normalweights they want to be, their weight would eventually stabilize at the desired point on the scale. So the first step on your program is determining your proper weight . . . then computing the calorie intake that can eventually bring you there.

Pick your weight. Shown is a "Desirable Weight Chart" which you can use as a guide. But it's only a guide. If you are overweight, you might choose a target above the "ideal," to make your goal more attainable. However, don't fall into the trap of overestimating your frame. *Frame* refers to skeleton, which can be small even if it's buried under mounds of fat. Unless you have very broad shoulders and wide wrists (due to bone structure, not accumulated fat or water), it's more likely that your frame is medium or possibly even small. (Many heavy people have tiny wrists and narrow shoulders, indications of a small frame.)

Multiply by 13. Thirteen is the magic number that can help you assess how many calories a day you can eat to be the weight you want to be. If you should weigh 125, multiply 125 by 13. The result is 1625 — and that's about how many calories a day you can eat to weigh 125. If you should weigh only 100, the right answer is 1300.

This is a generalization, of course, but a good enough guide for most overweights. According to general averages, the normal, moderately active person needs 15 calories per pound of body weight a day.

DESIRABLE WEIGHT CHART

Men

Height*	Small Frame	Medium Frame	Large Frame
5'2"	112-120	118-129	126-141
5'3"	115-123	121-133	129-144
5'4"	118-126	124-136	132-148
5'5"	121-129	127-139	135-152
5'6"	124-133	130-143	138-156
5'7"	128-137	134-147	142-161
5'8"	132-141	138-152	147-166
5'9"	136-145	142-156	151-170
5'10"	140-150	146-160	155-174
5'11"	144-154	150-165	159-179
6'0"	148-158	154-170	164-184
6'1"	152-162	158-175	168-189
6'2"	156-167	162-180	173-194
6'3"	160-171	167-185	178-199

*With shoes with 1-inch heels

Women

Height*	Small Frame	Medium Frame	Large Frame
4'10"	92-98	96-107	104-119
4'11"	94-101	98-110	106-122
5'0"	96-104	101-113	109-125
5'1"	99-107	104-116	112-128
5'2"	102-110	107-119	115-131
5'3"	105-113	110-122	118-134
5'4"	108-116	113-126	121-138
5'5"	111-119	116-130	125-142
5'6"	114-123	120-135	129-146
5'7"	118-127	124-139	135-150
5'8"	121-131	128-143	137-154
5'9"	126-135	132-147	141-158
5'10"	130-140	136-151	145-163
5'11"	134-144	140-155	149-168
6'0"	138-148	144-159	153-173

*With shoes with 2-inch heels

For them the magic number to multiply by is 15. But those who are overweight, underactive, or older need less, so the number 13 instead of 15 is more likely to apply to people with weight problems.

Naturally, cutting your calorie intake even lower will speed you towards your goal. But in no case should you attempt a reducing regimen below 1200 calories a day without medical supervision. At least 1200 calories a day has to be consumed in order to receive the minimum amounts of protein, fat, and carbohydrate. And also, a too-drastic cut in calories may leave you discouraged and defeated, ready to quit far short of your goal.

Designing a Diet to Fit Your Tastes

Weight control researchers have shown that the people most likely to succeed as "losers" are the ones who have worked out an eating plan that is tailored to their own tastes and life-styles, a custom-made diet that takes into account their likes and dislikes, as well as the demands on their day. What good is a printed diet sheet commanding you to eat broiled flounder and two vegetables for lunch when you usually eat at your desk in the office?

Designing a diet to suit yourself may seem like a complicated project, but the results are well worth the effort — like the difference between an exquisitely tailored outfit and an ill-fitting dress off the rack. Here's how:

1. Arm yourself with several calorie guides, including one which lists food by brand names. Have on hand a food scale, measuring cups, and measuring spoons.

2. Keep a record of what you eat every day for a week. Once a day look up and write down the calorie counts for each item and add up the totals. Don't guess at amounts — make use of your scale and measuring tools for more accurate estimates. (You may be surprised to learn that your usual calorie intake is nearly double what you should be eating!)

3. Go back over your daily food diary and:
   • eliminate any item you can easily do without — bread with dinner, for example.

- cut down, where possible — one slice of bread instead of two, for example.
- substitute a lower-calorie item — diet bread for example, or a slice of melba-thin bread at half the calories.

4. Check your daily food diary for balance. Are you getting enough green vegetables? Too much meat? Not enough milk? Can the items you're short on be added to your diet in place of fattening snacks?

Each Recipe Has Been Analyzed

At the end of each recipe there is an analysis of the calories, carbohydrate, protein, total fat, saturated fat and cholesterol for each recipe and for each serving. CONSUMER GUIDE Magazine's editors used the latest updated tapes from the U.S. Department of Agriculture, the U.S. Department of Agriculture's *Composition of Foods, Handbook 8,* and *Nutritive Value of Foods, Bulletin No. 72* to program a computer with every ingredient used in this book's recipes. Food processors and manufacturers provided additional statistics for the computer.

The analysis of nutrition at the end of each recipe is given in grams (gm) and milligrams (mg). Nutritional needs vary widely, so check the charts ("U.S. Recommended Daily Allowances"), at the back of the book for the nutritional requirements that are correct for you. Then you can accurately figure what percentage of your nutritional needs is filled by each serving. For instance, if you need 60 grams of protein a day and you use the recipe "Cheese-Scrambled Eggs" for breakfast you will eat 22.1 grams of protein, or over one-third of your daily protein requirement.

> Cholesterol *is one of many fat substances found in the food we eat. The American Heart Association suggests we cut down our level of cholesterol. By reducing your cholesterol intake you might help prevent a heart attack. Recommended daily allowances by the Food and Nutrition Board of the National Research Council is 300 mg. of cholesterol for moderately active people.*

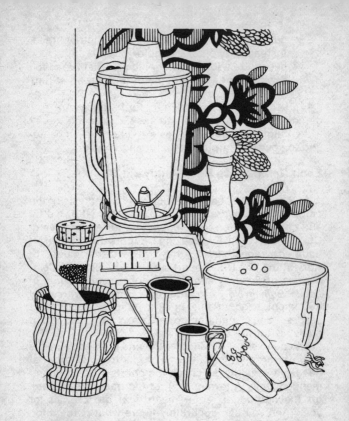

Slimming In The Kitchen

By providing yourself with special "diet" utensils and using some easy cooking, shopping, and eating hints, you can slash the calorie content of your favorite foods and daily intake, and lose weight in a painless and delicious way.

Equipment

• Equip yourself with non-stick pots and pans for cooking, baking, and "frying" without fat. Follow the manufacturers' directions for care. Inexpensive utensils can do the job if you keep them well-scrubbed. If a skillet loses its ability to cook without added fat, throw it out. You cannot afford to keep it!

• A pressure cooker is a handy gadget for cooks on the go because it cuts cooking time by one-third. The leanest, least fattening, less-expensive cuts of meat profit from pressure cookery. If you buy a new one, choose a model with a non-stick interior.

• A blender makes short work of many kitchen tasks. Dieters can turn a blender into a milk shake maker by combining skim milk powder, ice cubes, water, and flavoring — plus a few drops of sweetener. A handful of fresh berries or other fruit can be added for a garden-fresh flavor.

Cooking hints

• Use spray-on vegetable coating for no-fat frying. When used in conjunction with non-stick utensils, the spray eliminates the need for any added fat at all. The base of these products is lecithin, a natural food component much loved by health food fans.

• When making stews and other combination dishes, prepare them a day ahead and store them in the refrigerator — all day or overnight — until serving time. The flavors blend better, and all the fat rises to the surface where you can easily lift it off.

• Fat can be removed from the surface of stock, soup, or gravy by using a bulb-type baster.

• Keep your crisper well-stocked with shredded lettuce, chopped onion, and other greenery so that serving a salad at every meal is a snap.

• Keep your refrigerator's fruit compartment well-supplied with whatever fresh treats are in season. Fruit makes the perfect dessert. Freeze fruits in season for sugar-free treats during the winter.

• If time is at a premium (and when isn't it?), cook in double or triple quantities. Then package the leftovers into homemade low-calorie frozen dinners. Inexpensive aluminum pie pans can serve this purpose.

• Large roasts, casseroles, and other dishes meant for several meals should be packaged away in the freezer right after dinner. Don't keep leftovers around.

• Package meats and other foods for the freezer in serving-size quantities. Four to six ounces of boneless raw meat per person is about right. If you defrost and cook only what you need, you avoid waste — and "waist."

. . . In the Supermarket

Compare. Be a comparison shopper of calories. Check the nutritional label panel of competing products and choose the one with the lower calorie count. Smart label-readers can save calories the same way a cost-wise shopper saves money.

• Always look for the lowest fat content in dairy products. Cottage cheese that is labeled 99 percent fat free is only 160 to 180 calories a cup. Regular creamed cottage cheese is 240 to 260.

• Do not pay a premium price for fattening meat. Prime meat — the most expensive — has a higher ratio of fat and calories with less protein than do less costly grades.

• In choosing meat, always look for the leanest cuts. Have the butcher trim away all fat, or do it yourself. But trimmable exterior fat is less of a problem than fatty marbling (fat all through the meat).

Substitute. Play the substitution game. Look for diet-right versions of fattening products. Experiment, using them in recipes.

• Low-calorie cream cheese or part-skim Neufchatel cheese have the same flavor as fattening cream cheese, and perform the same way in recipes.

• Evaporated skim milk can take the place of cream in most sauces, casseroles, souffles, and desserts. It can even be whipped!

• Yogurt or buttermilk can take the place of sour

cream in many recipes. Or look for low-fat, non-dairy sour cream dressings that can serve the same function. But check the calorie count. Some non-dairy dressings contain just as much fat as real sour cream — vegetable fat instead of animal fat.

• Diet margarine is half the calories of regular margarine (or butter) because it is half water. Unfortunately it cannot replace ordinary margarine in regular recipes. However, many recipes in this book are adjusted to use this low-in-calories spread.

• Check the diet shelf for products that are sugar-free or fat-reduced. Low-sugar or sugar-free jam and jellies, sauces and toppings, pancake syrup, fruits canned in their own juices instead of in syrup, and other such items can be useful in preparing low-calorie desserts.

• Low-fat diet dressings and mayonnaise substitute can help keep salads slimming.

• Do not be put off by the word *imitation* on certain low-calorie, low-sugar, or low-fat products. The word doesn't mean that the product is made up of chemicals, but only that the lower sugar or fat content keeps the product from conforming to standard recipes. Often the imitations are more nutritious than the real thing. For example, low-sugar jams and preserves contain more fruit and less sugar, and the so-called "imitation" low-fat cheeses have a higher protein content.

• Beware the "Dietetic" product that does not list its calorie count! It may not be diet-wise at all, but simply salt-free. For example, some "dietetic" candies made for diabetics have just as many calories as regular candy.

• Bottled flavorings and extracts from the supermarket spice shelf are calorie bargains. Some to look for include butter flavoring, rum, brandy, banana, and chocolate. Most spices and seasonings add so few calories to a dish that they need not be counted.

Final shopping hints: Never go shopping when you are hungry. And leave the kids at home.

. . . In the Dining Room

One of the most successful new approaches to weight control is behavior modification. "Behavior mod" helps overweight people cut calories by forcing them to focus on unconscious eating habits. You can put these methods to work in the dining room by following a few simple rules:

- Never eat standing up. By following this rule, you preclude all nibbling, tasting, testing, and snacking.
- Always eat in the same place — the dining room, for example. Even if you are determined to eat that left-over half-donut, set yourself a place at the dining table, then sit down and eat it. By the time everything is set, you may have changed your mind.
- Always set your place properly. Use a placemat, napkin, waterglass — the whole bit. You'll enjoy your meal more in a pleasant setting, and the act of setting a place makes each meal into a ceremony.
- Never eat while reading or watching TV. Do not dilute the enjoyment of food by concentrating your attention on something else. Paperwork, crossword puzzles, business negotiations, and family arguments shouldn't cut into your eating pleasure either.
- Never prepare or put out more food than you need, lest you personally clean up the "leftovers" yourself. Leave the second helpings in the kitchen so you'll have to make a special trip to get them.
- Always compute the number of servings in any dish you make — main course, side dish, or dessert — and apportion it out accordingly. If a dish serves six, make it a point to serve yourself one-sixth of the total, and not a tablespoon more.
- Set out at one time everything you plan to eat at a meal from soup to dessert. With the finale in full view you'll be less likely to overeat at the main event.
- Equip yourself with smaller plates. Choose a restaurant-style design, with wide rims. A brimming luncheon-size plate is more eye-satisfying than a big expanse of china with lots of white space around modest servings of food. The same strategy applies to wine glasses and dessert dishes.
- Use the other tactic with salads and vegetable dishes. Serve your salad in big soup-size bowls to encourage yourself to fill up on non-fattening fare.
- Do not concentrate on easy-to-eat foods. Foods that take longer to consume are more satisfying than

boneless, bite-size swallows. Corn on the cob seems like more than the same amount of cut corn. Lobster in the shell will keep you busy longer than a boneless steak.

- Eat slowly; savor each bite.

And Away From It

- Once you are finished eating, leave the table. Do not keep others company.
- Do not "clean up" when you clean the table. If you cannot resist munching on the leftovers, put a piece of gum in your mouth before you start. Or better yet, turn the clean-up job over to somebody else.
- Keep busy. Get out of the house during those "crisis" hours when you're most inclined to succumb to a peanut butter frenzy. Go window shopping for the new clothes you'll buy when you're slim.
- Take up a hobby, preferably something that keeps your hands busy. It's hard to eat potato chips and refinish furniture at the same time. A good idea is to take up sewing — you'll need seamstress skills to create the new wardrobe in your thin future.
- Make a list of everything you hate about being fat, and post it prominently on the refrigerator. Or take the positive approach and list all the things you'd do if you were trim.

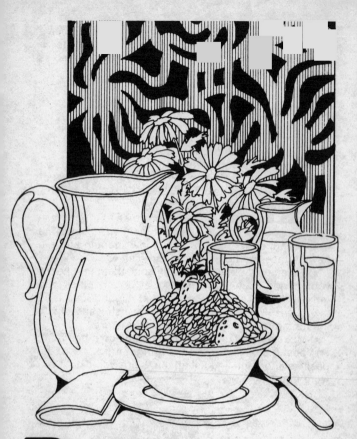

Better Breakfast Ideas

CONSUMER GUIDE

If skipping breakfast is your idea of saving calories, think again. Would-be skinnies who try to subsist without breakfast generally wind up giving into coffee-and-junk breaks at midmorning, or overeating at lunch — or both. The net result is more calories consumed than would have been had they eaten a decent morning meal.

Breakfast needn't be heavy or elaborate. In fact, if you're dieting, it should be light. But lightness in calories has nothing to do with shortchanging nutrition. Ideally, a dieter's breakfast should include:

• Fresh fruit for vitamins and bulk. Unsugared canned or frozen fruit can be used. High-in-vitamin-C choices like grapefruit, sliced strawberries, or melon are ideal.

• Grain — which can be either bread or cereal.

• Protein food. Meat or eggs or egg substitutes are the usual choices. High-protein cereals topped with protein-rich skim milk can also meet your morning protein requirement.

• Milk — preferably nonfat or lowfat, which can be a beverage by itself, poured on cereal or fruit, or used in coffee or tea.

Good Breakfast Combinations

• High-protein cereal, with skim milk, and sliced berries.

• Half grapefruit, toasted protein bread with low-calorie cream cheese.

• Melon wedge, cottage-cheese-filled omelet, and black coffee. Toast saved for a 10 o'clock snack.

• Blender-quick eggnog made with skim milk. Take an orange to the office for a 10 o'clock snack.

• Pancakes made with high-protein pancake mix, topped with sliced strawberries and diet syrup. Add a glass of skim milk.

If you're a confirmed coffee-breaker, there's no harm in saving part of your breakfast menu for a midmorning snack. However, postponing all food until 10 or 11 o'clock is a poor idea since it is likely that more than half a day has passed since your body took in any nourishment.

Bad Breakfast Bets

At the other extreme from breakfast-skippers are those who unwittingly load up on calories, often without redeeming nutritional value. Many traditional breakfast foods are exceedingly rich in sugar, starch, or fat. Some to watch for:

• **Sugar-coated cereals.** Most pre-sweetened cereals contain more sugar than anything else. When choosing cereal, pick a high-protein variety. Sweeten to taste, if necessary, with low-cal sugar substitute.

• **Bacon** is more than half fat, even after it has been broiled or fried and well-drained. Choose lean Canadian bacon instead, only 45 calories an ounce instead of 200.

• **Sausage** is generally 50 percent fat. Instead of buying packaged sausage make your own home-seasoned patties from lean ground pork.

• **Pastries** are simply empty-caloried concoctions of starch, sugar, and fat. Their low-protein means you'll be hungry by midmorning.

Recipes

Cooked Cereal

3 cups water	1 cup raw oatmeal or
1 tsp. butter-flavored	1½ cups quick
salt	cooking oatmeal

Bring the water to a rapid boil in a 2-quart saucepan over high heat. Add the salt. Gradually add the cereal, stirring constantly until it is blended. Reduce the heat to low, and cover the saucepan. Cook the cereal for 3 to 5 minutes or as directed on the package.

Makes 6 servings

	Calories	Carbo-hydrate (gm)	Protein (gm)	Total Fat (gm)	Saturated Fat (gm)	Choles-terol (mg)
Total	520.0	92.0	20.0	8.0	0.0	0.0
Per Serving	86.7	15.3	3.3	1.3	0.0	0.0

CONSUMER GUIDE

Florida Nog

1 cup orange or
   grapefruit juice
1 egg

sugar substitute to
   equal 2 tsp.

Combine all the ingredients, and beat them with a hand beater or in a blender until smooth. Pour the nog into a tall glass over ice and serve it immediately.

Makes 1 serving

	Calories	Carbo-hydrate (gm)	Protein (gm)	Total Fat (gm)	Saturated Fat (gm)	Choles-terol (mg)
Total	190.0	26.0	8.0	7.0	2.0	252.0

Cheese-Scrambled Eggs

6 eggs
¼ cup skim milk
¼ tsp. salt

dash of pepper
4 oz. low-fat
   American-style
   processed
   cheese

Before cooking: Shred the cheese.

Beat the eggs with the milk, salt, and pepper in a mixing bowl until they are frothy. Spray a non-stick skillet with vegetable coating for no-fat frying, and heat it for 2 minutes. Add the eggs, and cook them, stirring from the bottom of the skillet. While the eggs are still soft, sprinkle the shredded cheese over the top and stir or gently fold until the cheese begins to melt and the eggs are of the desired consistency. Garnish with parsley, if desired, and serve immediately.

Makes 3 servings

	Calories	Carbo-hydrate (gm)	Protein (gm)	Total Fat (gm)	Saturated Fat (gm)	Choles-terol (mg)
Total	742.5	7.0	66.3	48.0	20.0	1613.3
Per Serving	247.5	2.3	22.1	16.0	6.7	537.8

---

gm=grams; mg=milligrams. Nutritional figures are approximate. Figures are based on findings of U.S. Department of Agriculture.

Quick Fruit Syrup

$1/2$ cup low-sugar or
sugarless jam or
preserves (any
favorite flavor)

$1/2$ cup water

Combine the ingredients in a saucepan. Cook and stir them over low heat until they simmer. Serve with pancakes or French toast.

Makes 1 cup
(8 servings)

	Calories	Carbo-hydrate (gm)	Protein (gm)	Total Fat (gm)	Saturated Fat (gm)	Choles-terol (mg)
Total	96.0	24.0	0.0	0.0	0.0	0.0
Per Serving	12.0	3.0	0.0	0.0	0.0	0.0

Blintz Pancakes

1 cup flour
1 tsp. salt
1 cup skim milk
4 eggs, beaten

For Filling:
3 cups 99% fat-free
cottage cheese
sugar substitute to
equal 2 tbsp.
$1/2$ tsp. butter-flavored
salt
2 tsp. vanilla
$1/2$ tsp. grated lemon
peel
1 egg yolk

Combine the flour and salt in a bowl and gradually stir in the milk. Add the eggs and beat the mixture. Spray a 6-inch non-stick skillet with vegetable coating for no-fat frying, and heat it for 1 or 2 minutes. Pour about 2 tablespoons batter into the pan. Tip and roll the pan to cover the bottom with batter. Cook the pancake for about 1 minute until the top dries. Then turn it out on a towel, browned side up. Repeat this procedure until all the batter is used. You should have eighteen pancakes.

Mix all of the ingredients for the filling in a bowl and blend them well. Put 1 tablespoon of filling on each pancake. Fold in the sides, and roll the pancake to make an envelope. Place the blintzes in a baking pan, and reheat them in the oven before serving.

Makes 9 servings

Special hint: If you like, the blintzes can be served topped with your favorite low-calorie preserves, or with fresh fruit, or with cinnamon.

	Calories	Carbo-hydrate (gm)	Protein (gm)	Total Fat (gm)	Saturated Fat (gm)	Choles-terol (mg)
Total	1489.6	131.2	139.0	36.0	13.6	1323.2
Per Serving	165.5	14.6	15.4	4.0	1.5	147.0

Cornmeal Pancakes

¹/₂ cup flour	¹/₂ tsp. salt
¹/₂ cup yellow cornmeal	1 cup skim milk
1¹/₂ tsp. baking powder	2 eggs, slightly beaten

Before cooking: Sift the flour, and re-measure it so there is only ¹/₂ cup.

Sift the flour again with the baking powder and salt. Combine the milk with the beaten eggs in a bowl; then add the dry ingredients. Blend the mixture only until the larger lumps disappear. Spray a non-stick skillet with vegetable coating for no-fat frying. Preheat the skillet over medium heat for 1 to 2 minutes. With a tablespoon, drop the batter into the pan and cook the pancakes until the bubbles break and the edges are cooked. Then turn the pancakes to brown the other side. (This will make sixteen 4-inch pancakes.) Serve immediately.

Makes 8 servings

	Calories	Carbo-hydrate (gm)	Protein (gm)	Total Fat (gm)	Saturated Fat (gm)	Choles-terol (mg)
Total	699.2	105.5	33.0	15.0	4.5	509.0
Per Serving	87.4	13.2	4.1	1.9	0.6	63.6

gm=grams; mg=milligrams. Nutritional figures are approximate. Figures are based on findings of U.S. Department of Agriculture.

Baking Powder Biscuits

2 cups flour
3 tsp. baking powder
1 tsp. salt

2 tbsp. diet
    margarine
¾ cup skim milk

Before cooking: Sift the flour and re-measure it so there are only 2 cups.

Sift the flour again with the baking powder and salt. Cut in the margarine with a pastry blender. Add the milk. Stir the mixture quickly and lightly with a fork just until the dough clings together into a ball. Then turn the dough out onto a lightly floured board and knead it gently. Roll the dough or pat it out to ½-inch thickness. Cut the dough with a 2-inch biscuit-cutter and place the dough circles on an ungreased cookie sheet. Bake them for 12 to 15 minutes at 450°.

Makes 12 servings

	Calories	Carbo-hydrate (gm)	Protein (gm)	Total Fat (gm)	Saturated Fat (gm)	Choles-terol (mg)
Total	1084.8	200.8	32.8	14.0	2.0	3.8
Per Serving	90.4	16.7	2.7	1.2	0.2	0.3

Corn Bread

3 cups cornmeal
2 tsp. baking powder
1 tsp. baking soda

1½ tsp. salt
2 cups buttermilk
3 eggs, slightly
    beaten

Mix the cornmeal, baking powder, baking soda, and salt together. Add the buttermilk and eggs. If you want crisp corn bread, bake it in a shallow pan. Use a deep pan for thick servings. Bake the bread at 425° for 25 to 30 minutes.

Makes 10 servings

	Calories	Carbo-hydrate (gm)	Protein (gm)	Total Fat (gm)	Saturated Fat (gm)	Choles-terol (mg)
Total	1727.1	294.5	69.0	33.0	9.0	766.0
Per Serving	172.7	29.5	6.9	3.3	0.9	76.6

Low-Calorie Honey-Maple Syrup

1 tbsp. arrowroot or
     cornstarch
5 tbsp. honey
   pinch of salt

1 cup water
2 tsp. maple extract

Combine all of the ingredients except the maple flavoring in a saucepan. Cook and stir the mixture over moderate heat until it boils. Then lower the heat and simmer for 1 minute. Remove the pan from the heat, and stir in the maple flavoring. Store the syrup in the refrigerator.

*Makes 1 cup
(8 servings)*

	Calories	Carbo-hydrate (gm)	Protein (gm)	Total Fat (gm)	Saturated Fat (gm)	Choles-terol (mg)
Total	366.3	95.2	0.0	0.0	0.0	0.0
Per Serving	45.8	11.9	0.0	0.0	0.0	0.0

French Toast

4 eggs, slightly beaten
1¹/₃ cups skim milk

1 tsp. butter-flavored
     salt
12 slices day-old
     protein-enriched
     bread

Combine the eggs, milk, and salt in a shallow bowl. Dip the bread in the egg mixture 1 piece at a time, turning to coat both sides. Spray a non-stick skillet with vegetable coating for no-fat frying. Preheat the skillet over medium-low heat for 2 minutes. Brown the bread, turning the slices once.

Makes 6 servings

	Calories	Carbo-hydrate (gm)	Protein (gm)	Total Fat (gm)	Saturated Fat (gm)	Choles-terol (mg)
Total	1097.1	145.1	64.7	32.4	9.8	1025.5
Per Serving	182.9	24.2	10.8	5.4	1.6	170.9

gm=grams; mg=milligrams. Nutritional figures are approximate. Figures are based on findings of U.S. Department of Agriculture.

Blueberry Muffins

²/₃ cup diet margarine
sugar substitute to
equal ¹/₃ cup
2 eggs
1¹/₄ cups cornmeal
³/₄ cup flour

2¹/₂ tsp. double-acting
baking powder
³/₄ tsp salt
³/₄ cup skimmed milk
¹/₂ cup fresh
blueberries (or
unsweetened
frozen
blueberries,
thawed and
drained)

Before cooking: Sift the flour, and re-measure it so there is only ³/₄ cup.

Beat the diet margarine, sugar substitute, and eggs in a medium bowl. Stir in the cornmeal. Sift the flour again with the baking powder and salt. Stir ¹/₃ of this mixture into the cornmeal mixture. Then stir in ¹/₂ of the milk. Repeat this process, ending with the remaining ¹/₃ of flour mixture. Gently fold in the blueberries. Place a scant ¹/₄ cup of batter in each cup of a muffin tin that has been sprayed with vegetable coating. Bake the muffins at 350° for 20 to 25 minutes until they are golden brown. *Makes 15 servings*

	Calories	Carbo-hydrate (gm)	Protein (gm)	Total Fat (gm)	Saturated Fat (gm)	Choles-terol (mg)
Total	1194.3	204.8	42.9	23.6	6.0	507.8
Per Serving	79.6	13.7	2.9	1.6	0.4	33.9

Homemade Country Sausage

4 lbs. lean fresh pork,
trimmed of all fat
and ground
2 tbsp. sage
1 tbsp. salt

1 tsp. pepper
1 tsp. ground cloves
¹/₂ tsp. ground
nutmeg

Add the seasonings to the meat, and mix until they are well blended. Shape the meat into 3-oz. patties.

(This will make 20 patties.) Broil them 3 to 4 inches from the heat source until they are no longer pink inside. Or they may be pan-fried in a non-stick skillet.

Makes 20 servings

Special note: The raw patties may be frozen for later cooking and eating.

	Calories	Carbo-hydrate (gm)	Protein (gm)	Total Fat (gm)	Saturated Fat (gm)	Choles-terol (mg)
Total	4665.5	0.0	533.2	266.6	80.0	1599.6
Per Serving	233.3	0.0	26.7	13.3	4.0	80.0

Spicy Homemade Sausage

4 lbs. lean pork
    shoulder trimmed of
    all fat and ground
    twice
1 tbsp. onion salt
1 finely chopped garlic
    clove
1 tbsp. sage

1 tsp. ground cloves
1 tsp. mace
2 tsp. pepper
1 tbsp. minced
    parsley
1/4 tsp. ground
    allspice

Combine the ground pork with the other ingredients and mix them well. Shape the meat into 3-oz. patties. (This will make 20 patties.) The patties may be broiled or pan-fried in a non-stick skillet, and should be cooked until they are no longer pink inside.

Makes 20 servings

Special note: The raw patties may be frozen for later cooking and eating.

	Calories	Carbo-hydrate (gm)	Protein (gm)	Total Fat (gm)	Saturated Fat (gm)	Choles-terol (mg)
Total	4666.5	0.0	533.2	266.6	80.0	1599.6
Per Serving	233.3	0.0	26.7	13.3	4.0	80.0

gm=grams; mg=milligrams. Nutritional figures are approximate. Figures are based on findings of U.S. Department of Agriculture.

Veal Sausage

1½ lbs. ground veal
1 egg
4 tbsp. water
1 tsp. garlic salt
2 tsp. onion flakes

¼ tsp. pepper
2 tsp. fennel seeds
⅛ tsp. crushed red
pepper
2 tsp. oregano
1 tbsp. olive oil

Beat the egg and water together. Then combine it with all the rest of the ingredients except the olive oil. Shape the meat into 12 patties or meatballs. Heat the oil in a non-stick skillet, and pan-fry the patties.

Makes 12 servings

	Calories	Carbo-hydrate (gm)	Protein (gm)	Total Fat (gm)	Saturated Fat (gm)	Choles-terol (mg)
Total	1149.0	0.0	142.0	60.0	28.0	732.0
Per Serving	95.8	0.0	11.8	5.0	2.3	61.0

Hotcakes

1 cup flour
1 tsp. baking powder
¼ tsp. salt

1 cup skim milk
1 egg, slightly
beaten

Before cooking: Sift the flour and re-measure it so there is only 1 cup.

Sift the flour again with the baking powder and salt. In a mixing bowl, combine the milk with the beaten egg; then add the dry ingredients. Blend the mixture only until the larger lumps disappear. Spray a non-stick skillet with vegetable coating for no-fat frying and preheat the skillet over medium-low heat for 2 to 3 minutes or until a drop of water "sizzles" on the surface. With a tablespoon, drop the batter in the hot pan, and cook the hotcakes for about 1 minute per side. Serve immediately. This will make twelve 4-inch hotcakes.

Makes 6 servings

	Calories	Carbo-hydrate (gm)	Protein (gm)	Total Fat (gm)	Saturated Fat (gm)	Choles-terol (mg)
Total	627.1	107.5	28.0	7.0	2.0	257.0
Per Serving	104.5	17.9	4.7	1.2	0.3	42.8

Banana Hotcakes

For each hotcake place 3 to 4 thin banana slices in the preheated skillet. Pour the hotcake batter over the banana slices.

	Calories	Carbo-hydrate (gm)	Protein (gm)	Total Fat (gm)	Saturated Fat (gm)	Choles-terol (mg)
Total	660.1	116.1	28.3	7.0	2.0	257.0
Per Serving	110.0	19.4	4.7	1.2	0.3	42.8

Apple Hotcakes

To the batter, add $1/2$ cup grated, pared, cored tart apples that have been sprinkled with cinnamon.

	Calories	Carbo-hydrate (gm)	Protein (gm)	Total Fat (gm)	Saturated Fat (gm)	Choles-terol (mg)
Total	650.2	113.4	28.0	7.0	2.0	257.0
Per Serving	108.4	18.9	4.7	1.2	0.3	42.8

Pineapple Hotcakes

To the batter, add $1/4$ cup well-drained, juice-packed crushed pineapple and a dash of ground cloves.

	Calories	Carbo-hydrate (gm)	Protein (gm)	Total Fat (gm)	Saturated Fat (gm)	Choles-terol (mg)
Total	664.9	117.3	28.3	7.0	2.0	257.0
Per Serving	110.8	19.6	4.7	1.2	0.3	42.8

gm=grams; mg=milligrams. Nutritional figures are approximate. Figures are based on findings of U.S. Department of Agriculture.

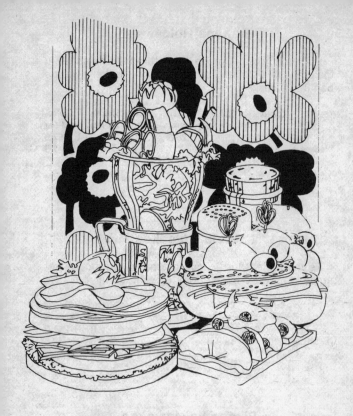

What's
For
Lunch?

Whether you brown-bag it to an office or lunch alone at home, munch on a carhop hamburger or an expense-account steak, un-thought-out lunches can pile on lots of extra calories. Worst of all, they often are not satisfying, and thus take an even higher toll when late-day hunger and fatigue bring on a "nibble-fit."

So plan ahead. Don't take lunch for granted.

How to slim down a sandwich

There are times when a sandwich is the only practical choice — if you carry your lunch, for example. Slimming down a sandwich without shortcutting protein takes some careful bargain-hunting among the possible ingredients.

Saving on bread. The fewer calories spent here, the more you'll have for the "meat" of the meal.

Ordinary white bread is around 65 calories per slice.

Slim sliced breads range from 43 to 53 calories per slice; their smaller size is what makes them lower.

Diet and protein breads range from 35 to 50 calories per slice, sometimes more, so be a label reader to get the best calorie buy for your money. (If the label won't say, why buy?) Protein-enriched breads are usually made from part soy flour, so they offer a nutrition boost and are more filling than ordinary breads. Gluten breads (made from high-protein flour) are among the least fattening — about 35 calories per slice. Do not be turned off by the name, they do not taste chewy-gluey.

Rye and pumpernickle breads are generally lower in calories than white bread, but the slices are larger, so they average around 65 calories a slice. Buy it unsliced and cut it superthin for a calorie bargain.

French and Italian breads will be lower in calories if no fat is used in the dough. Check the label.

Whole wheat and cracked wheat breads are lower, about 55 to 60 calories per slice.

Quality and premium-priced breads are usually richer and more fattening but the slices are slimmer than white bread so the calorie count is about the same, 65 per slice.

Toast is no lower in calories than the same bread untoasted.

Hard rolls or "Jewish" rolls average around 150 calories each. So do soft hamburger rolls. You can de-calorize a roll to around 100 calories by pulling out the doughy center.

Bakery or speciality breads are anybody's guess.

The meat of your sandwich

Sliced meats from homemade roasts can make the tastiest sandwiches — and the most economical in cost and calories. But choose with care. Dark meat turkey is 176 calories for a three-ounce serving while white meat turkey or roast veal add up to only 150 calories. Roast beef, ham, or lamb — if really lean and fat-trimmed — can be under 160 calories, but hidden or untrimmed fat can double the count. For example, lean roast round of beef is low, but three ounces of fatty rib roast can go as high as 375 calories. Leg of lamb is low, but fatty shoulder roast may be 250 calories or more. Lean smoked ham is relatively low, but a fatty pork roast or greasy glazed ham adds up to more than 300 calories. And don't forget: a calorie-conscious, non-greasy, homemade meatloaf of lean chopped beef makes a delicious sandwich, too.

Cold cuts can be a calorie bargain or a fatty disaster. Here are some of the popular choices found at the deli counter, given in three-ounce portions because "per slice" depends on the slice. These are averages only, based on government, industry or processors' data; individual brands may vary.

How different meats compare in calories

Meat	Calories per 3-ounce serving
Corned beef	204
Beef bologna	237
Turkey bologna	193
Braunschweiger	270
Smoked chicken	135
Cooked ("boiled") ham	120
Beef-pork loaf	297
Ham and cheese loaf	228
Head cheese	206

Meat	Calories per 3-ounce serving
Liverwurst	261
Olive loaf	156
Pickle-pimento loaf	234
Pastrami	171
Dry salami	384
Cooked salami	264
Turkey salami	176
Thuringer	254
Turkey loaf	100
Smoked turkey	136

What's "turkey bologna"? Or "turkey salami"? These calorie-shy newcomers may not yet be available in your area. A boon to cholesterol counters too, they are processed from low-calorie turkey, but they have the same spices, and the same color, taste, and texture as their more fattening namesakes.

Cheeses can make or break a low-cal sandwich. Are natural cheeses slimmer than the processed types? What about "cheese foods," "cheese spreads," and skim milk or "diet cheeses"? Here are some guidelines:

Cheese	Calories per Ounce
Most natural hard cheeses. (Cheddar, American, Swiss, Romano and other grating cheeses.)	110 or more
Most processed cheeses. Most soft cheeses. (Limburger, Bleu, Roquefort, etc., cream cheese.)	100 to 110
Most processed "cheese foods."	90 to 100
Most cheese spreads. Some part-skim cheeses. (Mozzarella, "pizza cheese," Scamorze, Sap Sago, Neufchatel.)	75 to 90

Cheese	**Calories per Ounce**
Farmer cheese, cottage cheese. Low calorie or diet cheeses such as "Imitation" cream cheese or "Imitation" processed American cheese slices. The word *Imitation* is used on the label because these products don't meet the federal standard of fat content (naturally!) although they generally contain more protein than the "real thing."	under 40

Recipes

Crab Meat Louis

1 small head of lettuce
1½ cups cooked or
    canned lump crab
    meat, chilled

1 large tomato
2 eggs
6 pimiento-stuffed
    olives

Before preparing: Hard-boil the eggs and cut them into slices. Cut the tomato into wedges. Slice the olives.

Arrange the lettuce in 4 salad serving bowls. Mound the crab meat on top and garnish with the tomato wedges, egg slices, and olives. Serve with Louis Dressing listed next. *Makes 4 servings*

	Calories	Carbo-hydrate (gm)	Protein (gm)	Total Fat (gm)	Saturated Fat (gm)	Choles-terol (mg)
Total	607.5	30.0	71.5	23.0	4.0	805.0
Per Serving	151.9	7.5	17.9	5.8	1.0	201.3

Louis Dressing

1 cup diet mayonnaise
1/2 cup chili sauce
1 1/2 tsp. grated onion
2 tsp. horseradish
1/4 tsp. pepper

1 tsp. fresh lemon
juice
1/4 tsp. tarragon
1/2 tsp. salt

Combine all of the ingredients and chill. Serve on chilled lobster, crabmeat, or shrimp. *Makes 1 1/2 cups (12 servings)*

	Calories	Carbo-hydrate (gm)	Protein (gm)	Total Fat (gm)	Saturated Fat (gm)	Choles-terol (mg)
Total	454.4	49.4	0.1	32.0	0.0	128.0
Per Serving	37.9	4.1	0.0	2.7	0.0	10.7

Chicken Liver Omelet

1/2 lb. chicken livers
1 cup water

1/2 tsp. salt
4 eggs

Simmer the chicken livers in 3/4 cup water for approximately 10 minutes until they are cooked through. Drain the livers, and cut them into small pieces. In a bowl, beat the eggs, and add the salt, the rest of the water, and the chicken liver pieces. Spray a non-stick skillet with vegetable coating for no-fat frying. Heat the pan for 1 or 2 minutes, and then add the egg mixture. Cook the eggs over low heat until the omelet is set. Cut across the center of the omelet with a spatula, and fold. Serve immediately. *Makes 4 servings*

	Calories	Carbo-hydrate (gm)	Protein (gm)	Total Fat (gm)	Saturated Fat (gm)	Choles-terol (mg)
Total	696.0	8.0	84.0	36.0	12.0	2708.0
Per Serving	174.0	2.0	21.0	9.0	3.0	677.0

gm=grams; mg=milligrams. Nutritional figures are approximate. Figures are based on findings of U.S. Department of Agriculture.

Hot Seafood Sandwiches

1 tbsp. diet margarine
1½ tsp. minced green
    pepper
1 tsp. minced onion
4 eggs, slightly beaten
¼ cup skim milk

½ tsp. salt
7 oz. can water
    packed tuna,
    lobster, or
    crabmeat
4 slices toasted
    protein bread

Preheat a non-stick saucepan over low heat for 2 minutes and melt the margarine. Add the green pepper and onion and sauté them for about 5 minutes. Remove the pan from the heat and add the eggs, milk, salt, and fish. Cook the mixture over low heat for about 10 minutes, stirring constantly, until it is thick and creamy. Serve the hot mixture over the toast.

Makes 4 servings

	Calories	Carbo-hydrate (gm)	Protein (gm)	Total Fat (gm)	Saturated Fat (gm)	Choles-terol (mg)
Total	868.7	46.8	92.0	34.8	9.6	1138.9
Per Serving	217.2	11.7	23.0	8.7	2.4	284.7

Lobster Salad Bowl

5 oz. can lobster
3 cups torn head lettuce
½ cup thinly sliced
    celery
¼ cup sliced green
    onions
¾ cup halved cherry
    tomatoes
1 grapefruit
5 pitted ripe olives

¼ cup fresh lemon
    juice
1½ cups 99% fat-free
    cottage cheese
⅓ cup yogurt
1 tsp. grated lemon
    peel
salt
pepper

Before preparing: Drain the lobster; peel and section the grapefruit; slice the olives.

Toss the lettuce, celery, and onions together. Arrange the lobster, tomatoes, grapefruit sections, and olive slices on top of the greens. Sprinkle the lemon juice over all. Cover the salad and chill it. In the meantime, prepare the dressing: whip the cottage cheese in a blender at the highest speed until it is smooth. Beat in the yogurt and lemon peel. Add salt and pepper according to your own taste. *Makes 1³/₄ cups (4 servings)*

	Calories	Carbo-hydrate (gm)	Protein (gm)	Total Fat (gm)	Saturated Fat (gm)	Choles-terol (mg)
Total	448.5	50.0	48.1	8.1	0.8	132.1
Per Serving	112.1	12.5	12.0	2.0	0.2	33.0

Seafood Salad

1 lb. frozen fish fillets
4 tbsp. diet Italian salad dressing
¹/₂ cup diced, pared cucumber
3 tbsp. yogurt

2 tbsp. capers
¹/₄ tsp. salt
dash of pepper
4 large lettuce leaves

Before cooking: Allow the fish to thaw.

Place the fish in a skillet and add just enough water to cover it. Cover the pan and simmer the fish for 8 to 10 minutes until it flakes easily. Flake the fish in a bowl and pour the Italian dressing over it. Marinate the fish in the refrigerator until it is chilled. Then combine the fish with the cucumber, yogurt, capers, salt, and pepper, mixing lightly. Serve on lettuce. *Makes 4 servings*

	Calories	Carbo-hydrate (gm)	Protein (gm)	Total Fat (gm)	Saturated Fat (gm)	Choles-terol (mg)
Total	992.4	7.1	140.8	42.1	11.1	414.2
Per Serving	248.1	1.8	35.2	10.5	2.8	103.6

gm=grams; mg=milligrams. Nutritional figures are approximate. Figures are based on findings of U.S. Department of Agriculture.

Egg Salad

10 eggs
1/2 cup diet mayonnaise
  or 1/2 cup yogurt (or
  1/4 cup of each)
3 tbsp. diced green
  peppers

3 tbsp. chopped
  celery
1 tbsp. prepared
  mustard
2 tbsp. finely
  chopped onion
1/4 tsp. salt
paprika

Before preparing: Hard-boil the eggs and then chop them.

Mix the chopped eggs with the remaining ingredients. Chill the mixture before serving.

Makes 6 servings

	Calories	Carbo-hydrate (gm)	Protein (gm)	Total Fat (gm)	Saturated Fat (gm)	Choles-terol (mg)
Total	989.0	38.6	64.4	62.0	21.0	2530.0
Per Serving	164.8	6.4	10.7	10.3	3.5	421.7

"Hawaiian" Open Face Turkey Sandwiches

4 slices leftover roasted
  turkey (about 2 oz.
  each)
4 slices juice-packed
  pineapple rings

4 slices Swiss
  cheese (1/2 oz.
  each)
4 slices high-protein
  toast

Arrange the toast on a baking sheet and lay a slice of turkey on each piece. Cover each slice of turkey with a pineapple ring, and top the pineapple with a slice of cheese. Bake the combination in a 350° oven for about 4 minutes until the cheese melts. *Makes 4 servings*

	Calories	Carbo-hydrate (gm)	Protein (gm)	Total Fat (gm)	Saturated Fat (gm)	Choles-terol (mg)
Total	775.9	77.1	62.1	24.7	10.5	161.8
Per Serving	194.0	19.3	15.5	6.2	2.6	40.5

Turkey Salad Sandwich Spread

1 cup cooked boned
turkey, diced
1 cup chopped or sliced
celery
1 tbsp. diet
mayonnaise

2 tbsp. finely
chopped onion
1 tsp. fresh lemon
juice
dash of pepper

Combine all of the ingredients and serve the mixture on crisp salad greens or as a sandwich filling.

Makes 3 servings

	Calories	Carbo-hydrate (gm)	Protein (gm)	Total Fat (gm)	Saturated Fat (gm)	Choles-terol (mg)
Total	508.4	8.6	78.9	16.8	4.9	226.9
Per Serving	169.5	2.9	26.3	5.6	1.6	75.6

Cottage Cheese Egg Salad Spread

3 eggs
1/2 cup 99% fat-free
cottage cheese
1 tbsp. yogurt
2 tsp. prepared mustard

1 1/2 tsp. chopped
chives
1/4 tsp. salt
1/8 tsp.
Worcestershire
sauce
1/4 tsp. dill

Before preparing: Hard-boil the eggs, and chop them finely.

Combine the eggs with the rest of the ingredients in a small bowl. Cover the bowl and chill the mixture to blend the flavors. Serve on rye bread or crisp crackers.

Makes 2 servings

	Calories	Carbo-hydrate (gm)	Protein (gm)	Total Fat (gm)	Saturated Fat (gm)	Choles-terol (mg)
Total	415.8	23.6	33.5	19.2	6.7	766.9
Per Serving	207.9	11.8	16.8	9.6	3.4	383.5

gm = grams; mg = milligrams. Nutritional figures are approximate. Figures are based on findings of U.S. Department of Agriculture.

Crab 'n' Apple Salad

1 cup cooked or canned
   crabmeat, drained
2 red apples
1 green pepper
6 pimiento stuffed
   olives

¹/₄ cup diet
   mayonnaise
1 tbsp. fresh lemon
   juice
lettuce

Before preparing: Dice the apples, but do not peel them. Cut the green pepper into narrow strips. Slice the olives.

Combine the crabmeat, apples, green pepper, and olives. Sitr in the diet mayonnaise and lemon juice. Chill the salad before serving it on the lettuce.

Makes 4 servings

	Calories	Carbohydrate (gm)	Protein (gm)	Total Fat (gm)	Saturated Fat (gm)	Cholesterol (mg)
Total	459.2	47.5	36.1	15.7	0.0	232.4
Per Serving	114.8	11.9	9.0	3.9	0.0	58.1

Melon Boat Salad

1 lb. cooked shrimp,
   crab meat, and/or
   lobster
¹/₂ cup diet salad
   dressing
¹/₄ tsp. dill
2 cups 99% fat-free
   cottage cheese
¹/₂ tsp. seasoned salt

¹/₂ tsp. fresh grated
   lime peel
1 tsp. fresh lime
   juice
2 medium
   cantaloupes
4 leaves romaine or
   leaf lettuce
4 lime wedges

Place the seafood in a bowl. Pour the dressing over it; sprinkle it with dill and chill it for several hours. Meanwhile, in another bowl, blend together the cottage cheese, seasoned salt, lime peel, and juice. Cover this mixture, and chill it. Cut the cantaloupes in half; remove the seeds; and chill them. To serve: Divide the cottage cheese mixture into fourths and spoon a fourth into each melon half. Drain the seafood from the marinade, and arrange it on lettuce next to the melon. Garnish each with a lime wedge. *Makes 4 servings*

	Calories	Carbo-hydrate (gm)	Protein (gm)	Total Fat (gm)	Saturated Fat (gm)	Choles-terol (mg)
Total	1019.7	73.7	144.0	9.3	2.4	721.0
Per Serving	254.5	18.4	36.0	2.3	0.6	180.3

Chicken Sandwich Spread

1 cup cooked white
   meat of chicken,
   ground
1/2 tsp. salt

1/4 cup diet
   mayonnaise
2 tbsp. yogurt

Combine all of the ingredients. Serve the spread on bread or crisp crackers. *Makes 4 servings*

	Calories	Carbo-hydrate (gm)	Protein (gm)	Total Fat (gm)	Saturated Fat (gm)	Choles-terol (mg)
Total	582.9	5.6	52.7	37.2	8.8	226.7
Per Serving	145.7	1.4	13.2	9.3	2.2	56.7

Classic Tuna Salad

2 (6 1/2-or 7-oz.) cans
   water-packed tuna
1 1/2 cups diced celery
1/2 tsp. fresh lemon juice

1/2 tsp. onion salt
1/8 tsp. pepper
6 tbsp. diet
   mayonnaise

Drain the tuna, and flake it apart. Combine the tuna with the rest of the ingredients. Chill the mixture before serving. *Makes 6 servings*

	Calories	Carbo-hydrate (gm)	Protein (gm)	Total Fat (gm)	Saturated Fat (gm)	Choles-terol (mg)
Total	651.1	15.2	112.0	16.0	0.0	300.0
Per Serving	108.5	2.5	18.7	2.7	0.0	50.0

---

gm=grams; mg=milligrams. Nutritional figures are approximate. Figures are based on findings of U.S. Department of Agriculture.

Tuna Rice Salad

2 (6½-or 7-oz.) cans
    water-packed tuna
1½ cups cold cooked rice
1½ cups diced celery
3 tbsp. raisins

1 tsp. lemon juice
½ tsp. curry
½ tsp. onion salt
⅛ tsp. pepper
½ cup diet
    mayonnaise

Drain the tuna, and flake it apart. Combine the tuna with the rest of the ingredients. Chill the mixture before serving.
Makes 8 servings

	Calories	Carbo-hydrate (gm)	Protein (gm)	Total Fat (gm)	Saturated Fat (gm)	Choles-terol (mg)
Total	1109.2	114.4	118.0	20.0	0.0	316.0
Per Serving	138.7	14.3	14.8	2.5	0.0	39.5

Tuna Macaroni Toss

3 cups cooked protein-
    enriched elbow
    macaroni
2 cans (7 oz.) water-
    packed tuna
½ cup green pepper
    strips
¼ cup thinly-sliced
    green onions

2 tbsp. diced
    pimiento
⅛ tsp. salt
½ cup diet French
    dressing
salad greens

Combine all the ingredients except the salad greens. Toss them well. Serve on crisp salad greens.
Makes 6 servings

	Calories	Carbo-hydrate (gm)	Protein (gm)	Total Fat (gm)	Saturated Fat (gm)	Choles-terol (mg)
Total	1007.4	102.5	128.3	7.3	0.0	252.0
Per Serving	167.9	17.1	21.4	1.2	0.0	42.0

gm=grams; mg=milligrams. Nutritional figures are approximate. Figures are based on findings of U.S. Department of Agriculture.

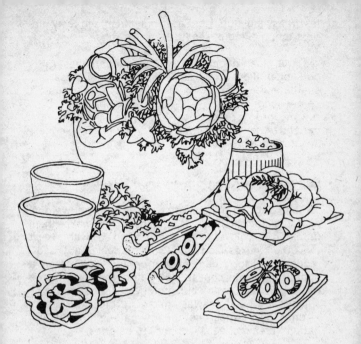

Let's Have A Party!

You do not have to sit on the sidelines when it's time to celebrate. Festive foods needn't be fattening. In fact, skinny stuff is standard fare at parties where the beautiful people circulate. How else would they keep their fashionable forms?

The prettiest — and most sophisticated — party trays start out at the vegetable stand. Chips for dips needn't be greasy kid stuff. Here are some crisp and tasty dippers that make diet sense.

red and green pepper rings	melon cubes
cucumber slices	zucchini strips
scallions	cauliflower buds
celery scoops	radish roses
raw mushroom caps	scallion sticks
canned water chestnut slices	raw turnip wedges
seedless orange sections	tiny pickles
fresh pineapple tidbits	

Quick Dips From Convenience Mixes

Most dips from packaged mixes pack a weighty wallop of calories. But it is not the mix that makes them fattening — it is what they're mixed with. Most packaged mixes add only 50 calories, but the directions call for a base of sour cream (485 calories a cupful) or cream cheese (850 calories in an 8-ounce package). You can cut calories dramatically by substituting plain unsweetened yogurt for sour cream — only 130 calories — or the low-calorie, low-fat "imitation" cream cheese — only 416 calories.

Recipes

Deviled Eggs

6 eggs	1/4 tsp. dry mustard
1/4 cup yogurt	paprika
1 tsp. fresh lemon juice	6 pitted black olives,
1/2 tsp. Worcestershire sauce	sliced

Hard-boil the eggs, peel them and slice them in half lengthwise. Remove the yolks and mash them with all the remaining ingredients except the paprika and olives. Then spoon the egg yolk mixture back into the egg white halves. Refrigerate the eggs until ready to

serve. Sprinkle them with paprika, and garnish with the
olive slices.   *Makes 12 servings*

	Calories	Carbo-hydrate (gm)	Protein (gm)	Total Fat (gm)	Saturated Fat (gm)	Cholesterol (mg)
Total	558.7	4.1	38.0	43.0	12.5	1517.0
Per Serving	46.6	0.3	3.2	3.6	1.0	126.4

Quick Curry Dip

1 cup plain yogurt   ¼ tsp. curry
1 tbsp. minced onion

Blend all of the ingredients together, and refrigerate
the mixture until ready to serve.   *Makes 1 cup*

	Calories	Carbo-hydrate (gm)	Protein (gm)	Total Fat (gm)	Saturated Fat (gm)	Cholesterol (mg)
Total	125.8	13.2	8.0	4.0	2.0	20.0
Per ½ cup	62.9	6.6	4.0	2.0	1.0	10.0

Horseradish Dip

1 cup 99% fat-free   ¼ tsp. dry mustard
  creamed cottage   2 drops
  cheese   Worcestershire
1 tbsp. horseradish   sauce
                             2 drops hot pepper
                               sauce

Combine all the ingredients. Using the high speed of
your mixer or blender, beat until smooth. Chill the dip
before serving.   *Makes 1 cup*

	Calories	Carbo-hydrate (gm)	Protein (gm)	Total Fat (gm)	Saturated Fat (gm)	Cholesterol (mg)
Total	186.0	7.0	30.0	2.0	1.2	19.4
Per ½ cup	93.0	3.5	15.0	1.0	0.6	9.7

---

*gm=grams; mg=milligrams. Nutritional figures are approximate. Figures
are based on findings of U.S. Department of Agriculture.*

Tuna-Cream Cheese Dip

8 oz. package low-
    calorie cream
    cheese
3 oz. can water-packed
    tuna
1 tsp. onion flakes

2 tsp. chicken
    bouillon
    granules
2 tbsp. water

Before preparing: Allow the cream cheese to reach room temperature. Drain the tuna, and flake it.

Combine the cream cheese, tuna, onion, and bouillon granules in a mixing bowl. Mix well. Then blend in the water. Cover the dip, and chill it for at least 1 hour. Serve it with fresh vegetables.   *Makes 1¹/₃ cups*

	Calories	Carbo-hydrate (gm)	Protein (gm)	Total Fat (gm)	Saturated Fat (gm)	Choles-terol (mg)
Total	685.5	45.8	59.6	62.9	36.0	222.2
Per ¹/₃ cup	171.3	11.5	14.9	15.7	9.0	55.6

Fruit Curry Dip

2 cups 99% fat-free
    cottage cheese
1 tsp. curry
¹/₂ tsp. garlic salt

8 oz. can juice-
    packed crushed
    pineapple, well-
    drained
²/₃ cup chopped
    unpeeled red
    apple

Using the highest speed of your mixer or blender, beat together the cottage cheese, curry and garlic salt until they are smooth. Then stir in the pineapple and apple. Cover the dip and chill it before serving.
                                    Makes 3 cups

	Calories	Carbo-hydrate (gm)	Protein (gm)	Total Fat (gm)	Saturated Fat (gm)	Choles-terol (mg)
Total	541.8	58.0	61.0	4.0	1.2	19.4
Per ¹/₂ cup	90.3	9.7	10.2	0.7	0.2	3.2

Bleu Cheese Dip

2 cups 99% fat-free
cottage cheese
1 cup (4 oz.) crumbled
bleu cheese
2 tbsp. chopped green
onion
1/4 tsp. garlic salt

1 tsp.
Worcestershire
sauce
2 tbsp. fresh lemon
juice
1 cup plain yogurt

Mix cottage cheese and bleu cheese, using the highest speed of your blender or mixer. Then beat in the onion, garlic salt, Worcestershire sauce, and lemon juice. Fold in the yogurt. Cover the dip and chill it before serving. Serve it with crackers or vegetable "dippers." Store the dip in the refrigerator.

Makes 4 cups

Special hint: The dip can also be used as a salad dressing or served on baked potatoes.

	Calories	Carbo-hydrate (gm)	Protein (gm)	Total Fat (gm)	Saturated Fat (gm)	Choles-terol (mg)
Total	917.0	32.9	92.4	44.0	24.4	154.8
Per 1/2 cup	114.6	4.1	11.6	5.5	3.1	19.4

Dilly Dip

1 cup plain yogurt
1 tsp. fresh lemon juice
1 tsp. grated onion or
onion juice

1/2 tsp. salt
1/2 tsp. dry mustard
1/4 tsp. dill weed

Combine all of the ingredients and mix them well. Chill the dip before serving. *Makes 1 cup*

	Calories	Carbo-hydrate (gm)	Protein (gm)	Total Fat (gm)	Saturated Fat (gm)	Choles-terol (mg)
Total	127.0	13.6	8.0	4.0	2.0	20.0
Per 1/2 cup	63.5	6.8	4.0	2.0	1.0	10.0

gm=grams; mg=milligrams. Nutritional figures are approximate. Figures are based on findings of U.S. Department of Agriculture.

Guacamole Dip

1 cup 99% fat-free
cottage cheese
2 tsp. grated onion
1 tsp. fresh lemon juice
1 crushed garlic clove

3/4 tsp. salt
1/8 tsp. pepper
1 ripe avocado
1 medium-size ripe
tomato

Combine the cottage cheese, onion, lemon juice, garlic, salt and pepper. Beat with the highest speed of your mixer or blender until smooth. Peel the avocado and remove the pit. Mash the avocado with a fork. Peel the tomato by first plunging it in boiling water; then mince it. Fold the avocado and tomato into the cottage cheese mixture. Cover the guacamole, and chill it before serving.   *Makes 2 cups*

	Calories	Carbo-hydrate (gm)	Protein (gm)	Total Fat (gm)	Saturated Fat (gm)	Choles-terol (mg)
Total	612.0	42.8	36.1	35.0	8.2	19.4
Per 1/2 cup	153.0	10.7	9.0	8.8	2.1	4.9

Chive Dip

1 cup 99% fat-free
cottage cheese
2 tsp. chicken bouillon
4 tbsp. water

1 tbsp. finely
chopped parsley
1 tbsp. chopped
chives (fresh,
frozen, or dried)
1/2 tsp. dill

Combine the cottage cheese, bouillon, and water in your blender container. Whip them until they are creamy. Then stir in the remaining ingredients. Chill dip for at least 1 hour before serving.   *Makes 1 cup*

	Calories	Carbo-hydrate (gm)	Protein (gm)	Total Fat (gm)	Saturated Fat (gm)	Choles-terol (mg)
Total	191.5	25.3	40.2	9.0	3.2	19.4
Per 1/2 cup	95.8	12.7	20.0	4.5	1.6	9.7

Peppery Olive Dip

1¼ cups 99% fat-free
cottage cheese
¼ cup skim milk
1 tbsp. instant minced
onion

⅛ to ¼ tsp. crushed
red pepper
flakes
¼ cup chopped
pimiento stuffed
olives

In a blender or mixer, blend the cottage cheese and milk until they are smooth. Then stir in the remaining ingredients. Chill the mixture until 30 minutes before serving time. *Makes 1½ cups*

	Calories	Carbo-hydrate (gm)	Protein (gm)	Total Fat (gm)	Saturated Fat (gm)	Choles-terol (mg)
Total	273.5	10.6	36.2	8.25	1.4	23.1
Per ½ cup	91.2	3.5	12.1	2.8	0.5	7.7

Cheddar Dip

2 cups 99% fat-free
cottage cheese
2 tsp. grated onion
1 tsp. celery salt

¼ tsp.
Worcestershire
sauce
1½ cups (6 oz.)
shredded extra-
sharp cheddar
cheese

Combine cottage cheese, onion, celery salt and sauce. Beat with the highest speed of your mixer or blender until smooth. Gradually add 1 cup of shredded cheese and continue beating at high speed until the mixture is smooth. Then fold in the remaining cheese. Serve the Cheddar Dip immediately. *Makes 3 cups*

	Calories	Carbo-hydrate (gm)	Protein (gm)	Total Fat (gm)	Saturated Fat (gm)	Choles-terol (mg)
Total	1051.6	18.4	102.1	58.0	32.4	206.8
Per ½ cup	175.3	3.1	17.0	9.7	5.4	34.5

gm=grams; mg=milligrams. Nutritional figures are approximate. Figures are based on findings of U.S. Department of Agriculture.

Romanian Chicken Liver Paté

2 lbs. chicken livers
1/2 cup sherry or dry
   vermouth
12 oz. low-calorie cream
   cheese

1 tsp. garlic salt
dash of hot pepper
   sauce
1 tsp.
   Worcestershire
   sauce

Simmer the chicken livers in the wine until they are tender. Then cut the chicken livers small enough to be chopped in a blender. Place the liver in the blender and add the cream cheese, garlic salt, hot pepper sauce, and Worcestershire sauce. Blend the ingredients until they are smooth. Chill the paté in the refrigerator for 1 hour. Garnish it with parsley, and serve it with crackers.   *Makes 7 1/2 cups*

	Calories	Carbo-hydrate (gm)	Protein (gm)	Total Fat (gm)	Saturated Fat (gm)	Choles-terol (mg)
Total	2485.4	50.1	267.0	120.7	64.2	7145.5
Per 1/2 cup	165.7	3.3	17.8	8.0	4.3	476.4

Liver Paté

1/2 lb. beef liver
1/4 cup diet mayonnaise
1/2 tsp. grated onion or
   onion juice

dash of salt
dash of pepper

Broil the liver about 6 inches from the heat source until it is cooked but still slightly pink inside. Then put it through a meat grinder. Combine the ground liver with the rest of the ingredients and blend well. Serve the paté with toast or crackers.   *Makes about 1 cup*

	Calories	Carbo-hydrate (gm)	Protein (gm)	Total Fat (gm)	Saturated Fat (gm)	Choles-terol (mg)
Total	600.4	16.1	60.0	32.0	0.0	1032.0
Per 1/2 cup	300.2	8.1	30.0	16.0	0.0	516.0

Chicken Liver Spread

1 lb. chicken livers
1 cup water
1 tbsp. instant minced
   onion

3 eggs
1/2 cup diet
   mayonnaise
1/2 tsp. hot pepper
   sauce

Hard-boil the eggs and chop them finely. Simmer the livers in water for approximately 10 minutes until cooked through; drain them. Crush the livers with a fork. Then add the onion, eggs, mayonnaise, and hot pepper sauce. Serve the spread on crackers.

Makes 3 cups

	Calories	Carbo-hydrate (gm)	Protein (gm)	Total Fat (gm)	Saturated Fat (gm)	Choles-terol (mg)
Total	1165.2	27.1	138.3	58.0	14.0	4220.0
Per 1/2 cup	194.2	4.5	23.1	9.7	2.3	703.3

Chicken Livers in Wine

1 lb. chicken livers
1 tbsp. diet margarine
1 1/2 tsp. salt

1/4 tsp. pepper
1/2 cup dry white wine

Melt the margarine in a non-stick skillet. Add the livers, season them with the salt and pepper and sauté them over medium heat for approximately 10 minutes, turning them occasionally. Add the wine, cover the pan and simmer the livers for about 5 minutes longer until they are done. Serve them on toothpicks.

Makes 12 servings

	Calories	Carbo-hydrate (gm)	Protein (gm)	Total Fat (gm)	Saturated Fat (gm)	Choles-terol (mg)
Total	898.9	20.6	120.0	30.0	9.0	3400.0
Per Serving	74.9	1.7	10.0	2.5	0.8	283.3

---

gm = grams; mg = milligrams. Nutritional figures are approximate. Figures are based on findings of U.S. Department of Agriculture.

Pickled Fresh Mushrooms

4 cups tiny fresh mushrooms
1 onion
3/4 cup tarragon vinegar
1/4 cup water
3 tbsp. corn or safflower oil

1 minced garlic clove
1 1/2 tsp. salt
1/4 tsp. pepper
1/8 tsp. cayenne

Slice the onion and separate it into rings. Combine it with the rest of the ingredients in a bowl. Cover the bowl and refrigerate the mixture for 24 hours. Drain the mushrooms and serve them with cocktail picks.

Makes 8 servings

	Calories	Carbo-hydrate (gm)	Protein (gm)	Total Fat (gm)	Saturated Fat (gm)	Choles-terol (mg)
Total	698.9	65.9	30.0	46.0	3.0	0.0
Per Serving	87.4	8.2	3.8	5.8	0.4	0.0

Lamb-Stuffed Mushroom Hors d'Oeuvres

1 lb. lean leg of lamb, trimmed of fat, and ground
2 tsp. prepared horseradish
1 tsp. chopped chives

1/2 tsp. garlic salt
coarse ground pepper to taste
1 lb. mushrooms (about 18)
2/3 cup dry sauterne

Mix the lamb, horseradish, chives, garlic salt, and pepper together. Remove the stems from the mushrooms and stuff the mushroom caps with the lamb mixture. Place the stuffed mushrooms in a shallow baking dish and pour the wine over them. Bake them at 350° for about 20 minutes until the meat is browned.

Makes 18 servings

	Calories	Carbo-hydrate (gm)	Protein (gm)	Total Fat (gm)	Saturated Fat (gm)	Choles-terol (mg)
Total	1305.5	61.9	163.1	37.0	19.2	454.4
Per Serving	72.5	3.4	9.1	2.1	1.1	25.2

Dried Beef Roulades

1 tsp. instant diced onions	1 tsp. horseradish
2 tsp. water	12 slices dried beef
4 oz. farmer cheese	

Add 2 teaspoons of water to the instant onions and allow them to stand for 5 to 10 minutes. Then blend the cheese, onion, and horseradish in a bowl. Spread some of the cheese mixture on each slice of dried beef. Roll the beef tightly around the cheese and secure each roll with a toothpick. *Makes 12 servings*

	Calories	Carbo-hydrate (gm)	Protein (gm)	Total Fat (gm)	Saturated Fat (gm)	Choles-terol (mg)
Total	388.5	18.3	103.9	64.4	34.0	177.0
Per Serving	32.4	1.5	8.7	5.4	2.8	14.8

Orange Cheese Spread

1/4 cup frozen orange juice concentrate	8 slices thinly-sliced bread
8 oz. low-calorie cream cheese	

Before preparing: Allow the orange juice to thaw, but don't dilute it. Allow the cream cheese to come to room temperature.

Blend the orange juice concentrate into the cream cheese and mix them well. Spread the mixture generously on the thinly sliced bread. Then cut each slice into thirds. *Makes 24 servings*

	Calories	Carbo-hydrate (gm)	Protein (gm)	Total Fat (gm)	Saturated Fat (gm)	Choles-terol (mg)
Total	1052.3	105.1	30.0	53.1	33.2	173.4
Per Serving	43.8	4.4	1.3	2.2	1.4	7.2

---

gm=grams; mg=milligrams. Nutritional figures are approximate. Figures are based on findings of U.S. Department of Agriculture.

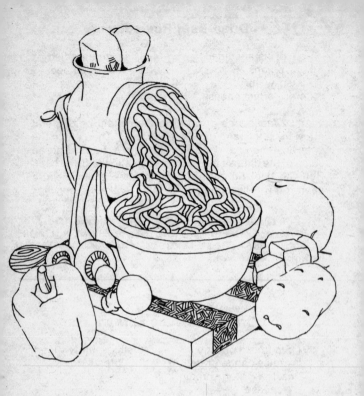

The Meat Of The Matter

Meat! What red-blooded American doesn't love it? If you're like most homemakers, meat is the most expensive item in your food budget. It may also be the most costly category in your calorie budget. Many well-intentioned but misinformed dieters are wasting their money and calories on meat — too much and the wrong kind — in the mistaken notion that a high-meat diet is necessary to achieve slimness. Meat is good, yes, but too much of a good thing is not only fattening, it's boring! If you've been subsisting on steak and hamburger in the hope of regaining a lost waistline, you are probably a victim of some commonly held misconceptions about the importance of lots of meat in the American diet.

How many of these fallacies do you believe?

Fallacy: Meat is all protein, and the more you eat, the thinner you'll be.

Fact: Meat is only part protein. Much of what's left is fat, and fat is the most fattening basic food there is. Some of the most popular cuts of meat have nearly five times as many fat calories as protein calories. And the more calories you eat, the fatter you'll be.

Fallacy: You need meat every day.

Fact: Other animal foods are an equal or better source of complete protein. Seafood, poultry, eggs, skim milk, cottage cheese, and yogurt are some examples of low-fat, low-calorie foods that are extra-rich in protein. Eight ounces of 99 percent fat-free cottage cheese alone is enough to satisfy most people's daily protein needs. Remember, the meat you eat is also balanced by the smaller amounts of less complete protein found in vegetable foods. Nuts and beans are especially rich in vegetable protein. And soy products — soy flours, protein-enriched mixes, meat extenders, etc. — are a particularly important source of inexpensive, low-calorie protein.

Fallacy: You can never eat too much meat.

Fact: Some steak-lovers may feel that way, but a super-abundance of protein, especially meat protein, can be harmful. Meat contains cholesterol and saturated fat which has been implicated in heart disease and certain forms of cancer. Too much protein in the diet is especially bad for anyone with latent kidney trouble. Recent studies have demonstrated that high-protein diets can upset calcium balance and accelerate osteoporosis, loss of bone tissue.

Fallacy: Simple steaks and roasts are better for calorie counters than combination dishes, like stews or casseroles.

Fact: The cuts of meat most amenable to simple broiling or roasting are generally the most expensive — in calories as well as cost — while the leanest and least costly cuts are ideally suited to imaginative combinations and "gourmet" creations. And, since most of the other ingredients in casseroles are less fattening than meat, combination dishes allow dieters to satisfy their appetites with fewer calories. (Of course it's necessary to prepare these dishes in a way that eliminates excess fat.)

Fallacy: Rare meat is less fattening than meat that is well-done.

Fact: The longer meat is cooked, the more fat is melted out and eliminated (presuming, of course, that the fat is drained away or skimmed off). We're not suggesting that you overcook an expensive porterhouse, but rather that you concentrate on the less expensive, less fattening cuts — the kind that are usually slow-simmered to a well-done tenderness.

Fallacy: Fat meat is juicy; lean meat is dry.

Fact: Fat meat is greasy, and because of its greasiness, fatty meat is better able to withstand the mishandling of too-high temperatures. Too-quick cooking at too-high temperatures robs lean meat of its juiciness.

Fallacy: Beef is less fattening than most other meats.

Fact: Many cuts of lamb, pork, and ham are lower in fat and calories then the most popular cuts of beef. And veal is the leanest of all.

How to Cook Meat

Broiling is the dry-heat method for quick cooking. When broiling, the heat source is above the meat.

1. Set your oven regulator for broiling.

2. Place the meat on a rack in your broiler pan, 3 to 6 inches from the heat. (Place a thick cut of meat further away from the heat.)

3. Broil the meat until the top side is brown.

4. Sprinkle the browned surface with salt, pepper, and whatever other seasonings you desire.

5. Turn the meat and brown the other side. Make a small cut in the center of the meat to see if the desired "doneness" has been reached.

Barbecuing is another form of dry-heat cookery, usually done outdoors, over glowing charcoals. Electric and gas barbecues are also available; some are built right into the kitchen. When barbecuing, the source of heat is beneath the meat. For best results, the meat should not be closer than 3 inches to the heat. When the meat is brown on one side, turn it with tongs and brown the other side.

Panbroiling is another dry-heat method of cooking.

1. Place the meat in an uncovered non-stick skillet.

2. The pan may be sprinkled with a thin layer of salt to prevent sticking, or spray it with vegetable coating for non-stick cooking. Do not add fat or water. Do not cover the pan.

3. Cook slow over low heat, turning occasionally.

4. Pour off or remove all fat as it accumulates.

5. Brown the meat on both sides, being careful not to overcook it.

6. Season the meat and serve it at once.

Oven roasting is the slow method of dry cooking.

1. To achieve tenderness with lean cuts, treat the meat with meat tenderizer according to package directions, or for a more interesting flavor marinate the meat for several hours. (Check the index for a variety of marinade recipes.)

2. Place the meat on a rack in an open shallow roasting pan.

3. Insert a meat thermometer so that the tip of the thermometer — the bulb — is in the center of the meat.

4. Do not add water, and do not cover the pan.

5. Roast the meat in a slow oven — approximately 325° — to the desired degree of doneness. If you like your beef rare, roast it until the thermometer reads 140°; if medium is your taste, the thermometer should read 160°. Never allow the thermometer to reach more than 170°. Lamb is rare at 165°-170°; medium at 174°, and well-done at 180°. Pork should be roasted to an internal temperature of 170°.

HOW DIFFERENT MEATS COMPARE IN CALORIES

Compare the typical calories in similar cuts from different animals. All calorie counts are for one pound of boneless meat, uncooked, and are derived from U.S. Department of Agriculture data for "choice" or "medium-fat" grades of meat, the kind most frequently found in supermarkets. Individual cuts will vary.

	BEEF	VEAL	LAMB	PORK AND HAM
From the shoulder	Chuck	Shoulder	Shoulder	Boston Butt
Meat and fat	1,597	785	1,275	1,302
Lean only	853	*	671	816
From the rib	Rib Steak	Rib Chop	Rib Chop	Rib or Loin Chop
Meat and fat	1,819	939	1,252	1,352
Lean only	875	*	612	857
From the leg				
Meat and fat	894	744	1,007	1,397
Lean only	612	*	590	694

*Per 100 grams (approximately 3½ ounces). All data approximate, adapted from U.S. Department of Agriculture information.

Braising or pot-roasting is the preferred method for moist-heat cooking. It is particularly suitable for less tender cuts of beef.

1. Brown the meat slowly on all sides in a heavy non-stick utensil with no fat added. One low-cal method of browning is to add a tablespoon of water to the meat, cover the utensil, and heat it slowly over moderate heat. The water will evaporate, and the steam will cause the meat to release its own inner fat. Then, uncover the pot and let the meat brown in its own fat. The meat may also be browned under the broiler.

2. Season the meat with salt, pepper, herbs, and spices, if you like.

3. Add a small amount of liquid — water, wine, tomato juice, or fruit juice — to the meat.

4. Cover the pot tightly, and cook the meat at a low temperature until it is tender.

5. You can make a sauce or gravy from the liquid in the pot, if you like, but first skim the fat from the pan juices.

6. Pot roast is best made a day ahead, then refrigerated until about a half hour before serving time. The refrigeration will cause the fat that rises to the top to harden so it can be lifted off and discarded before the meat is reheated.

Simmering is another method of moist-heat cooking. This method requires more liquid than others and is used with cuts of meat that need longer cooking and more moisture to make them fork tender.

1. If desired, brown the meat on all sides in a non-stick utensil with no fat added. (For directions, see step 1 under Braising.)

2. Cover the meat with water or some other liquid.

3. Season with salt, pepper, herbs, and spices.

4. Cover the pot and simmer — do not boil — the meat until it is tender.

5. For best results, cook the meat the day before serving and chill it overnight in the stock in which it was cooked. The fat will float to the top and harden so it can be easily removed before heating and serving.

6. When vegetables are to be cooked with the meat, add them whole or in pieces after the fat has been removed, and cook them just long enough before serving to be tender.

Beef

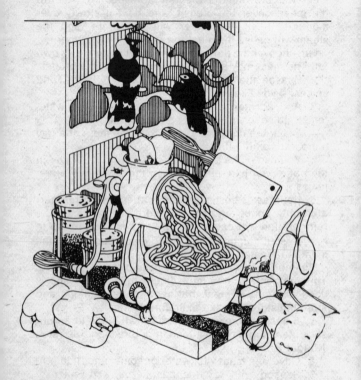

Beef is America's favorite food. From filet mignon to hamburger to stew, beef proves its great versatility. You can boil it, broil it, braise it, fry it, and even eat it raw.

And it is available in a wide range of prices. Fortunately for the weight-conscious millions, it is the less expensive cuts of beef that are the calorie bargains. Part of what makes prime beef "prime" is the marbling of fat throughout the meat — great for flavor, lousy for waistlines.

Recipes

Chinese Pepper Steak

1 lb. boneless round
   steak or roast
1 tbsp. diet margarine
2 tbsp. finely chopped
   onion
1 garlic clove
2 large green peppers
1/2 cup celery, diagonally
   sliced

1/2 cup beef
   consommé
salt
pepper
2 tbsp. chopped
   pimiento
2 tsp. cornstarch
3 tbsp. water
1 tsp. soy sauce

Before cooking: Trim the meat of all visible fat and cut it into thin strips. Chop the onion, garlic, and pimiento. Cut the green pepper into strips.

Place the diet margarine in a non-stick skillet and heat it over low heat. When the margarine is melted, add the strips of beef and brown them on both sides. Before going any further, pour off any drippings that have accumulated in the pan. Then add the onion, garlic, green peppers, and celery. Add the consomme and season the whole mixture with salt and pepper. Cover the skillet tightly and simmer the meat for 20 minutes. Do not boil it. Add the pimiento. Thicken the mixture with the cornstarch which has been blended with the water and soy sauce. Simmer, covered, for an additional 5 minutes. *Makes 4 servings*

	Calories	Carbo-hydrate (gm)	Protein (gm)	Total Fat (gm)	Saturated Fat (gm)	Choles-terol (mg)
Total	1001.4	17.9	145.2	32.8	14.3	424.9
Per Serving	250.4	4.5	36.3	8.2	3.6	106.2

gm=grams; mg=milligrams. Nutritional figures are approximate. Figures are based on findings of U.S. Department of Agriculture.

Burgundy Pot Roast

5 lbs. boneless bottom round or rolled rump	1 tsp. peppercorns
2 cups sliced onion	4 or 5 sprigs of parsley
2 crushed garlic cloves	1 tsp. salt
1 bay leaf	2 cups dry Burgundy wine
$1/2$ tsp. thyme	$10^1/2$ oz. can beef broth
	3 tbsp. flour

Before cooking: Trim meat of all visible fat. Put the meat in a stainless steel or glass bowl just large enough to hold the meat and onions. In a separate bowl combine the onions, herbs, salt, and wine. Pour this mixture over the meat. Cover the meat, and refrigerate it for 10 to 12 hours, turning it occasionally. Skim fat from liquid of broth using a bulb-type baster.

Remove the meat from the marinade and pat it dry. Separate the onions from the liquid of the marinade. Place the meat on a rack in a shallow roasting pan. Insert a meat thermometer so that the bulb is in the center of the roast. Roast the meat for 30 minutes at 475°, basting once or twice with the reserved marinade. Reduce the heat to 400°. Add the reserved onions to the pan and continue to roast the meat for 40 to 45 minutes, basting occasionally with the marinade. When the thermometer reaches 140°-150°, remove the meat to a warm platter. Let it stand for about 15 minutes before carving.

Pour the pan drippings from the roasting pan into a container. Put the container in the freezer to cool it quickly and bring the fat to the surface. Skim off the fat. On the top of the range, heat the pan drippings to boiling and boil them for 1 minute. In a separate bowl combine the broth and flour, and add this mixture to the hot drippings. Continue to cook, stirring constantly, until the sauce is thick. Serve this over the sliced beef. *Makes 15 servings*

	Calories	Carbo-hydrate (gm)	Protein (gm)	Total Fat (gm)	Saturated Fat (gm)	Choles-terol (mg)
Total	4300.3	60.3	724.1	89.1	29.6	2134.9
Per Serving	286.7	4.0	48.3	5.9	2.0	142.3

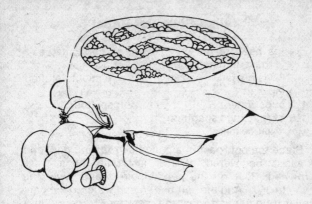

Spicy Pot Roast

3 lbs. boneless top
    round roast, bottom
    or eye
1/4 cup cider vinegar
1 cup water

3 whole cloves
1 bay leaf
3/4 tsp. salt
3/4 tsp. sugar

Before cooking: Trim the meat of all visible fat. Place the meat in a bowl. Combine all the ingredients and pour this mixture over the meat. Cover the bowl and place it in the refrigerator for 24 hours.

Transfer the meat and liquid into a heavy pot or Dutch oven. Simmer it over low heat, covered, for about 2 1/2 hours until the meat is tender — or roast it, covered, in a 350° oven for about 2 1/2 hours. Remove the meat to a serving platter. Using a bulb-type baster, skim all of the fat from the pan drippings. Simmer the remaining liquid, uncovered, until it is reduced to just enough to pour over the meat. Pour the reduced liquid over the meat and serve. *Makes 10 servings*

	Calories	Carbo-hydrate (gm)	Protein (gm)	Total Fat (gm)	Saturated Fat (gm)	Choles-terol (mg)
Total	2226.5	4.0	426.7	53.3	17.8	1262.4
Per Serving	222.7	0.4	42.7	5.3	1.8	126.2

gm=grams; mg=milligrams. Nutritional figures are approximate. Figures are based on findings of U.S. Department of Agriculture.

Italian-Style Pot Roast

4 lbs. beef arm pot
    roast, trimmed of all
    visible fat
1/2 tsp. salt
1 1/2 cups water
1 1/2 oz. package spaghetti
    sauce mix

16 oz. can tomatoes
1/4 cup sliced
    pimiento-stuffed
    olives
2 tbsp. flour

Place the pot roast in a non-stick roasting pan, and roast it, uncovered, at 475° just until the meat is browned. Pour off the pan drippings and lower the oven to 350°. Add the salt and 1/4 cup water to the pan, cover it tightly and roast the meat for 1 1/2 hours. In a separate bowl, combine the spaghetti sauce mix, tomatoes, olives, and 1 cup water. Add this mixture to the meat. Cover the pot, and continue cooking the meat for another 1 1/2 hours or until it is tender. Remove the meat to a heated platter. Using a bulb-type baster, skim all the fat from the pan drippings. Blend together the flour and 1/4 cup water and add this mixture to the sauce, stirring constantly until the mixture has thickened. Serve the sauce around the pot roast.

Makes 12 servings

	Calories	Carbo-hydrate (gm)	Protein (gm)	Total Fat (gm)	Saturated Fat (gm)	Choles-terol (mg)
Total	3166.7	32.4	574.5	79.2	23.7	1682.7
Per Serving	263.9	2.7	47.9	6.6	2.0	140.2

Mexican Pot Roast

4 lbs. lean boneless
    bottom round,
    trimmed of all
    visible fat and
    rolled for pot roast
2 tsp. diet margarine
1/2 cup water

1 tsp. chili powder
1 tbsp. paprika
2 tsp. onion salt
1/8 tsp. ground clove
1/2 tsp. cinnamon
2 tbsp. flour

Melt the diet margarine over low heat in a heavy, non-stick Dutch oven. Brown the meat slowly on all sides in the melted margarine. Add the seasonings and $^1/_2$ cup water to the pot, and simmer the meat slowly, covered, for $2^1/_2$ to 3 hours — until it is tender. Remove the meat to a platter, and keep it warm.

Pour the pan drippings into a large measuring cup. Add water and ice cubes to bring it to 2 cups. When the ice cubes have melted and the fat has risen to the surface, skim off all the fat. Stir the flour into the cold drippings, and return it to the pot. Over low heat, cook and stir the liquid, scraping the pan well, until it simmers and thickens.   *Makes 12 servings*

	Calories	Carbo-hydrate (gm)	Protein (gm)	Total Fat (gm)	Saturated Fat (gm)	Choles-terol (mg)
Total	3121.7	12.4	570.5	83.2	25.7	1682.7
Per Serving	260.1	1.0	47.5	6.9	2.1	140.2

Roast Beef in Beer

3 lbs. lean boneless top round, bottom round, or eye of round
2 tsp. garlic salt
$^1/_8$ tsp. pepper
$^1/_4$ tsp. poultry seasoning
12 oz. low-calorie, low-carbo-hydrate beer

Before cooking: Trim the meat of all visible fat.

Sprinkle the meat with the seasonings and place it in a heavy Dutch oven. Add the beer. Roast the meat, covered, in a 350° degree oven for $2^1/_2$ hours or more — until it is tender — basting occasionally. Skim off all the fat from the pan drippings by using a bulb-type baster. Continue to roast the meat, uncovered, until most of the liquid has evaporated and the roast is nicely browned. After the meat has been sliced, pour the remaining pan juices over it.   *Makes 12 servings*

	Calories	Carbo-hydrate (gm)	Protein (gm)	Total Fat (gm)	Saturated Fat (gm)	Choles-terol (mg)
Total	2318.5	2.8	427.6	53.3	17.8	1262.4
Per Serving	193.2	0.2	35.6	4.4	1.5	105.2

gm=grams; mg=milligrams. Nutritional figures are approximate. Figures are based on findings of U.S. Department of Agriculture.

Italian Steak

2½ lbs. top round steak
½ cup water
¼ cup cider vinegar
1 tbsp. salt

2½ tsp. Italian
    seasoning
¼ tsp. pepper
¼ tsp. garlic powder
1 tbsp. instant
    chopped onion

Before cooking: Trim the meat of all visible fat. Place the meat in a bowl just large enough to hold it. Combine the rest of the ingredients and pour this mixture over the meat. Cover the bowl, and place the meat in the refrigerator overnight; or let it sit uncovered, at room temperature, for 6 hours. Turn the meat 2 or 3 times during the marinating.

Place the meat in a roasting pan and pour half the marinade over it. Roast the meat at 300° for 1 hour. Add the remaining marinade, and continue to roast the meat for about 30 minutes — or until it is done to your taste. *Makes 10 servings*

	Calories	Carbo-hydrate (gm)	Protein (gm)	Total Fat (gm)	Saturated Fat (gm)	Choles-terol (mg)
Total	2181.6	6.5	350.4	66.7	33.3	1033.5
Per Serving	218.2	0.7	35.0	6.7	3.3	103.4

Zesty Steak Bake

1½ lbs. lean, ½-inch
    thick round steak,
    trimmed of all fat
1 tbsp. diet margarine
12 small white onions
1 tsp. salt
½ tsp. pepper

⅛ tsp. allspice
1 cup water
¼ cup vinegar
1 tbsp. sugar
1 cup canned
    tomatoes

Before cooking: Cut the round steak into six equal slices. Combine the seasoning, vinegar, sugar, tomatoes, and allspice in a bowl with 1 cup water.

Place the diet margarine in a non-stick skillet and heat it over low heat. Add the steak and onions to the skillet and sauté them in the diet margarine until they are brown. Then transfer the meat and onions to a roasting pan. Pour the tomato mixture over the meat and onions. Place the roasting pan in the oven, uncovered, and roast the meat at 325° for one hour and 15 minutes.   *Makes 6 servings*

	Calories	Carbo-hydrate (gm)	Protein (gm)	Total Fat (gm)	Saturated Fat (gm)	Choles-terol (mg)
Total	1690.2	85.9	224.0	47.0	21.0	620.0
Per Serving	281.7	14.3	37.3	7.8	3.5	103.3

Rare Flank Steak

1¼ lbs. flank steak
   meat tenderizer
   garlic powder

coarsely-ground
   pepper
2 tbsp. soy sauce or
   Worcestershire
   sauce

Before cooking: Make shallow criss-cross cuts on both sides of the steak with a sharp knife, being careful not to slice too deeply. Sprinkle the meat liberally with meat tenderizer, garlic powder, and pepper. Then leave the meat out, uncovered, at room temperature for about 30 minutes. Or refrigerate it, covered, for several hours.

Heat 1 tablespoon soy sauce or Worcestershire sauce in a non-stick skillet over a high temperature. Add the steak and brown it quickly on one side. Add the second tablespoon of sauce and turn the steak. Continue to cook the meat over high heat; remember that it should be served quite rare. When done, remove the meat from the skillet and serve it immediately.

Makes 5 servings

	Calories	Carbo-hydrate (gm)	Protein (gm)	Total Fat (gm)	Saturated Fat (gm)	Choles-terol (mg)
Total	1102.9	2.0	176.9	33.3	16.7	516.5
Per Serving	220.6	0.4	35.4	6.7	3.3	103.3

---

gm=grams; mg=milligrams. Nutritional figures are approximate. Figures are based on findings of U.S. Department of Agriculture.

Skinny Swiss Steak

2 lbs. boneless round
steak
1 tbsp. diet margarine
1 tsp. garlic salt
1/8 tsp. pepper

1 cup chopped
onions
3 cups canned
stewed tomatoes
1 cup chopped
celery

Before cooking: Trim the round steak of all visible fat.
Place the margarine in a non-stick skillet and heat it
over moderate heat. When the margarine is melted,
add the steak to the pan. Season the meat with the
garlic salt and pepper. Raise the heat under the pan to
high and brown the meat quickly on both sides. Lower
the heat, and before going any further, pour off any fat
that has accumulated in the pan. Then add the onions,
tomatoes, and celery to the meat and cover the skillet
tightly. Simmer — do not boil — the meat mixture over
very low heat for 1 1/2 hours or more until the meat is
tender and the sauce is thick.   *Makes 8 servings*

	Calories	Carbo-hydrate (gm)	Protein (gm)	Total Fat (gm)	Saturated Fat (gm)	Choles-terol (mg)
Total	1987.9	46.0	287.9	62.3	27.7	826.5
Per Serving	248.5	5.8	36.0	7.8	3.5	103.3

Soy-Barbecued Round Steak

3 lbs. lean round steak,
1 1/2-inches thick
1 tbsp. Italian
seasoning
1/2 tsp. pepper

1 tbsp. catsup
3 tbsp. soy sauce
2 tsp. meat
tenderizer

Before cooking: Trim the meat of all visible fat. Blend
together the Italian herbs, pepper, catsup, soy sauce,
and meat tenderizer. Brush this mixture all over the
steak. Place the steak in a shallow dish, pouring any
leftover marinade over it. Cover the dish and place it in
the refrigerator over night.
    When you are ready to cook the steak, the grill

should be lightly coated with oil to prevent the meat from sticking. Or the grill can be sprayed with spray-on vegetable coating before the coals are lighted. Place the grill 4 to 5 inches above hot coals. Grill the meat for about 40 minutes on each side until the desired doneness is reached. Turn the meat only once. (This dish may also be oven-broiled.) To serve, carve the meat into ¼-inch slices.   *Makes 10 servings*

	Calories	Carbohydrate (gm)	Protein (gm)	Total Fat (gm)	Saturated Fat (gm)	Cholesterol (mg)
Total	2645.0	7.0	423.0	80.0	40.0	1240.0
Per Serving	264.5	0.7	42.3	8.0	4.0	124.0

Trim Teriyaki

2 lbs. lean round steak,
1-inch thick
1 small onion
½ cup soy sauce

½ cup orange juice
1 tsp. ground ginger
1 garlic clove

Before cooking: Slice the onion and chop the garlic. Cut the round steak into thin slices (¼-inch thick or less) and place it, with the onion slices, in a shallow baking dish. In a separate bowl combine the soy sauce, orange juice, ginger, and garlic. Pour this mixture over the meat, coating slices thoroughly. Cover the dish and refrigerate meat overnight.

Drain off and reserve the marinade. Weave the strips of beef back and forth on bamboo or metal skewers. Place the skewers on a rack on the broiler pan so the meat is 4 inches from the heat. Broil the meat about 3 minutes, turn it, brush it with reserved marinade and continue to broil until the meat has reached the desired doneness.   *Makes 8 servings*

	Calories	Carbohydrate (gm)	Protein (gm)	Total Fat (gm)	Saturated Fat (gm)	Cholesterol (mg)
Total	1887.9	26.0	289.9	53.8	26.7	826.5
Per Serving	236.0	3.3	36.2	6.7	3.3	103.3

gm=grams; mg=milligrams. Nutritional figures are approximate. Figures are based on findings of U.S. Department of Agriculture.

Steak Diane

1½ lbs. lean boneless sirloin steak, ½-inch thick
2 tsp. peanut oil
½ tsp. dry mustard
⅛ tsp. coarse freshly ground pepper
¼ tsp. garlic salt
1 tbsp. chopped chives
1 tbsp. lemon juice
2 tsp. Worcestershire sauce
3 tbsp. brandy

Before cooking: Trim the steak of all visible fat. Mix the dry mustard, salt, and pepper together. Sprinkle this mixture over one side of the steak and rub it in.

Pour the oil into a non-stick skillet and heat it over medium heat. Rotate the pan to spread the oil evenly. Add the steak to the skillet and brown the meat for about 1½ minutes on each side. Sprinkle the chives, lemon juice and Worcestershire sauce into the skillet.

Heat the brandy in a small saucepan over a low heat. Or it can be heated at the table over a candle warmer. Bring the steak to the table in the skillet. Pour the brandy over the steak and ignite it. When the flame goes out, transfer the steak to a serving platter.

Makes 6 servings

	Calories	Carbo-hydrate (gm)	Protein (gm)	Total Fat (gm)	Saturated Fat (gm)	Cholesterol (mg)
Total	1619.6	2.0	216.4	57.2	26.0	612.0
Per Serving	269.9	0.3	36.1	9.5	4.3	102.0

Chinese Beef and Asparagus

1 lb. flank steak
2 tbsp. soy sauce
1 tbsp. dry white wine
1 garlic clove
¼ tsp. ground ginger
1 tbsp. diet margarine
1 lb. asparagus
1 cup beef broth
1½ tbsp. cornstarch

Before cooking: Slice the flank steak diagonally, across the grain, into 1-inch wide strips. Slice the asparagus diagonally into 2-inch pieces. Mince the garlic. In a ceramic bowl, mix together the soy sauce, wine, garlic, ginger, and beef. Let this mixture sit uncovered at room temperature for 1 hour.

Melt the diet margarine in a non-stick skillet over moderate heat. Add the meat, and brown it quickly on all sides. (Save the marinade that the beef was sitting in.) Add the asparagus to the skillet, and stir-fry the asparagus and meat for 3 minutes. In a bowl, mix together the broth, cornstarch, and reserved marinade; stir this mixture into the skillet. Cook the entire mixture over moderate heat, stirring constantly, until the sauce has thickened. *Makes 4 servings*

	Calories	Carbo-hydrate (gm)	Protein (gm)	Total Fat (gm)	Saturated Fat (gm)	Choles-terol (mg)
Total	1139.7	45.3	154.6	32.4	14.2	433.2
Per Serving	284.9	11.3	38.7	8.1	3.6	108.3

Beef-Harvest Stew

2 lbs. boneless round steak	¹/₂ lb. zucchini
1 tbsp. diet margarine	1 small eggplant
3 tbsp. sweet paprika	2 onions
1 lb. can tomatoes	2 green peppers
1 lb. green beans	2 bay leaves
	3 tsp. garlic salt

Before cooking: Cut the meat into 1-inch cubes, trimming off all visible fat. Cut the green beans and zucchini into slices. Peel and slice the eggplant. Chop the onions and green pepper.

Melt the diet margarine in a heavy Dutch oven. Brown the meat on all sides in the melted margarine. Add the vegetables to the pot in layers and sprinkle the paprika and garlic salt over all. Add the bay leaves. Cover the pot tightly and roast the meat in a 350° oven for 2 hours or more — until it is tender. Remove the bay leaves before serving. *Makes 8 servings*

	Calories	Carbo-hydrate (gm)	Protein (gm)	Total Fat (gm)	Saturated Fat (gm)	Choles-terol (mg)
Total	1909.5	80.2	307.6	43.5	12.9	852.0
Per Serving	238.7	10.0	38.5	5.4	1.6	106.5

gm=grams; mg=milligrams. Nutritional figures are approximate. Figures are based on findings of U.S. Department of Agriculture.

Beef Stroganoff

2 lbs. filet of beef	2 onion bouillon
2 tbsp. diet margarine	cubes
½ lb. fresh mushrooms,	1 tbsp. catsup
sliced	⅛ tsp. pepper
2 tbsp. flour	1½ cups water
	1 cup plain yogurt

Before cooking: Trim the beef of all visible fat. With a sharp knife, cut the filet into thin strips, about 2 inches long and ½ inch wide.

Melt 1 tablespoon margarine in a large skillet over high heat. Add the beef and brown it quickly on all sides. Remove the meat from the skillet. Add the remaining tablespoon of margarine and melt it over moderate heat. When the margarine is melted, add the mushrooms to the skillet and saute them for about 5 minutes. Then add the flour, bouillon cubes, catsup, and pepper. Stir this mixture until smooth. Gradually add the water and bring the mixture to a boil, stirring. Reduce the heat and simmer for 5 minutes. Keeping the cooking heat low, blend in the yogurt. Add the beef and cook slowly just until the meat is heated.

Makes 8 servings

	Calories	Carbo-hydrate (gm)	Protein (gm)	Total Fat (gm)	Saturated Fat (gm)	Choles-terol (mg)
Total	2346.5	62.6	318.0	83.7	36.0	842.0
Per Serving	293.3	7.8	39.8	10.5	4.5	105.3

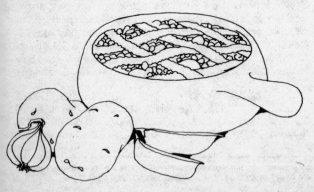

Sweet and Sour Stew

2 lbs. lean round steak
1 tsp. salt
dash pepper
1 tbsp. diet margarine
1 cup boiling water
5 tbsp. catsup
2 tbsp. vinegar

1 tbsp. Worcester-
shire sauce
1 cup chopped
onion
6 large carrots
2 tbsp. all-purpose
flour
¼ cup cold water
sugar substitute to
equal 2 tbsp.

Before cooking: Cut the meat into 1-inch cubes, trimming off all visible fat. Cut the carrots into 3/4-inch
pieces (to make 3 cups).

Season the meat with salt and pepper. Melt the diet
margarine in a large non-stick skillet. Add the meat,
and brown it well. Combine the boiling water, catsup,
vinegar, and Worcestershire sauce in a separate bowl.
Pour this mixture over the browned meat. Add the
onion. Cover the skillet tightly. Simmer the meat over
low heat for 45 minutes, stirring it once or twice. Add
the carrots and simmer the meat for an additional 45
minutes or so until the meat and carrots are tender. In
a separate bowl, combine the flour, cold water and
sugar substitute. Stir this mixture into the skillet and
continue to cook over low heat, stirring constantly, until the sauce has thickened.   *Makes 8 servings*

	Calories	Carbo-hydrate (gm)	Protein (gm)	Total Fat (gm)	Saturated Fat (gm)	Choles-terol (mg)
Total	2077.8	74.4	289.5	59.3	27.6	825.8
Per Serving	259.7	9.3	36.2	7.4	3.5	103.2

---

*gm=grams; mg=milligrams. Nutritional figures are approximate. Figures
are based on findings of U.S. Department of Agriculture.*

Lazy Day Chuck Roast

3 lbs. boneless chuck
   shoulder, trimmed
   of all fat
2 tbsp. Worcestershire
   sauce

3 tbsp. prepared
   mustard
coarse freshly
   ground pepper
salt (or onion salt
   or garlic salt)

Spread the mustard liberally over the surfaces of the meat. Sprinkle the Worcestershire sauce, salt, and pepper all over. Place the meat on a rack in a roasting pan. Slow-roast it, uncovered, at 225° for 5 hours or more — until the meat is tender. (If you want a browner roast, you can place it under the broiler briefly just before serving — or you can raise the oven temperature to 450° for the last 20 minutes of roasting.)

Makes 9 servings

	Calories	Carbo-hydrate (gm)	Protein (gm)	Total Fat (gm)	Saturated Fat (gm)	Choles-terol (mg)
Total	2570.5	87.0	426.7	53.3	17.8	1262.4
Per Serving	285.6	9.7	47.4	5.9	2.0	140.3

Beef Parmigiana

6 "minute steaks," 4 oz.
   each
4 tbsp. grated
   Parmesan cheese
1/3 cup bread crumbs
1 tbsp. olive oil

8 oz. tomato sauce
garlic salt
   (optional)
1 tsp. oregano
3 (1-oz.) slices part-
   skim mozzarella
   cheese

Before cooking: Combine the grated Parmesan and the bread crumbs in a paper bag. Put the steaks in the bag, one at a time, and shake the bag until the steaks are well-coated with the crumb mixture.

Heat the oil in a non-stick skillet over high heat. Add the meat and quickly brown it on both sides. Arrange the meat in a baking dish, and pour the tomato sauce over all. Sprinkle the meat with garlic salt according to your own taste. Cut the mozzarella slices in half and place one half atop each steak. Sprinkle the oregano all over. Bake the meat in a preheated 375° oven for about 10 minutes — until the cheese is bubbly.

Makes 6 servings

Diet hint: Olive oil is the favorite of Italian cooks. But calorie-conscious cooks can save 75 calories (about 12 per serving) by substituting diet margarine for olive oil.

	Calories	Carbo-hydrate (gm)	Protein (gm)	Total Fat (gm)	Saturated Fat (gm)	Choles-terol (mg)
Total	2168.4	44.6	291.3	92.7	37.3	740.5
Per Serving	361.4	7.4	48.6	15.5	6.2	123.4

Pot Roast with Cheese Sauce

3 lbs. beef arm pot roast
2 tsp. salt
$1/8$ tsp. pepper
2 medium onions
$1/2$ can (11 oz.)
    condensed cheddar
    cheese soup

8 oz. can tomato
    sauce
4 oz. can mushroom
    stems and
    pieces,
    undrained
$1/4$ tsp. oregano
$1/4$ tsp. basil

Before cooking: Trim meat of all visible fat. Cut the onions into slices.

Place the pot roast in a non-stick roasting pan and roast it, uncovered, at 475° just until the meat is browned. Pour off the pan drippings that have accumulated and lower the oven temperature to 325°. Season the meat with the salt and pepper, and add the onions, cheese soup, tomato sauce, mushrooms, oregano, and basil to the pan. Cover the pan tightly, and roast the meat slowly for about 2$1/2$ hours until it is tender. To serve, slice the meat thinly.

Makes 10 servings

	Calories	Carbo-hydrate (gm)	Protein (gm)	Total Fat (gm)	Saturated Fat (gm)	Choles-terol (mg)
Total	2574.9	51.5	442.4	65.7	23.8	1292.4
Per Serving	257.5	5.2	44.2	6.6	2.4	129.2

gm=grams; mg=milligrams. Nutritional figures are approximate. Figures are based on findings of U.S. Department of Agriculture.

Stuffed Rolled Beef

2 lbs. round steak or
flank steak (if round
used, buy thin
piece)
1/4 cup fresh lemon juice
2 tbsp. soy sauce
2 garlic cloves
1/2 tsp. pepper
1/2 lb. cooked smoked
ham

2 hard-boiled eggs
2 tbsp. raisins
6 green olives
2 cups water
1 medium onion
1/4 cup cider vinegar
8 oz. can plain
tomato sauce

Before cooking: Pound the meat to a thickness of 1/4 inch. Mince the garlic, slice the smoked ham, hard-boiled eggs, and onion, and pit and chop the olives.

Spread the pounded beef out flat. Sprinkle the surface with the lemon juice, soy sauce, minced garlic, and pepper. Spread the ham strips and egg slices evenly over the meat. Sprinkle the raisins and chopped olives over all. Beginning at a narrow end, carefully roll up the beef, tucking in the ends. Tie the roll with string. Place the rolled beef in a deep skillet or pan, and add the water, sliced onions, vinegar, and tomato sauce. Cover the pan tightly, and simmer the meat slowly for about one hour, or until it is tender when a fork is inserted into it. To serve, slice the rolled beef crosswise and serve it with the sauce from the pan.

Makes 10 servings

	Calories	Carbo-hydrate (gm)	Protein (gm)	Total Fat (gm)	Saturated Fat (gm)	Choles-terol (mg)
Total	2779.2	52.1	347.3	120.2	49.3	1532.7
Per Serving	277.9	5.2	34.7	12.0	4.9	153.3

Roast Tenderloin With Onion Sauce

2 lbs. beef tenderloin
10 1/2 oz. can condensed
onion soup

salt
pepper

Before cooking: Trim beef of all visible fat. Separate the liquid from the onions of the onion soup. Skim fat from liquid using a bulb-type baster.

Season the meat well with salt and pepper. Insert a meat thermometer so that the tip (the bulb) is in the center of the meat. Place the meat on a rack in a nonstick roasting pan. Roast the meat in a hot, preheated 450° oven until the meat is done to your taste. During roasting, baste the meat every 10 minutes with the liquid from the onion soup. When the meat is done, remove it to a serving platter. Skim all the fat from the pan drippings by using a bulb-type baster. Stir the onions from the onion soup into the pan and return the pan to the oven to heat the drippings through. If the roasting pan is flame-proof, the drippings can be heated on the top of the range. Slice the meat thinly, and serve it with the onion sauce. Do not let the meat sit a long time before slicing, as it will continue to cook in its own hot juices.   *Makes 8 servings*

	Calories	Carbo-hydrate (gm)	Protein (gm)	Total Fat (gm)	Saturated Fat (gm)	Choles-terol (mg)
Total	2011.0	13.2	301.2	69.3	32.0	879.1
Per Serving	251.4	1.7	37.7	8.7	4.0	109.9

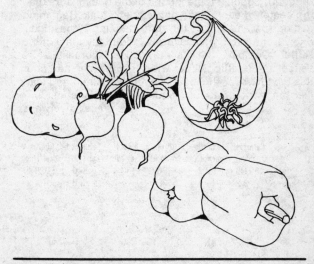

gm=grams; mg=milligrams. Nutritional figures are approximate. Figures are based on findings of U.S. Department of Agriculture.

Beef Roll-Ups

1½ lbs. beef round steak,
 ¼-inch thick
¼ cup chopped onion
¼ cup chopped green
 pepper
2 tbsp. water
1 cup cooked rice

¼ tsp. oregano
8 oz. can tomato
 sauce
1 tbsp. Worcester-
 shire sauce
2 beef bouillon
 cubes
½ cup boiling water

Before cooking: Cook the rice according to package directions to yield 1 cup. Trim the round steak of all visible fat. Cut the steak into 6 equal pieces and pound it thin.

Place the chopped onions, green pepper, and 2 tablespoons water in a non-stick skillet. Cook the vegetables in the water until they are tender. In a bowl combine the cooked vegetables with the rice and oregano. Spoon 2 tablespoons of the rice mixture onto the center of each piece of pounded steak. Beginning at a narrow end, roll up the steak, tucking in the edges. Skewer the meat rolls securely, and place them in the skillet. Combine the tomato sauce, Worcestershire sauce, and boullion cubes with ½ cup water, and pour this mixture over the meat. Cover the skillet, and simmer the meat for about 1 hour or until it is tender.

Makes 6 servings

	Calories	Carbo-hydrate (gm)	Protein (gm)	Total Fat (gm)	Saturated Fat (gm)	Choles-terol (mg)
Total	1621.3	69.8	220.0	40.4	20.0	626.0
Per Serving	270.2	11.6	36.7	6.7	3.3	104.3

---

gm=grams; mg=milligrams. Nutritional figures are approximate. Figures are based on findings of U.S. Department of Agriculture.

Veal

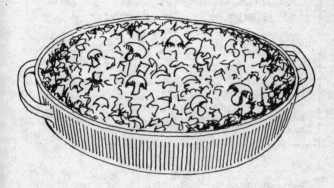

Luxurious veal! Did you know that it's the leanest and least-fattening of all meats? Differing from many luxury foods, veal is one extravagance the calorie counter can "afford" — if the budget permits. Veal, unfortunately, is expensive, and in many sections of the country, hard to find. If veal isn't on display in your supermarket meat case, don't give up. Most likely it's available on special order, or in the butcher shop.

While the price per pound is high compared with other meats, veal is actually a better bargain than simple price comparisons indicate. Veal's relative lack of fat (and fat calories) means a corresponding increase in protein content. And protein, after all, is why you feed your family meat in the first place.

Veal, of course, is "baby beef." The best veal comes from animals 4 to 14 weeks old, weighing 100 pounds or less. Because of its tender age, veal is naturally tasty and tender without the fatty marbling of mature beef.

HOW VEAL AND BEEF COMPARE

	Protein	Fat	Calories*
Veal chuck	19%	10%	173
Beef chuck	16%	31%	352
Veal rib chops	19%	14%	207
Beef rib steak	14%	43%	444
Veal loin chops	19%	11%	181
Beef porterhouse	15%	36%	390
Veal shank	20%	8%	156
Beef shank	18%	23%	289
Veal rump	19%	9%	164
Beef rump	17%	25%	303

*Per 100 grams (approximately 3¹/₂ ounces). All data approximate, adapted from U.S. Department of Agriculture Information.

Compare the calorie, fat, and protein content of similar cuts of beef and veal and you see why veal is often a better buy for dieters.

How to Cook Veal

Veal's sophisticated flavor is subtly accented by the judicious use of lemon or wine and herbs — or garlic, cheese, and tomato for more robust dishes.

Because of its leanness, veal is at its best when gently cooked; scaloppini sautéed lightly in a nonstick skillet, for example, or a tender, rolled rump slow-roasted at low temperature. The less tender cuts of veal can be creatively seasoned and slow-simmered in wine or tomato juice. Under no circumstances, however, should veal be carelessly tossed into a hot frying pan, seared in a hot oven, or scorched under the broiler. Only the tiniest, most tender chops can be broiled or barbecued and then only with patience and care.

Recipes

Baked Veal Chops with Rice

6 lean veal loin chops,
   ³/₄-1-inch thick
1 tbsp. diet margarine
6 tbsp. uncooked rice
1 medium onion
1 medium green pepper
1 large tomato or 16 oz.
   can tomatoes

garlic salt
pepper
water or liquid
   from canned
   tomatoes
¹/₄ tsp. oregano

Before cooking: Trim the chops of all visible fat. Cut the onion into 6 slices and the green pepper into 6 strips. If you are using a fresh tomato, cut it into 6 slices. If you are using canned tomatoes, separate the tomatoes from the liquid, reserving the liquid.

Melt the margarine in a large non-stick skillet. Add the chops and brown them slowly on both sides. Remove the chops from the skillet and place them in a large baking dish. On top of each chop put 1 tbsp. of uncooked rice, 1 slice of tomato, 1 slice of onion, and 1 piece of green pepper. Sprinkle with garlic salt, pepper, and oregano. If you have used a fresh tomato, cover the chops with water; if you have used canned tomatoes, cover the chops with the liquid from the can. Cover the baking dish and bake the chops at 350° for 1¹/₂ hours. *Makes 6 servings*

	Calories	Carbo-hydrate (gm)	Protein (gm)	Total Fat (gm)	Saturated Fat (gm)	Choles-terol (mg)
Total	1878.7	90.6	193.0	83.1	33.0	640.2
Per Serving	313.1	15.1	32.2	13.9	5.5	106.7

gm=grams; mg=milligrams. Nutritional figures are approximate. Figures are based on findings of U.S. Department of Agriculture.

Veal Marlene

2 lbs. boneless veal
2 tbsp. diet margarine
2 tbsp. all-purpose flour
1/2 tsp. salt
1/4 tsp. pepper

1 cup boiling water
1 chicken bouillon
cube
2 tbsp. instant
onions
2 strips lemon peel
1/2 cup evaporated
skim milk

Before cooking: Cut the veal into 1-inch cubes, trimming it of all visible fat.

Melt the margarine in a large non-stick skillet. Add the veal and brown it slowly. Then sprinkle the flour, salt, and pepper over the veal. Add the bouillon cube, onion, lemon peel, and 1 cup of boiling water. Cover the skillet and simmer the mixture for 30 to 45 minutes until the meat is tender. Remove the lemon peel and discard it. Add the evaporated milk, and continue to cook the mixture until the milk is heated through.

Makes 8 servings

	Calories	Carbo-hydrate (gm)	Protein (gm)	Total Fat (gm)	Saturated Fat (gm)	Choles-terol (mg)
Total	1548.6	48.9	202.4	71.9	30.8	679.2
Per Serving	193.6	6.1	25.3	9.0	3.9	84.9

Veal Marengo

1 lb. lean boneless
veal, cut from leg or
shoulder
garlic salt
pepper
10 1/2 oz. can onion soup

1/2 cup dry sherry
8 oz. can stewed
tomatoes
1 cup water
1 tbsp. lemon juice
4 oz. can
mushrooms,
drained

Before cooking: Cut the veal into 1 1/2-inch cubes, trimming away all visible fat. Skim off the fat of the onion soup by using a bulb-type baster.

94   CONSUMER GUIDE

Spray a non-stick skillet with spray-on vegetable coating. Season the meat with garlic salt and pepper and brown it in the skillet over moderate heat. Add all the remaining ingredients, except the mushrooms. Cover the skillet and simmer the contents over low heat for 50 to 60 minutes until the meat is tender. Then uncover the pan and add the mushrooms. Raise the heat to moderate and continue to cook the mixture, uncovered, until the liquid has been reduced to a thick sauce. *Makes 4 servings*

	Calories	Carbo-hydrate (gm)	Protein (gm)	Total Fat (gm)	Saturated Fat (gm)	Choles-terol (mg)
Total	995.2	36.3	108.4	27.5	10.7	382.6
Per Serving	248.8	9.1	27.1	6.9	2.7	95.7

Easy Veal and Mushroom Casserole

2 lbs. lean veal shoulder
4 oz. can sliced mushrooms, drained

1 tbsp. diet margarine
10½ oz. can condensed cream of chicken soup

Before cooking: Cut the veal into 1½-inch cubes, trimming away all visible fat.

Melt the margarine in a heavy oven-safe pan. Add the veal and mushrooms and brown them slowly. Pour off any fat that has accumulated in the pan before going any further. Then add soup. Cover the pan and bake the veal at 350° for 1 hour or more until the meat is tender. *Makes 8 servings*

	Calories	Carbo-hydrate (gm)	Protein (gm)	Total Fat (gm)	Saturated Fat (gm)	Choles-terol (mg)
Total	1503.4	24.0	191.7	64.5	24.9	666.4
Per Serving	188.0	3.0	24.0	8.1	3.1	83.3

---

gm=grams; mg=milligrams. Nutritional figures are approximate. Figures are based on findings of U.S. Department of Agriculture.

South Seas Veal Spareribs

2¹/₂ lbs. lean breast of
veal
¹/₄ cup cider vinegar
1¹/₂ cups salt-free tomato
juice

1 cup unsweetened
applesauce
3 tbsp. soy sauce

Before cooking: Trim the veal of all fat and cut it into individual ribs.

Place the ribs in a roasting pan in a single layer. Bake them, uncovered, in a 425° oven for 20 to 25 minutes — just to brown them and remove the excess fat. Pour off all the fat that accumulates in the pan. Then combine the remaining ingredients and pour them over the ribs. Lower the oven temperature to 350°, return the meat to the oven and bake it, covered, for about 1¹/₂ hours until the veal is tender, basting occasionally.   *Makes 8 servings*

	Calories	Carbo-hydrate (gm)	Protein (gm)	Total Fat (gm)	Saturated Fat (gm)	Choles-terol (mg)
Total	1681.1	48.0	233.6	53.3	26.7	799.8
Per Serving	210.1	6.0	29.2	6.7	3.3	100.0

Budapest Veal Chops

6 veal loin chops, ³/₄-
inch thick
1 tbsp. diet margarine
¹/₂ cup sliced onion
1 cup chicken broth

1 tbsp. paprika
1¹/₂ tsp. butter-flavored
salt
¹/₄ tsp. pepper
²/₃ cup plain yogurt

Before cooking: Trim the chops of all visible fat. Chill the chicken broth until the fat has risen to the top, hardened, and can be lifted off, or skim off the fat, using a bulb-type baster.

Melt the margarine in a large non-stick skillet. Add the chops and brown them well on both sides. Add the onion and sauté the meat and onion a few minutes longer. Pour the chicken broth over the chops and sprinkle the paprika, salt, and pepper over all. Cover the skillet and simmer the chops for 20 to 30 minutes until they are nearly tender. Uncover the skillet and continue to simmer the veal for about 10 minutes until most of the liquid has evaporated. Then stir in the yogurt. Cook the mixture for 1 or 2 minutes longer until the yogurt is heated, but be careful not to let it boil.

Makes 6 servings

	Calories	Carbo-hydrate (gm)	Protein (gm)	Total Fat (gm)	Saturated Fat (gm)	Choles-terol (mg)
Total	1238.5	15.6	145.3	64.6	26.3	506.7
Per Serving	206.4	2.6	24.2	10.8	4.4	84.5

Bavarian Veal Steak

1½ lbs. veal round steak,
  ¾-inch thick
2 tbsp. diet margarine
1 envelope chicken
  bouillon or beef
  bouillon, or 1
  bouillon cube

½ cup boiling water
3 tbsp. lemon juice
½ tsp. butter-flavored
  salt
⅛ tsp. pepper
¼ cup chopped
  parsley

Melt the margarine over moderate heat in a large non-stick skillet. Add the veal and brown it on both sides. Dissolve the bouillon in ½ cup boiling water and add this to the skillet. At the same time, add the lemon juice, salt, and pepper. Cover the pan and bring the mixture to boiling. Lower the heat and simmer the meat for about 30 minutes until it is tender. Then stir in the parsley. Remove the steak to a serving platter, and pour the pan juices over it.

Makes 6 servings

	Calories	Carbo-hydrate (gm)	Protein (gm)	Total Fat (gm)	Saturated Fat (gm)	Choles-terol (mg)
Total	1008.4	3.8	137.2	44.0	18.0	483.0
Per Serving	168.0	0.6	22.9	7.3	3.0	80.5

---

gm=grams; mg=milligrams. Nutritional figures are approximate. Figures are based on findings of U.S. Department of Agriculture.

Goulash

2 lbs. lean veal shoulder	1½ tsp. salt
1 tbsp. diet margarine	1 tbsp. paprika
2 onions	¼ tsp. pepper
16 oz. can whole peeled Italian tomatoes in puree	1 tsp. caraway seeds

Before cooking: Cut the meat into 1-inch cubes, trimming off all the fat. Slice the onions.

Melt the margarine in a large non-stick skillet. Brown the meat slowly in the melted margarine; then add the remaining ingredients. Heat the mixture to boiling. Then lower the heat, cover the pan and simmer the contents for 1¼ hours, or until the meat is tender.

Makes 8 servings

	Calories	Carbo-hydrate (gm)	Protein (gm)	Total Fat (gm)	Saturated Fat (gm)	Choles-terol (mg)
Total	1414.4	40.0	189.4	50.7	22.3	640.2
Per Serving	176.8	5.0	23.7	6.3	2.8	80.0

Veal Stroganoff

1½ lbs. veal for scaloppini, cut from the leg	½ cup sliced onion
2 tbsp. flour	½ cup dry white wine
1½ tsp. salt	1 tsp. prepared mustard
¼ tsp. pepper	2 tbsp. catsup
1 tbsp. diet margarine	1 tsp. parsley flakes
	½ cup plain yogurt

Before cooking: Cut the veal into 1-inch strips.

Mix the flour, salt, and pepper in a paper bag. Add the veal strips a few at a time and shake the bag until the meat is completely coated with the flour mixture. Melt the margarine in a non-stick skillet. Add the veal pieces and quickly brown them on both sides. Add the onion, wine, mustard, catsup, and parsley flakes.

CONSUMER GUIDE

Cover the skillet and simmer the veal for about 10 minutes until it is tender. Then stir in the yogurt. Continue to cook the mixture over low heat until the yogurt is heated through.   *Makes 6 servings*

	Calories	Carbo-hydrate (gm)	Protein (gm)	Total Fat (gm)	Saturated Fat (gm)	Choles-terol (mg)
Total	1206.6	36.5	142.7	40.1	18.0	490.0
Per Serving	201.1	6.1	23.8	6.7	3.0	81.7

Veal Parmigiana

1½ lbs. lean veal round, thinly-sliced
¼ cup bread crumbs
1 tbsp. diet margarine
16 oz. can tomato sauce
2 tsp. Italian seasoning or oregano
1½ tsp. garlic salt
⅛ tsp. pepper
3 oz. part-skim mozzarella cheese

Before cooking: Cut the veal into 6 serving pieces, trimming off all visible fat. Cut the mozzarella cheese into slices.

Dip the veal in the bread crumbs until they are lightly coated. Melt the margarine in a large non-stick skillet. Add the coated veal and brown it slowly, turning once. Remove the veal from the skillet, and arrange it in a single layer in a shallow baking dish. Spoon the tomato sauce over the veal. Then season it with Italian seasoning, garlic salt, and pepper. Top the veal with the mozzarella slices. Bake the veal uncovered at 350° for 20 to 25 minutes — until the cheese is melted and bubbly.   *Makes 6 servings*

	Calories	Carbo-hydrate (gm)	Protein (gm)	Total Fat (gm)	Saturated Fat (gm)	Choles-terol (mg)
Total	1411.3	52.9	190.7	55.1	20.3	535.3
Per Serving	235.2	8.8	31.8	9.2	3.4	89.2

---

gm=grams; mg=milligrams. Nutritional figures are approximate. Figures are based on findings of U.S. Department of Agriculture.

Veal Stroganoff Stew

1½ lbs. boneless veal shoulder	1 medium onion
1 tsp. salt	⅓ cup Sauterne
¼ tsp. pepper	2 potatoes
1 tbsp. diet margarine	1 tbsp. flour
½ lb. fresh mushrooms	⅔ cup buttermilk

Before cooking: Cut the veal into thin strips, trimming off all visible fat, and season them with the salt and pepper. Slice the mushrooms and onion thinly and peel and thinly slice the potatoes.

Melt the margarine in a large non-stick skillet. Add the veal, mushrooms, and onions, and brown them slowly. Then add the Sauterne and potatoes. Cover the pan and simmer the contents for 10 or 15 minutes — until the potatoes are tender. In a separate bowl mix together the flour and buttermilk. Add this to the skillet and continue cooking and stirring until the mixture has thickened. Then simmer for 3 more minutes.

Makes 6 servings

	Calories	Carbo-hydrate (gm)	Protein (gm)	Total Fat (gm)	Saturated Fat (gm)	Choles-terol (mg)
Total	1459.3	90.1	166.2	40.6	17.0	483.3
Per Serving	243.2	15.0	27.7	6.8	2.8	80.6

Veal "Cordon Bleu"

1 lb. veal for scaloppini, cut from the leg	3 oz. Canadian bacon, thinly sliced
3 oz. part-skim pizza cheese, thinly sliced	¼ cup seasoned bread crumbs
	1 tsp. corn oil

Before cooking: Cut the veal into 8 equal slices.

Pound the veal slices with a meat pound to make them as thin as possible. Top each piece with a slice of cheese and a slice of bacon. Then top each with another slice of veal to make 4 veal "sandwiches" with cheese and bacon in the middle. Combine the bread crumbs with the oil, and brush the mixture lightly on both sides of the sandwiches. Place them on a cookie sheet. Bake the veal in a 350° oven for about 25 minutes until the veal is cooked and the cheese melts.

Makes 4 servings

	Calories	Carbo-hydrate (gm)	Protein (gm)	Total Fat (gm)	Saturated Fat (gm)	Choles-terol (mg)
Total	1196.4	19.9	161.9	57.3	18.3	446.1
Per Serving	299.1	5.0	40.5	14.3	4.6	111.5

Veal Piccata

1¹/₂ lbs. lean veal for
    scaloppini, cut from
    the leg
1 tbsp. diet margarine
1 envelope chicken
    bouillon

¹/₄ cup water
¹/₂ cup dry white wine
1 lemon
    fresh parsley

Before cooking: Cut the veal into 6 equal serving pieces, trimming off all visible fat. Cut the lemon in half. Cut one half into slices for a garnish and squeeze the juice from the other half.

Melt the margarine in a large non-stick skillet. Add the veal and brown it quickly on both sides. Remove the veal to a platter. Stir the bouillon, wine, lemon juice, and ¹/₄ cup water into the skillet, scraping the pan to loosen the brown bits. Return the veal to the pan and cook it over high heat for about 5 minutes until it is tender. Return the veal to the serving platter and garnish it with lemon slices and parsley sprigs.

Makes 6 servings

	Calories	Carbo-hydrate (gm)	Protein (gm)	Total Fat (gm)	Saturated Fat (gm)	Choles-terol (mg)
Total	1041.9	23.1	145.0	45.0	19.0	480.0
Per Serving	173.7	3.9	24.2	7.5	3.2	80.0

gm=grams; mg=milligrams. Nutritional figures are approximate. Figures are based on findings of U.S. Department of Agriculture.

"Can Opener" Veal Provencal

1 lb. lean boneless veal
2 tsp. diet margarine
  salt
  pepper
10½ oz. can chicken
  consommé
2 tbsp. Worcestershire
  sauce

1 bay leaf
½ cup dry white wine
8 oz. can boiled
  whole onions
8 oz. can small
  carrots
8 oz. can potatoes
4 oz. can mushroom
  caps

Before cooking: Cut the veal into 1-inch cubes, trimming off all visible fat. Chill the consomme until the fat rises to the top, hardens, and can be lifted off, or skim off the fat by using a bulb-type baster. Reserve liquid from the canned vegetables.

Melt the margarine in a large non-stick skillet. Season the veal with salt and pepper and brown it in the melted margarine. Add the consommé, bay leaf, Worcestershire sauce, wine, and the liquid from all the canned vegetables. Cover the skillet and simmer the mixture over very low heat for 1 hour or more until the meat is tender. Then uncover the pan and add the vegetables. Raise the heat to moderate and continue to simmer the mixture, uncovered, until nearly all of the liquid is evaporated.   *Makes 4 servings*

Diet hint: If you are particularly calorie-conscious, you can save an extra 50 calories (about 12 calories per serving) by eliminating the diet margarine and browning the meat with spray-on vegetable coating. See the cooking tips in "Slimming in the Kitchen" for directions.

	Calories	Carbo-hydrate (gm)	Protein (gm)	Total Fat (gm)	Saturated Fat (gm)	Cholesterol (mg)
Total	1039.1	68.7	108.5	25.3	11.4	356.4
Per Serving	259.8	17.2	27.1	6.3	2.9	89.1

gm=grams; mg=milligrams. Nutritional figures are approximate. Figures are based on findings of U.S. Department of Agriculture.

Lamb

Once upon a time lamb was a seasonal meat — available mainly in the spring and hard to find the rest of the year. Today lamb is here the year round and is a versatile choice whether you're planning a patio cookout or a fireside supper.

Lamb is a lean and luscious main course for dieters. It wears most of its fat on the outside, where it is easily trimmable by the calorie-wise cook. Because lamb is young and succulent, it doesn't need fatty marbling to provide tenderness.

Europeans have been wise to the ways of lamb much longer than Americans have. They enjoy it often, and serve it slightly pink in the middle. Stateside home-makers, on the other hand, tend to overcook young lamb as if it were a tough piece of mutton. If you've served lamb well-done and have been disappointed in its taste or texture, next time try it European-style. Broil or sauté it so there's still a tinge of inner pinkness — or roast it to an internal temperature of only about 165°. Lamb is rare at 165°-170°, medium at 174°, and well done at 180°.

Lamb is just as versatile as beef. Large tender cuts — like leg, sirloin, loin, rack, crown, and shoulder — can be oven roasted. And smaller cuts — leg or sirloin steaks, chops, and ground fat-trimmed patties — can be broiled, barbecued, or sautéed. (Steaks are the lowest in calories.) The less tender, less expensive cuts of lamb can be braised or simmered to scrumptious tenderness. To check on how to use any of these cooking methods, turn to the introduction of "The Meat of the Matter."

Recipes

Chinese Sweet 'N Sour Lamb

1 lb. boneless lean lamb, cut from the leg
unseasoned meat tenderizer
2 tbsp. soy sauce
2 onions
8½ oz. can water chestnuts
1 green pepper

8 oz. can pineapple chunks or tidbits, packed in juice
2 tbsp. catsup
1 tbsp. wine vinegar
1 tbsp. cornstarch
3 tbsp. cold water
2 firm, ripe tomatoes

Before cooking: Cut the lamb across the grain into thin slices with a sharp knife, removing all visible fat. Moisten the meat with water, and sprinkle it with meat tenderizer. Cut the onion into thin wedges; drain and slice the water chestnuts; cut the green pepper into 1½-inch squares; and cut the tomatoes into eighths.

Heat the soy sauce in a non-stick skillet. Add the lamb and brown it over high heat, stirring rapidly until the liquid evaporates. Add the onion, water chestnuts, and green pepper, and continue stir-frying for about 3 minutes. Then add the undrained pineapple, catsup, and vinegar; and heat the contents of the skillet to boiling. In a cup, mix the cornstarch with the cold water until it is smooth. Add this mixture to the sauce in the skillet and continue heating, stirring constantly, until the sauce clears and thickens.   *Makes 6 servings*

	Calories	Carbo-hydrate (gm)	Protein (gm)	Total Fat (gm)	Saturated Fat (gm)	Choles-terol (mg)
Total	1302.6	113.3	141.3	32.0	19.2	454.4
Per Serving	217.1	18.9	23.6	5.3	3.2	75.7

Lamb Stew Silverton

1 lb. lean lamb
    shoulder
1 tbsp. diet margarine
1 cup sliced onion
2 tsp. salt
1/4 tsp. coarse freshly
    ground pepper

3/4 tsp. ground
    allspice
1/4 tsp. ground ginger
1 tbsp. flour
8 oz. can tomato
    sauce
1 lb. can carrots,
    undrained
1 cup and 2 tbsp.
    cold water

Before cooking: Cut the lamb into 2-inch cubes, trimming off all fat.

Melt the margarine in a large non-stick skillet or saucepan. Add the meat and brown it on all sides. Add the onion and brown lightly. Drain off any fat that has accumulated in the pan. Then stir in the salt, pepper, allspice, ginger, and 1/2 cup water. Cover the pot tightly, and simmer the mixture for about 2 hours. If necessary, add more water during the simmering period. Using a bulb-type baster, skim the fat from the pan juices. Blend 2 tablespoons cold water into the flour and add this mixture to the meat. Also add the tomato sauce and carrots. Continue to cook the stew, uncovered, until it has thickened (about 15 minutes).

Makes 6 servings

Diet hint: The calorie-conscious cook can save an extra 50 calories by browning the meat in its own fat instead of using margarine (that's about 8 calories per serving). For directions, see the second cooking hint in "Slimming in the Kitchen."

	Calories	Carbo-hydrate (gm)	Protein (gm)	Total Fat (gm)	Saturated Fat (gm)	Choles-terol (mg)
Total	1158.8	64.2	138.6	38.5	20.2	454.4
Per Serving	193.1	10.7	23.1	6.4	3.4	75.7

gm=grams; mg=milligrams. Nutritional figures are approximate. Figures are based on findings of U.S. Department of Agriculture.

Barbecued "Ribs"

3 lbs. breast of lamb,
trimmed of fat and
sliced into ribs
6 oz. can tomato paste
1/2 cup catsup
2 tbsp. cider vinegar

1 medium onion,
sliced
1 tsp. salt
1/4 tsp. pepper
1/8 tsp. hot pepper
sauce

Place the lamb riblets on a rack in a shallow roasting pan. Bake them at 325° for about 1 1/2 hours. Drain off the fat that has accumulated in the pan before going any further. Then combine the remaining ingredients in a bowl and mix them well. Brush some of this sauce over the riblets, and continue baking them for 1 1/2 hours more, basting occasionally with the sauce. Turn the riblets twice to coat the underside.

Makes 9 servings

	Calories	Carbo-hydrate (gm)	Protein (gm)	Total Fat (gm)	Saturated Fat (gm)	Choles-terol (mg)
Total	2309.7	74.5	249.7	108.0	63.0	900.0
Per Serving	256.6	8.3	27.7	12.0	7.0	100.0

Lamb Salonika

2 lbs. lean boneless
leg of lamb
1 tsp. salt
1/8 tsp. pepper
1 tbsp. diet margarine
1 minced garlic clove
1/2 cup chopped onion

1/3 cup water
1/2 oz. can condensed
cream of celery
soup
1 cup sliced
mushrooms
1/2 cup plain yogurt
3 tbsp. chopped
parsley

Before cooking: Cut the lamb into 1-inch cubes, trimming it of all fat.

Season the lamb cubes with salt and pepper. Melt the diet margarine in a large non-stick skillet. Add the lamb, garlic, and onions to the melted margarine.

Sauté them over low heat until the lamb is browned on all sides. If any fat has accumulated in the skillet, drain it before going any further. Then add the water, celery soup, and mushrooms. Cook the entire mixture over very low heat for 45 minutes, stirring occasionally. Gradually add the yogurt to the hot mixture, being careful not to let the mixture boil. Add the parsley before serving, or sprinkle it over the top as a garnish.

Makes 8 servings

	Calories	Carbo-hydrate (gm)	Protein (gm)	Total Fat (gm)	Saturated Fat (gm)	Choles-terol (mg)
Total	2093.7	46.2	273.3	86.2	40.4	937.2
Per Serving	261.7	5.8	34.2	10.8	5.1	117.2

Lamb Teriyaki

1³/₄ lbs. slice of lean leg
   of lamb
2 tsp. ground ginger
2 garlic cloves

1 medium onion
   sugar substitute to
    equal 2 tbsp.
¹/₂ cup soy sauce
¹/₄ cup water

Before cooking: Cut the lamb into 6 equal pieces, trimming them of all visible fat. Mince the garlic and chop the onion finely. Place the meat in a large baking dish. In a separate bowl combine the ginger, garlic, onion, sugar substitute, soy sauce, and ¹/₄ cup water. Pour this mixture over the meat and let it stand at room temperature, uncovered, for 2 hours.

Drain the meat well. Place it on a rack in the broiler and broil it for 3 to 5 minutes on each side.

Makes 6 servings

	Calories	Carbo-hydrate (gm)	Protein (gm)	Total Fat (gm)	Saturated Fat (gm)	Choles-terol (mg)
Total	1573.9	18.0	233.7	55.9	33.6	794.0
Per Serving	262.3	3.0	38.9	9.3	5.6	132.3

---

gm=grams; mg=milligrams. Nutritional figures are approximate. Figures are based on findings of U.S. Department of Agriculture.

Lamb Chops with Rice

8 lamb shoulder chops,	2 medium green
1-inch thick	peppers
1 cup uncooked rice	16 oz. can tomatoes
2 medium onions	10½ oz. can beef
	bouillon

Before cooking: Trim the chops of all visible fat. Slice the onions and green peppers.

Place the lamb chops under the broiler until they are just brown. Place the rice in a baking dish. Then cover the rice with chops, onion, green pepper, and tomatoes. Pour the bouillon over all. Cover the baking dish, and bake the meat and vegetables at 350° for 1½ hours.   *Makes 8 servings*

	Calories	Carbo- hydrate (gm)	Protein (gm)	Total Fat (gm)	Saturated Fat (gm)	Choles- terol (mg)
Total	4159.2	204.9	235.2	267.0	144.0	1135.4
Per Serving	519.9	25.6	29.4	33.4	18.0	141.9

Lamb and Artichoke Kebabs

1½ lbs. lean boneless leg	¼ cup fresh lemon
of lamb	juice
2 packages (9 oz. each)	2 tsp. salt
frozen artichoke	1 tsp. marjoram or
hearts	oregano leaves
½ cup low-calorie	¼ tsp. pepper
French salad	2 large tomatoes
dressing	

Before cooking: Cook the artichokes according to the package directions, drain them, and allow them to cool. Cut the lamb into 1½-inch cubes, trimming away all visible fat. In a large bowl mix together the French dressing, lemon juice, and seasonings. Add the lamb and artichokes and mix lightly. Cover the bowl and put it in the refrigerator for several hours or overnight.

Place the lamb on skewers. Cut each of the

tomatoes into 6 wedges and alternate the artichokes and tomatoes on another set of skewers. Brush the lamb and vegetables with the marinade. Broil the lamb 3 to 5 inches from the heat source for 5 to 7 minutes on each side, or until they have reached the desired doneness. Broil the artichoke kebabs for 3 to 4 minutes on each side. *Makes 6 servings*

	Calories	Carbo-hydrate (gm)	Protein (gm)	Total Fat (gm)	Saturated Fat (gm)	Cholesterol (mg)
Total	1484.6	74.4	211.7	48.0	28.8	681.6
Per Serving	247.4	12.4	35.3	8.0	4.8	113.6

Lamb and Bean Sprouts

1¹/₂ lbs. lean boneless leg
   of lamb
1 tbsp. diet margarine
4 green onions
1¹/₂ tsp. crushed garlic
   cloves

2 tbsp. flour
2 tbsp. soy sauce
1¹/₂ lbs. fresh bean
   sprouts
boiling salted
   water

Before cooking: Cut the lamb into strips, about 1 inch wide and 2¹/₂ inches long, trimming off all visible fat. Cut the green onions into ¹/₄-inch pieces.

Melt the diet margarine in a non-stick skillet. Add the lamb strips and brown them lightly. Then mix the onions and garlic with the meat and continue to cook them for about 5 minutes, stirring constantly. Sprinkle the flour over this mixture, cooking and stirring, until it is well blended with the lamb and onions. Add the soy sauce and continue cooking and stirring until the lamb is tender. Cook the bean sprouts in boiling salted water until they are just tender. Drain them well. Serve the meat mixture on a bed of bean sprouts.

Makes 6 servings

	Calories	Carbo-hydrate (gm)	Protein (gm)	Total Fat (gm)	Saturated Fat (gm)	Cholesterol (mg)
Total	1580.8	55.8	218.2	54.1	29.8	681.6
Per Serving	263.5	9.3	36.4	9.0	5.0	113.6

---

gm=grams; mg=milligrams. Nutritional figures are approximate. Figures are based on findings of U.S. Department of Agriculture.

Shish Kebab

1¹/₂ lbs. lean boneless leg
of lamb
1 green pepper
1 red pepper
3 tomatoes

4 onions
¹/₃ cup fresh lemon
juice
1¹/₂ tsp. garlic salt
1 tbsp. soy sauce
water

Before cooking: Cut the lamb into 1-inch cubes, trimming away all visible fat. Cut the peppers and onions into 2-inch chunks and cut the tomatoes into wedges. Place the lamb cubes into a glass or ceramic bowl. Add the lemon juice, garlic salt, soy sauce, and enough water to cover the meat. Marinate the meat at room temperature, uncovered, for 2 hours.

Drain the meat, reserving the marinade. Thread the meat onto 6 skewers, alternating it with the pieces of peppers, tomato, and onion. Broil the kebabs for about 15 minutes over hot coals or in a broiler, turning them frequently and brushing them with the reserved marinade. *Makes 6 servings*

	Calories	Carbo-hydrate (gm)	Protein (gm)	Total Fat (gm)	Saturated Fat (gm)	Choles-terol (mg)
Total	1595.8	83.6	209.3	48.0	28.8	681.6
Per Serving	266.0	13.9	34.9	8.0	4.8	113.6

Acorn Squash-Lamb Bake

1 lb. lean leg of lamb,
trimmed of fat and
ground
3 small acorn squash
2 tbsp. grated onion
1 garlic clove
1 tsp. salt

¹/₄ tsp. ginger
¹/₄ tsp. allspice
1 egg, slightly
beaten
²/₃ cup frozen green
peas
¹/₂ cup crushed high-
protein cereal,
unsweetened

Before cooking: Cut the squash in half. Crush or mince the garlic. Allow the peas to defrost.

Place the squash cut side down on a baking sheet and bake them at 350° for 35 minutes. In the meantime, heat a large non-stick skillet and add the lamb, onion, and garlic. Brown the meat. Do not add any oil to the pan because the meat will release enough of its own fat for frying. Stir in the salt, ginger, and allspice. Allow the mixture to cool slightly; then stir in the beaten egg, peas, and cereal crumbs. Remove the squash from the oven and turn them cut sides up. Pack the lamb mixture firmly into the squash cups and cover the filling in each squash with a small piece of aluminum foil. Continue baking the squash for about another 25 minutes until they are tender.

Makes 6 servings

	Calories	Carbo-hydrate (gm)	Protein (gm)	Total Fat (gm)	Saturated Fat (gm)	Choles-terol (mg)
Total	1628.2	168.1	160.4	42.7	21.2	706.4
Per Serving	271.4	28.0	26.7	7.1	3.5	117.7

Herb-Coated Lamp Chops

8 loin lamb chops, 1-inch thick	¹/₂ tsp. salt
2 tbsp. flour	¹/₄ tsp. thyme
1 tsp. dry mustard	¹/₈ tsp. oregano

Before cooking: Trim the chops of all visible fat.

Mix the flour, mustard, salt, thyme, and oregano together in a paperbag. Add the lamb chops, a few at a time and shake the bag until they are coated with the flour mixture. Place the coated chops on a rack on a broiling pan placed 3 to 4 inches from the heat source. Broil them about 7 minutes on each side, or until the desired doneness is reached. *Makes 8 servings*

	Calories	Carbo-hydrate (gm)	Protein (gm)	Total Fat (gm)	Saturated Fat (gm)	Choles-terol (mg)
Total	3259.2	12.4	201.7	264.1	144.0	1072.0
Per Serving	407.4	1.6	25.2	33.0	18.0	134.0

gm=grams; mg=milligrams. Nutritional figures are approximate. Figures are based on findings of U.S. Department of Agriculture.

Pork

The expletive "fat pig" no longer applies to pork. Once upon a time pork was plenty pudgy, but thanks to modern breeding techniques, today's pork contains only half as much fat as in the olden days, and far fewer calories. Although not as trim as veal, pork does beat out many cuts of beef in the calorie sweepstakes. (Check the comparison chart in the introduction to "The Meat of the Matter" to see how some cuts of pork and beef compare.) Another point in pork's favor: it's always served well-done, which eliminates even more fat. Comparable cuts of beef which have been broiled or roasted are generally served rare.

Which brings us to another point about pork. Many homemakers, aware that pork must be cooked through, habitually overcook it and thereby ruin its delightful taste and texture. Many old cookbooks and meat thermometers suggest an internal temperature of 185°, but research shows that pork is more tender and tasty when served at 170° — which is perfectly safe, since all trichinae are killed at 140°. When cooking pork, a meat thermometer is doubly important — to avoid either undercooking or overcooking!

Smoked or Cured Pork and Ham

Much of the cured ham available in supermarkets is "fully cooked" or "ready to eat," which means that it needs only sufficient cooking to warm it through and improve its flavor. Such meat should always be properly identified on the can, label, or wrapper. Reheat ready-to-eat whole or half hams to an internal temperature of 130 degrees in a preheated 300° or 325° oven for the best flavor. Ready-to-eat ham slices can be sautéed in a non-stick skillet, or barbecued, or broiled until heated through.

Cured or smoked pork that is labeled "cook before eating" must, of course, be cooked. Follow the label directions. Or, roast an uncooked ham to an internal temperature of 160° in a preheated 300° or 325° oven. Uncooked picnic roast (shoulder) or boneless butt (cottage roll) should be roasted to 170° or simmered in liquid until tender.

The Substitution Game

Of course, some cuts of pork are still exceedingly high in fat and calories and should be avoided by the committed calorie-counter. Included are bacon (69 percent fat and 3,016 per pound), sausage (50 percent fat and 2,259 calories per pound), and spareribs (33 percent fat and 1,637 calories per pound).

Canadian bacon (only 980 calories) can be sliced and served in place of fatty bacon, and homemade sausage patties can be prepared from lean ground pork. Veal or lamb ribs cut from the breast make an interesting stand-in for fatty pork spareribs.

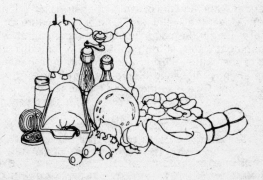

Recipes

Pork Pepper Steak

1½ lbs. lean boneless
    pork shoulder
1 crushed garlic clove
1 lb. can tomatoes,
    undrained
1 green pepper
1 cup chopped onion

½ cup diced celery
2 tbsp. cornstarch
6 tbsp. soy sauce
1 tsp. Worcester-
    shire sauce
¼ tsp. coarse freshly
    ground pepper
1¼ cups water

Before cooking: Cut the meat across the grain into ½-inch thick slices, trimming off all fat with a sharp knife. Then slice the meat again, lengthwise, into strips. Cut the green pepper into strips.

Spray a non-stick skillet with vegetable spray for no-fat frying and brown the pork strips over low heat. Or you can brown the meat in its own fat which can be released with steam. See the second cooking hint in "Slimming in the Kitchen" for directions. Add the garlic, tomatoes (with juice), ground pepper, sauces and 1 cup water to browned meat. Cover the pan, and simmer the mixture for about 45 minutes until the meat is tender. Then add the green pepper strips, onion, and celery. Cover the skillet, and simmer the mixture for 15 minutes longer. In a cup, combine the cornstarch with ¼ cup cold water, stirring until smooth. Add this mixture to the skillet, stirring and cooking until contents have slightly thickened. Serve the Pork Pepper Steak over Skinny Rice (see the index for the recipe).

Makes 6 servings

	Calories	Carbo-hydrate (gm)	Protein (gm)	Total Fat (gm)	Saturated Fat (gm)	Choles-terol (mg)
Total	1593.2	55.3	213.0	50.0	24.0	600.0
Per Serving	265.5	9.2	35.5	8.3	4.0	100.0

CONSUMER GUIDE

Pork Mandarin

1½ lbs. lean boneless
    pork shoulder
2 beef bouillon cubes
1 cup hot water
11 oz. can mandarin
    oranges, packed in
    juice
¼ cup soy sauce
1 tbsp. instant minced
    onion
½ tsp. ground ginger

2 tbsp. cornstarch
¼ cup cold water
4 oz. can water
    chestnuts,
    drained
2 green peppers
1 cup sliced
    mushrooms
1 cup sliced celery
    cabbage (cut
    diagonally ½- to
    ¾- inch thick)

Before cooking: Cut the meat into 1-inch cubes, trimming off all fat. Slice the water chestnuts and cut the green peppers into ¼-inch strips. Drain the mandarin oranges, reserving the liquid.

Spray a non-stick skillet with vegetable spray for no-fat frying. Add the meat and brown it slowly. Or you can brown the meat in its own fat. See the second cooking hint in "Slimming in the Kitchen" for directions. Dissolve the bouillon cubes in 1 cup hot water. Add this — with the liquid from the oranges, the soy sauce, minced onion, and ginger — to the pork. Bring the mixture to a boil; then cover the pan, reduce the heat, and simmer the contents for about 30 minutes. In a separate bowl blend the cornstarch with ¼ cup cold water. Gradually add the cornstarch mixture to the meat, cooking and stirring constantly until the sauce has thickened and is clear. Then add the water chestnuts, green pepper, mushrooms, and celery cabbage. Cover the skillet again, and continue to cook over low heat for 7 minutes. Fold in the mandarin oranges just before serving. *Makes 8 servings*

	Calories	Carbo-hydrate (gm)	Protein (gm)	Total Fat (gm)	Saturated Fat (gm)	Choles-terol (mg)
Total	1714.1	80.7	219.0	49.3	24.0	606.0
Per Serving	214.3	10.1	27.3	6.2	3.0	75.8

gm=grams; mg=milligrams. Nutritional figures are approximate. Figures are based on findings of U.S. Department of Agriculture.

Country Pork Roast

4 lbs. lean pork
    shoulder, boned
    and rolled
    seasoned meat
    tenderizer

For Glaze:
1/3 cup apple butter
1/3 cup apple juice or
    cider
1/8 tsp. thyme
1/8 tsp. cinnamon
1/8 tsp. ground cloves

Before cooking: Trim the meat of all visible fat. Prepare it with meat tenderizer according to the directions on the bottle.

Place the meat on a rack in an open roasting pan. Insert a meat thermometer so that the tip (the bulb) is in the center of the meat. Roast the meat at 325° for about 4 hours until the thermometer reads 170°. In a bowl mix together the ingredients for the glaze. Cover the entire roast with the glaze for the last half hour of cooking.

Makes 14 servings

	Calories	Carbohydrate (gm)	Protein (gm)	Total Fat (gm)	Saturated Fat (gm)	Cholesterol (mg)
Total	3771.1	63.5	533.3	129.1	64.0	1599.8
Per Serving	269.4	4.5	38.1	9.2	4.6	114.3

Pork and Sauerkraut

1 1/2 lbs. boneless lean
    pork, cut from leg
3 cups drained
    sauerkraut
1 cup peeled and
    chopped apples

1 cup chopped
    onion
2 tsp. caraway seeds
1 1/2 cups water
1 tbsp. water

Before cooking: Cut the pork into 6 serving pieces, trimming off all fat. Rinse the sauerkraut in water to eliminate some of the strong salt and vinegar flavors.

Place the meat with 1 tablespoon water in a large non-stick skillet. Cover the skillet, and heat it over a moderate temperature until the water has evaporated and the steam has caused the meat to release its own inner fat. Then uncover the skillet and brown the meat slowly on both sides in the fat. Or you may brown the meat by first spraying the pan with spray-on vegetable coating. In a separate bowl mix together the rinsed sauerkraut, apples, onions, caraway seeds, and 1½ cups water. Pour this mixture over the pork. Cover the skillet, and simmer the meat over low heat until the meat is very tender — about 1½ hours.

Makes 6 servings

	Calories	Carbo-hydrate (gm)	Protein (gm)	Total Fat (gm)	Saturated Fat (gm)	Choles-terol (mg)
Total	1971.2	48.9	208.0	100.0	30.0	600.0
Per Serving	328.5	8.1	34.7	16.7	5.0	100.0

Baked Tomato Pork Chops

6 lean pork chops, 1-inch thick
salt
pepper

6 onion slices, 1-inch thick
6 tbsp. uncooked rice
16 oz. can tomatoes, undrained

Before cooking: Trim the chops of all visible fat.

Season the chops with salt and pepper and place them in a baking dish. Bake them at 450° for about 20 minutes — just until they are brown. Drain off all the fat that has accumulated in the dish before going any further. Then place one slice of onion and 1 table-spoon of uncooked rice on each chop. Pour the can of tomatoes with the juice over all. Season with salt and pepper again. Cover the dish, and bake the chops at 350° for 1 hour.

Makes 6 servings

	Calories	Carbo-hydrate (gm)	Protein (gm)	Total Fat (gm)	Saturated Fat (gm)	Choles-terol (mg)
Total	1994.6	96.6	108.6	128.4	48.0	522.0
Per Serving	332.4	16.1	18.1	21.4	8.0	87.0

---

gm=grams; mg=milligrams. Nutritional figures are approximate. Figures are based on findings of U.S. Department of Agriculture.

Apricot Stuffed Pork Chops

6 lean pork chops, 1-
   inch thick
salt
pepper
16 oz. can juice-packed
   apricot halves
1 tbsp. diet margarine

1/4 cup catsup
1/2 cup apricot juice
   (from can)
2 tbsp. chopped
   onion
1 tbsp. lemon juice
1/2 tsp. dry mustard

Before cooking: Trim the chops of all fat. With a sharp knife make a slit in the side of each chop as a pocket for the stuffing. Drain the can of apricot halves, saving 1/2 cup of juice.

Season the pockets with a little salt and pepper and put 2 apricot halves in each one. Pin the pockets closed with wooden picks. Cut the remaining apricots in 1/2-inch pieces and set them aside. Melt the margarine in a non-stick skillet. Add the stuffed pork chops, and brown them slowly, turning them once. Then add the chopped apricots, reserved apricot juice, catsup, onion, lemon juice, and mustard to the skillet. Bring this mixture to a boil; then reduce the heat, cover the pan, and simmer the contents for 1 hour or more — until the meat is tender.   *Makes 6 servings*

	Calories	Carbo-hydrate (gm)	Protein (gm)	Total Fat (gm)	Saturated Fat (gm)	Choles-terol (mg)
Total	1925.6	80.7	101.0	132.0	49.0	522.0
Per Serving	320.9	13.5	16.8	22.0	8.2	87.0

Ham Patties Hawaiian

1 1/2 lbs. cooked smoked
   ham, trimmed of all
   fat and ground
1 tsp. grated onion
1 tbsp. chopped parsley
1 tbsp. prepared
   mustard

2 tbsp. pineapple
   juice (from pine-
   apple slices)
1 egg, beaten
8 tbsp. crushed corn
   flakes
8 pineapple slices,
   juice-packed

Before cooking: Drain the pineapple, saving 2 tablespoons of the juice.

Mix the ground ham with the onion, parsley, mustard, egg, and the 2 tablespoons of juice. Shape the meat into 8 patties and roll them in the crushed corn flakes. Arrange the pineapple slices in a shallow baking dish. Place 1 patty on each pineapple slice. Bake the patties at 375° for 25 to 30 minutes.

Makes 8 servings

	Calories	Carbo-hydrate (gm)	Protein (gm)	Total Fat (gm)	Saturated Fat (gm)	Choles-terol (mg)
Total	2390.5	107.6	151.0	158.0	58.0	860.0
Per Serving	298.8	13.5	18.9	19.8	7.3	107.5

B.B.Q. Pork Chops

8 pork chops about 1-inch thick
salt
pepper

Sauce:
1 cup tomato puree
1/4 cup vinegar
2 tbsp. brown sugar substitute
2 tsp. Worcestershire sauce
2 tbsp. prepared mustard
1/4 cup hot water

Before cooking: Trim the chops of all visible fat.

Season the pork chops with salt and pepper according to your own taste, and place them in a baking dish. Cover the dish, and bake them at 350° for 45 minutes. Pour off the fat that accumulates in the dish. Combine the sauce ingredients and mix them well. Pour the sauce over the chops, and cook them for an additional 30 minutes.

Makes 8 servings

	Calories	Carbo-hydrate (gm)	Protein (gm)	Total Fat (gm)	Saturated Fat (gm)	Choles-terol (mg)
Total	3299.2	83.0	186.7	239.8	91.4	993.5
Per Serving	412.4	10.4	23.3	30.0	11.4	124.2

gm=grams; mg=milligrams. Nutritional figures are approximate. Figures are based on findings of U.S. Department of Agriculture.

Hawaiian Ham Skillet

1½ lbs. lean cooked
    smoked ham
2 large onions
2 large green peppers
1 tbsp. diet margarine
2 cups pineapple
    chunks, packed in
    their own juice

2 tbsp. cornstarch
¾ tsp. salt
¼ tsp. pepper
1 tbsp. soy sauce
water

Before cooking: Cut the ham into 1-inch strips, trimming off all fat. Slice the onions and cut the green peppers into strips. Drain the pineapple, reserving the juice. Add enough water to the juice to make ¾ of a cup of liquid.

Melt the margarine in a large, non-stick skillet. Add the ham, onions, and green pepper, and cook them over moderate heat until the ham is browned. Combine the cornstarch, salt, pepper, soy sauce, and pineapple liquid in a separate bowl. Add this to the ham and vegetables, and continue cooking over low heat, stirring constantly, until the sauce has thickened.

Makes 6 servings

	Calories	Carbo-hydrate (gm)	Protein (gm)	Total Fat (gm)	Saturated Fat (gm)	Choles-terol (mg)
Total	1954.7	119.3	217.0	70.0	25.0	600.0
Per Serving	325.8	19.9	36.2	11.7	4.2	100.0

Bavarian Pork Steak

1 lb. lean pork leg steak
    (fresh ham slice)
1½ tsp. salt
½ tsp. pepper
1 lb. 11 oz. can
    sauerkraut

1 lb. can whole
    tomatoes,
    undrained
2½ tbsp. instant onion
1 green pepper
¼ tsp. thyme

Before cooking: Trim the meat of all visible fat. Drain the sauerkraut. Cut the green pepper into 1-inch strips.

Spray a non-stick skillet with vegetable spray for no-fat frying and brown the meat slowly. Or you can brown the meat in its own fat. See the second cooking hint in

"Slimming in the Kitchen" for directions. Season the browned meat, on both sides, with the salt and ¼ tsp. of pepper. In a bowl, combine the other ¼ tsp. of pepper with the sauerkraut, tomatoes (with the juice), onion, green pepper, and thyme. Mix them together well, and pour them into a 7½ x 11¾-inch baking dish. Place the meat on top of the mixture. Cover the dish with aluminum foil and place it in a 325° oven for 30 minutes. Then uncover the dish and bake for another 30 minutes until the pork is tender. *Makes 4 servings*

	Calories	Carbo-hydrate (gm)	Protein (gm)	Total Fat (gm)	Saturated Fat (gm)	Choles-terol (mg)
Total	1556.0	52.0	106.4	103.4	37.3	405.1
Per Serving	389.0	13.0	26.6	25.9	9.3	101.3

Ham and Cheese Casserole

1 lb. cooked lean ham
½ cup finely chopped onions
1 tbsp. diet margarine
1 cup grated American or Cheddar cheese
½ cup finely crushed cracker crumbs
1½ cups skim milk
3 eggs, slightly beaten
2 tsp. prepared mustard

Before cooking: Trim the ham of all fat and chop it into small pieces.

Melt the margarine in a non-stick skillet. Saute the onions in the melted margarine until they are lightly browned. In an oven-safe casserole combine the rest of the ingredients. Mix the onions into this mixture. Bake the casserole at 350° for 30 to 40 minutes — until a knife blade inserted in the center of the casserole comes out clean. *Makes 6 servings*

	Calories	Carbo-hydrate (gm)	Protein (gm)	Total Fat (gm)	Saturated Fat (gm)	Choles-terol (mg)
Total	2445.7	58.1	228.1	139.6	57.0	1387.3
Per Serving	407.6	9.7	38.0	23.3	9.5	231.2

gm=grams; mg=milligrams. Nutritional figures are approximate. Figures are based on findings of U.S. Department of Agriculture.

Sausage Patties in Chili Sauce

1 lb. lean pork
  shoulder, ground
³/₄ cup soft bread crumbs
¹/₂ cup evaporated skim
  milk
2 onions
1 tsp. garlic salt
¹/₈ tsp. pepper

¹/₂ cup chili sauce or
  catsup
¹/₂ cup water
¹/₂ cup diced celery
2 tbsp. horseradish
1 tbsp. lemon juice

Before cooking: Mix the bread crumbs and evaporated milk together and let them stand for 4 minutes. Chop the onions.

Add to the bread crumb mixture the meat, onions, garlic salt, and pepper. Mix them thoroughly and then shape the meat into 8 patties. Place the patties in an oven-safe, non-stick pan, and brown them over low heat. Do not add any oil to the pan because the meat will release enough of its own fat for browning. (If you like, you can spray the pan with vegetable coating for no-fat frying.) When the patties are brown, drain off the fat that has accumulated in the pan. In a separate bowl mix together the chili sauce (or catsup), celery, horseradish, and lemon juice. Add ¹/₂ cup water and pour the mixture over the patties. Cover the pan and bake the meat at 350° for 50 minutes, turning the patties once during the baking period. *Makes 8 servings*

	Calories	Carbohydrate (gm)	Protein (gm)	Total Fat (gm)	Saturated Fat (gm)	Cholesterol (mg)
Total	1575.6	125.0	156.2	45.8	22.3	442.6
Per Serving	197.0	15.6	19.5	5.7	2.8	55.3

Florida Orange-Glazed Ham

12 lbs. smoked or ready-
  to-eat lean whole
  ham
whole cloves
6 oz. can frozen orange
  juice concentrate

4 tbsp. prepared
  mustard
sugar substitute to
  equal 4 tbsp.

Before cooking: If you are using a ready-to-eat ham, trim off all the fat. Allow the orange juice to defrost, but don't mix it with water.

Insert a meat thermometer into the ham so the tip is in the center of the meat. Place the ham in a shallow pan, and bake it slowly (at 325°). If you are using a smoked ham, bake it 18 to 20 minutes per pound — or until the meat thermometer registers 160°. If you're using a ready-to-eat ham, bake it 12 minutes per pound — or until the meat thermometer registers 130°. Take the ham from the oven 45 minutes before it is done. If it is a smoked ham, remove the rind. Drain the pan of all the fat that has accumulated there. Score the surface of the meat, and stud it with cloves by sticking the pointed end of the clove into the meat. In a separate bowl combine the orange juice concentrate, mustard, and sugar substitute, and brush part of this mixture on the ham. Return the ham to the oven, and continue baking it until it is done, brushing it frequently with the remaining glaze.   *Makes 30 servings*

	Calories	Carbo-hydrate (gm)	Protein (gm)	Total Fat (gm)	Saturated Fat (gm)	Choles-terol (mg)
Total	7984.0	203.0	1045.0	320.0	120.0	3000.0
Per Serving	266.1	6.8	34.8	10.7	4.0	100.0

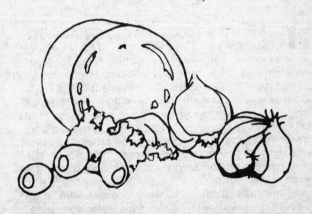

gm=grams; mg=milligrams. Nutritional figures are approximate. Figures are based on findings of U.S. Department of Agriculture.

Hip Hamburger Dishes

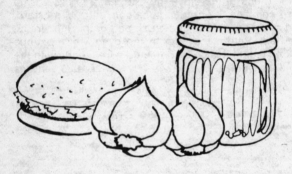

Hamburger is one of America's favorite meats. The typical American eats in excess of 50 pounds of ground meat a year, much of it, unfortunately, calorie-contaminated with excess fat. Most pre-packaged ground meat contains close to the legal limit of fat — 30 percent — and weighs in at more than 1600 calories per pound. Fat-trimmed beef, by contrast, is less than 700 calories per pound. You can eliminate more than 50,000 excess calories this year by switching from pre-packaged hamburger to fat-trimmed beef which has been custom-ground to your order. Simply pick out a piece of lean bottom round and ask the butcher to trim away the fat and grind the lean to order. Almost all supermarkets will perform this service for you, especially when you explain that you have to eliminate as much fat as possible from your diet. Rest assured that you won't be the first customer to request custom-ground, fat-trimmed beef; many heart-smart cholesterol watchers shop for it as a matter of prudence.

Isn't lean hamburger more expensive? The price tag for boneless bottom round is generally at least one-third higher than ready-ground hamburger. But the price differential is really not as great as it appears. Lean hamburger won't shrink the way fatty hamburger will, so one pound will give you four servings, instead of three or less. And the nutritive value is much higher, because the fat in the packaged ground meat is replaced with protein in the lean meat. Here's how fatty hamburger and lean ground round compare:

One Pound, Raw	Fat	Protein	Calories
Hamburger, 29% fat	148 grams	73 grams	1,647
Lean ground round, trimmed of fat	21 grams	98 grams	612

Isn't lean hamburger dry? Only if you overcook it. Like all lean meat, fat-trimmed hamburger can't stand up to blast-furnace temperatures and prolonged cooking times. The best way to broil lean burgers is to mix the meat with crushed ice, season it, and broil it only until it is well-browned on the outside. The inside should remain pink and juicy.

What else can you do with lean hamburger? Anything you'd do with fatty hamburger. Meat loaf and casserole dishes are particularly well-suited to the use of lean meat. On the other hand, a casserole dish made with fatty hamburger will be greasy and undigestible (as well as fattening) because the fat has nowhere to escape. Meat loaf made with lean meat is delicious hot or cold, while fatty meat loaf is unpleasantly greasy when chilled!

What about other meats? Any meat can be fat-trimmed and ground to order. Try pork, lamb, or veal for a change. If you're fortunate enough to live in an area where the stores stock and sell raw ground turkey-burger, be sure to take advantage of this non-fattening treat — only 736 calories a pound!

Recipes

Juicyburgers

2 lbs. round steak,
trimmed of fat, and
ground
2 tbsp. snipped chives

¼ cup crushed ice
1 tsp. bitters

Combine all the ingredients and mix them well. Shape the meat into 8 patties and place them on a rack in the broiler, 4 inches from the heat source. Broil them for about 10 minutes, turning them once during the broiling.

Makes 8 servings

	Calories	Carbo-hydrate (gm)	Protein (gm)	Total Fat (gm)	Saturated Fat (gm)	Choles-terol (mg)
Total	1488.3	1.5	284.4	35.6	11.9	841.4
Per Serving	186.0	0.2	35.6	4.5	1.5	105.2

Basic Broiled Burgers

2 lbs. lean round steak,
trimmed of fat, and
ground
½ tsp. salt or garlic salt

¼ tsp. pepper
½ cup crushed ice

Toss the ingredients together lightly and shape the meat into 8 patties. Place the patties on a rack in the broiler, 4 inches from the heat source. Broil them for a total of 10 to 15 minutes, turning them once.

Makes 8 servings

	Calories	Carbo-hydrate (gm)	Protein (gm)	Total Fat (gm)	Saturated Fat (gm)	Choles-terol (mg)
Total	1481.3	0.0	284.4	35.6	11.9	841.4
Per Serving	185.2	0.0	35.6	4.5	1.5	105.2

CONSUMER GUIDE

Hamburger Chop Suey

2 lbs. lean round steak,
    trimmed of fat, and
    ground
1 onion
2 beef bouillon cubes
$\frac{1}{2}$ cup hot water
4 oz. can whole
    mushrooms
$\frac{1}{3}$ cup soy sauce

2 tbsp. cornstarch
5 to $6\frac{1}{2}$ oz. can
    water chestnuts
16 oz. can bean
    sprouts
16 oz. can Chinese
    vegetables
$\frac{1}{4}$ cup pimiento strips

Before cooking: Cut the onion into eighths. Drain the mushrooms, reserving the juice from the can, and drain the bean sprouts and vegetables. Drain the water chestnuts and cut them in half. Dissolve the bouillon cubes in $\frac{1}{2}$ cup hot water.

Brown the ground meat in a large non-stick skillet. Do not add any oil to the pan because the meat will release enough of its own fat. Add the onion to the browned meat and continue to cook over low heat for 5 minutes. Before going any further, pour off all the fat that has accumulated in the pan. Then combine the liquid from the mushrooms with the bouillon and add this to the meat along with the soy sauce and corn starch. Bring the liquid to a boil, then reduce the heat and simmer the mixture, stirring constantly, until it thickens. Stir in the mushrooms, water chestnuts, bean sprouts, and Chinese vegetables, cooking just until they are heated through. Stir in the pimiento strips just before serving. *Makes 8 servings*

	Calories	Carbo-hydrate (gm)	Protein (gm)	Total Fat (gm)	Saturated Fat (gm)	Choles-terol (mg)
Total	1964.4	95.4	312.9	36.1	11.9	847.4
Per Serving	245.6	11.9	39.1	4.5	1.5	105.9

gm=grams; mg=milligrams. Nutritional figures are approximate. Figures are based on findings of U.S. Department of Agriculture.

Basic Meat Loaf

2 lbs. lean round steak, trimmed of fat, and ground
2 tsp. salt or garlic salt
1/4 tsp. pepper
2 eggs
1/2 cup high-protein cereal, unsweetened
1/2 cup skim milk
1/4 cup chopped onion
1/4 tsp. dried sage

Mix all of the ingredients together thoroughly and form the meat into a loaf in a shallow baking pan. Bake the meat loaf at 350° for about 1 hour, basting it occasionally. *Makes 8 servings*

Diet hint: The calorie-wise cook can save a whopping 100 calories (that's 12 1/2 per serving) by using 4 egg whites instead of 2 whole eggs. Egg whites are also kinder to your heart — with hardly a trace of saturated fat or cholesterol.

	Calories	Carbo-hydrate (gm)	Protein (gm)	Total Fat (gm)	Saturated Fat (gm)	Choles-terol (mg)
Total	1739.9	16.8	303.7	47.7	15.9	1347.9
Per Serving	217.5	2.1	38.0	6.0	2.0	168.5

Meat Loaf Italiano

1 1/2 lbs. lean round steak, trimmed of fat, and ground
10 3/4 oz. can tomato soup
1/4 cup finely chopped onion
1 egg, slightly beaten
1 tsp. salt
1/2 tsp. oregano
generous dash pepper
1 tbsp. grated Parmesan cheese
1/4 cup water

Mix the beef, onion, egg, salt, oregano, pepper, and 1/2 cup soup together in a large bowl. Shape the meat mixture into a loaf and place it in a shallow baking pan. Bake the loaf at 350° for 1 hour. During the last 15 minutes, put the remaining soup in a saucepan. Blend into it the cheese and $1/4$ cup water. Heat the soup just until boiling, and serve it over the meat loaf.

Makes 6 servings

Diet hint: The super calorie-watcher can use 2 egg whites instead of 1 whole egg — a savings of 50 calories (about 8 per serving!).

	Calories	Carbo-hydrate (gm)	Protein (gm)	Total Fat (gm)	Saturated Fat (gm)	Choles-terol (mg)
Total	1513.8	45.1	232.0	45.8	13.9	898.7
Per Serving	252.3	7.5	38.6	7.6	2.3	149.8

Saucy Hamburger Steak

1 lb. lean round steak, trimmed of all fat, and ground
$1/2$ cup high-protein cereal, unsweetened
$1/2$ tsp. salt
$1/4$ tsp. pepper
8 oz. can tomato sauce
1 tbsp. chopped green onion
1 tsp. Worcestershire sauce
1 tsp. prepared mustard

Mix the ground steak, cereal, salt, and pepper together, and shape the mixture into 4 patties. Brown the patties slowly in a non-stick skillet. Do not add any fat to the pan; if you cook the meat slowly, enough of its own inner fat will be released. In a separate bowl blend together the tomato sauce, onion, Worcestershire sauce, and mustard, and pour this mixture over the patties. Cover the pan and simmer the meat for 10 minutes.

Makes 4 servings

	Calories	Carbo-hydrate (gm)	Protein (gm)	Total Fat (gm)	Saturated Fat (gm)	Choles-terol (mg)
Total	898.2	35.1	147.9	18.3	5.9	421.0
Per Serving	224.6	8.8	37.0	4.6	1.5	105.3

gm=grams; mg=milligrams. Nutritional figures are approximate. Figures are based on findings of U.S. Department of Agriculture.

Oriental Pepper-Burgers

2 lbs. lean round steak,
trimmed of fat, and
ground
1/2 tsp. salt
1/8 tsp. pepper
2 large onions

2 medium green
peppers
2 (8 oz.) cans tomato
sauce
1/2 tsp. ground ginger
or dry mustard
3 tbsp. soy sauce

Before cooking: Slice the onions, and cut the green peppers into 1-inch squares.

Season the meat with the salt and pepper and shape it into 8 oval steaks. Place the steaks in a large non-stick skillet over low heat until they are just lightly brown. Do not add any oil to the pan because the meat will release enough of its own fat. Drain off this fat after the meat has browned. Then add the onions and green peppers to the pan. Pour the tomato sauce over all and blend in the ginger (or mustard) and soy sauce. Cover the pan, and simmer the meat for 15 to 25 minutes — or until it has reached the desired doneness.   *Makes 8 servings*

	Calories	Carbo-hydrate (gm)	Protein (gm)	Total Fat (gm)	Saturated Fat (gm)	Choles-terol (mg)
Total	1879.1	84.0	303.8	36.4	11.9	841.4
Per Serving	234.9	10.5	38.0	4.6	1.5	105.2

Italian Beef Sausage

2 1/2 lbs. lean round steak,
trimmed of fat and
ground
1/2 tsp. coriander
1 tsp. oregano
1 tsp. basil

1 tsp. sage
1 tsp. meat
tenderizer
1/2 tsp. thyme
1/2 tsp. marjoram

Mix all of the ingredients together lightly. Shape the mixture into small flat patties, using 1 heaping tbsp. for each sausage. Place the patties on a rack on the

broiler pan and broil them about 4 inches from the heat
source for about 3 minutes on each side.

Makes 20 sausages

	Calories	Carbo-hydrate (gm)	Protein (gm)	Total Fat (gm)	Saturated Fat (gm)	Choles-terol (mg)
Total	2165.8	0.0	349.9	66.6	33.3	1032.9
Per Serving	108.3	0.0	17.5	3.3	1.7	51.6

Lamb Patties Hawaiian

1¹/₂ lbs. lean lamb from
    leg or shoulder,
    trimmed of fat, and
    ground
1 egg

1¹/₄ tsp. salt
    dash black pepper
2 tbsp. skim milk
6 slices juice-
    packed
    pineapple

Before cooking: Drain the pineapple slices, discarding
the juice.

Mix the meat with the egg, salt, pepper, and milk,
and divide it into 6 portions. Form the meat into patties
about the same size as the pineapple slices. Place the
patties on a rack in the broiler, about 4 inches from the
heat source, and broil them for 5 to 7 minutes until the
top side is brown. At the same time, spread the pineapple slices on a non-stick baking sheet and broil them
until they are golden. When the patties are brown on
top, turn each of them onto a pineapple slice, and broil
them for about another 5 minutes. *Makes 6 servings*

Diet hint: The calorie-smart cook will use 2 egg whites
instead of 1 whole egg — a savings of 50 calories
(about 8 per serving).

	Calories	Carbo-hydrate (gm)	Protein (gm)	Total Fat (gm)	Saturated Fat (gm)	Choles-terol (mg)
Total	1535.1	52.1	200.4	54.0	30.8	934.2
Per Serving	255.9	8.7	33.4	9.0	5.1	155.7

---

*gm=grams; mg=milligrams. Nutritional figures are approximate. Figures
are based on findings of U.S. Department of Agriculture.*

Savory Lamb Loaf

1½ lbs. lean lamb from
    leg, trimmed of fat,
    and ground
1 egg, beaten
1 onion
1 green pepper
2 stalks of celery

1 tbsp. parsley
½ cup catsup
1 tsp. dry mustard
1 minced garlic
    clove
1 tsp. salt
½ tsp. coarse freshly
    ground pepper

Before cooking: Chop the onion and celery into fine pieces. Cut 2 or 3 rings from the green pepper to use as garnish and chop the rest of the green pepper into fine pieces.

Mix all of the ingredients together except the green pepper rings. Form the meat into a loaf and place it on a rack in a shallow baking dish. Garnish the top of the loaf with the green pepper rings. Bake the meat at 325° for about 1 hour. *Makes 6 servings*

Diet hint: The super calorie-watcher can use 2 egg whites instead of 1 whole egg — a savings of 50 calories (about 8 per serving!).

	Calories	Carbo-hydrate (gm)	Protein (gm)	Total Fat (gm)	Saturated Fat (gm)	Choles-terol (mg)
Total	1514.0	50.0	201.0	54.0	30.8	933.6
Per Serving	252.3	8.3	33.5	9.0	5.1	155.6

Veal Meat Loaf

2 lbs. lean veal leg,
    rump, or shoulder,
    ground
2 eggs, beaten
⅔ cup bread crumbs
3 tbsp. dried onion
    flakes
2 stalks celery, minced

¼ cup water
½ tsp. poultry
    seasoning
2 tsp. salt
⅛ tsp. pepper
⅛ tsp. garlic powder

Combine all of the ingredients and mix them

carefully in a bowl. Shape the meat into a loaf and place it in a shallow baking dish. Bake the meat at 350° for about 1 hour. *Makes 10 servings*

Diet hint: You can save 100 calories (10 per serving!) by using 4 egg whites instead of 2 eggs.

	Calories	Carbo-hydrate (gm)	Protein (gm)	Total Fat (gm)	Saturated Fat (gm)	Choles-terol (mg)
Total	1642.2	59.6	202.6	58.0	26.0	1146.9
Per Serving	164.2	6.0	20.3	5.8	2.6	114.7

Sloppy Turkey Joes

1 lb. fresh ground turkey
1 tbsp. diet margarine
1½ cups chopped onion
1½ cups chopped celery
½ cup chopped green pepper

10½ oz. can condensed tomato soup
1 tsp. salt
dash of pepper
12 toasted buns

Melt the margarine in a large non-stick skillet. Add the ground turkey and cook it over low heat until it has browned. Then add the chopped vegetables and continue to cook until they are tender. Stir in the soup, salt, and pepper, cover the skillet, and simmer the mixture for about 30 minutes. Serve the Sloppy Turkey Joe on a toasted bun. *Makes 12 servings*

Special note: If ground turkey isn't available in your area, buy a turkey thigh that weighs about 1¼ lbs. Trim the meat from the bone, discarding the skin, and put the meat through a grinder.

	Calories	Carbo-hydrate (gm)	Protein (gm)	Total Fat (gm)	Saturated Fat (gm)	Choles-terol (mg)
Total	2684.1	320.0	190.9	65.2	22.1	430.7
Per Serving	223.7	26.7	15.9	5.4	1.8	35.9

gm=grams; mg=milligrams. Nutritional figures are approximate. Figures are based on findings of U.S. Department of Agriculture.

Turkey Loaf

2 lbs. fresh ground
turkey
3 slices protein bread
2 eggs, slightly beaten
1 medium onion,
minced
1/4 cup minced green
pepper ·

2 tbsp. prepared
horseradish
2 tsp. salt
1 tsp. dry mustard
1/4 cup evaporated
skim milk
3/4 cup catsup

Before cooking: Toast the protein bread.

Lightly mix all of the ingredients together except 1/2 cup catsup. Mold the meat into a 9 x 5 x 3-inch loaf pan and spread the top with the 1/2 cup catsup. Bake the loaf at 350° for about 1 1/4 hours. Drain the juices from the pan and unmold the loaf onto a heated platter.

If you like, you can make a gravy from the pan juices. Check "The Flavor-Uppers" for directions.

Makes 8 servings

	Calories	Carbo-hydrate (gm)	Protein (gm)	Total Fat (gm)	Saturated Fat (gm)	Choles-terol (mg)
Total	2383.7	99.4	318.5	73.9	25.6	1339.7
Per Serving	298.0	12.4	39.8	9.2	3.2	167.5

Turkey Chili

1 1/4 lbs. raw ground turkey
1 tbsp. diet margarine
1 cup chopped onion
1/2 cup chopped green
pepper
1/2 cup chopped red
pepper

16 oz. can chopped
tomatoes
2 tsp. salt
1 tsp. chili powder
1/2 tsp. black pepper
1/4 tsp. red pepper

Melt the margarine in a heavy non-stick skillet. Add the turkey, onion, and peppers, and brown them slowly. Then add the tomatoes (with the juice) and the seasonings. Cover the pan, and simmer the mixture for about 15 minutes.

Makes 6 servings

Special note: If ground turkey isn't available in your area, a large turkey thigh (about 1½ lbs.) will yield 1¼ lbs. ground turkey. Don't forget to throw away the skin before you grind the meat.

	Calories	Carbohydrate (gm)	Protein (gm)	Total Fat (gm)	Saturated Fat (gm)	Cholesterol (mg)
Total	1293.9	34.5	189.7	42.3	13.4	508.2
Per Serving	215.6	5.8	31.6	7.1	2.2	84.7

Stuffed Turkey Loaf

2 lbs. ground turkey
½ cup chopped onion
¾ cup chopped celery
2 tsp. oil

3 cups prepared stuffing mix
2 eggs, slightly beaten
½ cup water
½ cup tomato juice

Heat the oil in a non-stick skillet, and sauté the onion and celery. When the onion and celery are brown, add them to the stuffing mix, along with the eggs and ½ cup water, to make a stuffing. Add half of the stuffing to the ground turkey, mixing them well. Pat half of the meat mixture into a 2-quart loaf pan (4½ x 8½ x 3 inches). Spread the stuffing mixture on top, and then pat on the rest of the meat. Pour the tomato juice over the loaf, and bake it at 350° for 1½ hours.

Makes 8 to 10 servings

Special note: If ground turkey isn't available in your area, buy 3 large frozen turkey thighs. Defrost them, remove the meat from the bones (discarding the skin), and put the meat through a grinder.

	Calories	Carbohydrate (gm)	Protein (gm)	Total Fat (gm)	Saturated Fat (gm)	Cholesterol (mg)
Total	3145.9	230.5	345.5	88.0	26.0	1329.5
Per Serving	349.5	25.6	38.4	9.8	2.9	147.7

gm=grams; mg=milligrams. Nutritional figures are approximate. Figures are based on findings of U.S. Department of Agriculture.

Chicken

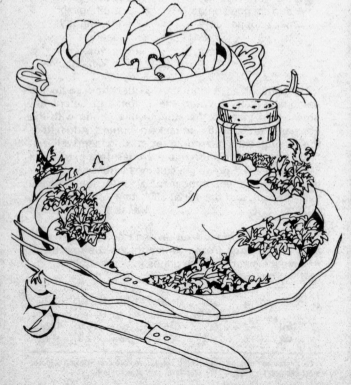

This is truly a nation of meat-eaters. The United States grows and consumes more meat than any other nation in the world. But even the most enthusiastic meat-and-potatoes person needs a change once in a while, and that change is usually in the form of poultry. Poultry is tasty, relatively inexpensive, easy to prepare, and — best of all — low in calories.

Of all the main course choices available to dieters, chicken is the unchallenged champion in terms of popularity, availability, versatility, and affordability. Chicken is lower in calories than any other "meat," it's also cholesterol-wise because of its relative lack of saturated fat.

Chicken is easy to digest and simple to prepare, so it's the ideal choice for beginning cooks, or those who have to prepare food for picky appetites or plain-food fans. On the other hand, chicken is a favorite in nearly every cuisine, so there's an endless variety of elegant or exotic dishes waiting for the culinary adventurer — "gourmet delights" that won't break either the dollar or calorie budget. The universal availability of "chicken in parts" serves to widen the repertoire of chicken fans at very little additional cost.

The popularity of chicken and its congenial calorie count are due to modern farming methods that make young "spring chickens" the least expensive and most available. These prize broiler-fryer chickens are also the prime choice nutritionally. Check the comparison chart and you will see that young frying chickens offer the most protein and the least fat and calories.

Although it is clear that you will get the most nutritional value and least calories by choosing a young frying chicken over an older roasting chicken, you can give yourself even greater control over the calories you eat by choosing the leanest parts of the chicken to eat.

From the following chart, it is easy to see that chicken breasts are a nutrition bargain. They are only 21 percent bones; the rest is meat. No other part of the chicken is as meaty. And in all that meat, there are only 7 grams of fat and a giant 75 grams of protein, which makes them a calorie bargain, too.

CHICKEN COMPARISON CHART

per pound	fat	protein	calories
Fryers 9 weeks 1½-3½ lbs.	15 grams	57 grams	382
Roasters 12 weeks 3½-5 lbs.	59 grams	43 grams	564
Hens 1½ years 4½-6 lbs.	82 grams	41 grams	703
Capons 4 - 7 pounds	53 grams	50 grams	668

HOW CUT-UP PARTS COMPARE
(Young Frying Chicken)

	bones	fat	protein
Back	46%	24 grams	40 grams
Breast	21%	7 grams	75 grams
Drumstick	40%	11 grams	51 grams
Neck	52%	21 grams	34 grams
Rib	49%	13 grams	41 grams
Thigh	25%	19 grams	62 grams
Wing	51%	17 grams	41 grams

How to Cook a Chicken

Broiling. Because of the fat in chicken skin, broiler-fryer chickens can be broiled without additional fat. Simply:

1. Sprinkle the chicken halves, quarters, or pieces with salt, pepper, lemon juice, and an herb such as tarragon, thyme, or basil.

2. Place the pieces skin side down on the broiler

rack. In the broiler of a gas range, the chicken should be 3 to 6 inches from the heat source; in an electric range, the distance should be 6 to 9 inches.

3. Broil the chicken for 20 to 25 minutes. Then turn it over and broil it for 15 to 20 minutes longer.

4. If you like, you can baste the chicken with barbecue sauce near the end of the cooking time.

Frying. One of the most popular ways to cook chicken is to fry it. It's also the most fattening way. What makes frying so fattening, of course, is the oil used in the frying process. So a simple way of decalorizing fried chicken is to eliminate the oil.

1. Cut a broiler-fryer chicken into serving pieces — or buy one that is already cut up. A 2-pound chicken will serve 4 people.

2. In a paper bag mix 3 tbsp. flour with 1 tsp. salt, $\frac{1}{2}$ tsp. pepper, and 1 tsp. paprika.

3. Add the chicken, a few pieces at a time, to the bag, and shake them until the chicken is coated.

4. Place the chicken in a non-stick baking dish, skin side down.

5. Bake the chicken for about 25 minutes at 400°.

6. Turn the chicken over and continue baking it for 20 to 25 minutes more — until it is tender, brown, and crisp.

7. Before serving, blot chicken with paper toweling.

Simmering. Chicken simmered in water and seasonings makes a great beginning for other dishes.

1. Use a broiler-fryer chicken, whole or cut into serving pieces.

2. Put the chicken in a kettle and add 2 cups of water, 1 small sliced onion, 3 celery tops, 1 tsp. salt, and $\frac{1}{2}$ tsp. pepper.

3. Bring the water to a boil.

4. Cover the kettle, reduce the heat and simmer the chicken for about 1 hour until it's tender.

5. Strain the broth.

6. Refrigerate the chicken and broth in separate containers.

7. When the chicken is cool, remove the meat from the skin and bones, and cut it into chunks.

8. Skim the fat from the surface of the broth.

Roasting. Another healthy and low-calorie way of preparing chicken is roasting it. In this dry-heat method, the chicken is cooked to juicy tenderness while the bird's excess fat is melted away.

1. Even though it may seem more appropriate to use a roasting chicken, buy a broiler-fryer. It is lower in calories and faster to cook.

2. Sprinkle the neck and body cavities with 1 tsp. salt.

3. If you like, stuff the body cavity with your favorite stuffing. (Several stuffing recipes are in this chapter.)

4. Hook the wing tips onto the chicken's back to hold the neck skin. Tie the legs together; then tie them to the tail.

5. Place the chicken in a shallow roasting pan. Do not brush the chicken with fat.

6. Roast the chicken according to the following timetable. If you have stuffed the chicken, add 15 minutes to the total roasting time.

7. When the chicken is done, the drumstick meat will feel soft when pressed between your fingers, and the leg will twist easily out of the thigh joint. Another way of testing the chicken for doneness is to pierce the skin of the breast with a fork. If the liquid that seeps out is clear, not yellow, the chicken is done.

TIMETABLE FOR BROILER-FRYER AND YOUNG ROASTING CHICKEN

Weight	Time Per Pound	Temperature	Approx. Amt. Stuffing	Approx. Total Time*
1½ lbs.	40 min.	400°	¾ cup	1 hour
2 lbs.	35 min.	400°	1 cup	1 hr. 10 min.
2½ lbs.	30 min.	375°	1¼ cups	1 hr. 15 min.
3 lbs.	30 min.	375°	1½ cups	1 hr. 30 min.
3½ lbs.	30 min.	375°	1¾ cups	1 hr. 45 min.
4 lbs.	30 min.	375°	2 cups	2 hours
4½ lbs.	30 min.	375°	2¼ cups	2 hrs. 15 min.
5 lbs.	30 min.	375°	2½ cups	2 hrs. 30 min.

*If the chicken is stuffed, add 15 min. to the total roasting time.

CONSUMER GUIDE

Recipes

Spiced Pineapple Chicken

2¹/₂ lbs. broiler-fryer
    chicken pieces
³/₄ cup unsweetened
    pineapple juice

¹/₄ cup vinegar
¹/₄ cup soy sauce
¹/₄ tsp. cinnamon

Arrange the chicken pieces, skin side up, in a single layer in a shallow roasting pan. Combine the pineapple juice, vinegar, soy sauce, and cinnamon, and pour this mixture over the chicken. Bake the chicken at 350° for 50 to 60 minutes until it is tender, basting frequently with the pineapple liquid. *Makes 6 servings*

	Calories	Carbo-hydrate (gm)	Protein (gm)	Total Fat (gm)	Saturated Fat (gm)	Choles-terol (mg)
Total	1225.1	33.5	167.6	42.9	17.1	694.2
Per Serving	204.2	5.6	27.9	7.2	2.9	115.7

Easy Orange Chicken

2 lbs. broiler-fryer
    chicken pieces

³/₄ cup orange juice
1 tsp. garlic salt

Place the chicken pieces, skin side up, in a non-stick baking dish. Season them with garlic salt. Pour the orange juice over the chicken, cover the dish with foil, and bake it for about 1 hour at 350° until it is very tender. *Makes 4 servings*

	Calories	Carbo-hydrate (gm)	Protein (gm)	Total Fat (gm)	Saturated Fat (gm)	Choles-terol (mg)
Total	946.9	19.5	131.8	35.1	13.7	555.7
Per Serving	236.7	4.9	33.0	8.8	3.4	138.9

gm=grams; mg=milligrams. Nutritional figures are approximate. Figures are based on findings of U.S. Department of Agriculture.

Herb-Broiled Chicken

1 lb. broiler-fryer
chicken, split in half
lengthwise
1 tsp. salt
3 tbsp. lemon juice
2 tbsp. water

1 tsp. rosemary
1 tsp. thyme
2 tsp. dried tarragon
leaves

Before cooking: Make a basting sauce by combining the salt, water, lemon juice, and seasonings.

Place the chicken on a broiler rack, skin side up, and brush it with the basting sauce. Broil the chicken 8 to 10 inches from the heat source for approximately 45 minutes, until it is tender, basting it as needed.

Makes 4 servings

	Calories	Carbo-hydrate (gm)	Protein (gm)	Total Fat (gm)	Saturated Fat (gm)	Choles-terol (mg)
Total	875.8	3.8	130.5	34.3	13.7	555.7
Per Serving	219.0	1.0	32.6	8.6	3.4	138.9

Moroccan Chicken

2 lbs. broiler fryer
chicken, quartered
1 tbsp. grated lemon
peel
1/2 cup water
1/4 cup lemon juice
1 tsp. thyme

1 tsp. garlic salt
1/2 tsp. black pepper
1 lemon
1/4 cup chopped
parsley

Before cooking: Combine the grated lemon peel, water, lemon juice, thyme, garlic salt, and pepper. Spoon this mixture over the chicken, coating it well. Refrigerate the chicken for 3 to 4 hours, turning it in the marinade several times.

Arrange the chicken in a single layer in a shallow baking dish. Save the marinade. Bake the chicken, uncovered, at 425° for 25 minutes. Pour off the fat that accumulates in the pan. Lower the oven to 350°. Brush the chicken with the reserved marinade and bake it for an additional 25 to 35 minutes until it is tender and brown. Cut the lemon into thin slices, and serve the chicken with lemon slices as garnish and with the parsley spinkled over it. *Makes 4 servings*

	Calories	Carbo-hydrate (gm)	Protein (gm)	Total Fat (gm)	Saturated Fat (gm)	Choles-terol (mg)
Total	886.6	5.8	130.7	34.3	13.7	555.7
Per Serving	221.7	1.5	32.7	8.6	3.4	138.9

Lemon Chicken

1 lb. broiler-fryer
  chicken pieces
¹/₂ tsp. salt
¹/₂ tsp. onion salt
¹/₂ tsp. crushed thyme
¹/₂ tsp. crushed
  marjoram

2 tsp. grated lemon
  peel
¹/₃ cup fresh lemon
  juice
¹/₂ cup water
  lemon quarters
  dash of paprika
  snipped parsley

Season the chicken with salt and place it in a non-stick baking pan, skin side down. In a separate bowl, combine the seasonings, lemon peel, and lemon juice with ¹/₂ cup water. Pour this mixture over the chicken and bake it, uncovered, at 350° for about 30 minutes, basting once or twice with the pan liquid. Then turn the chicken over, and continue to bake it, basting with the pan liquid, for another 30 minutes — until the chicken is done and the skin is crispy. Remove the chicken to a heated platter and garnish it with lemon quarters and parsley. *Makes 4 servings*

	Calories	Carbo-hydrate (gm)	Protein (gm)	Total Fat (gm)	Saturated Fat (gm)	Choles-terol (mg)
Total	886.8	7.2	130.7	34.3	13.7	555.7
Per Serving	221.7	1.8	32.7	8.6	3.4	138.9

gm=grams; mg=milligrams. Nutritional figures are approximate. Figures are based on findings of U.S. Department of Agriculture.

No-Fat-Added Fried Chicken

2 lbs. broiler-fryer   salt
   chicken pieces   pepper

Place the chicken pieces in a large non-stick skillet. Do not add any shortening or oil to the pan. Season the chicken with salt and pepper. Fry the chicken, uncovered, over moderate heat for 20 to 30 minutes. Turn the chicken over, season it again, and continue to fry it for 20 or 30 minutes more until it is tender.

Makes 4 servings

	Calories	Carbo-hydrate (gm)	Protein (gm)	Total Fat (gm)	Saturated Fat (gm)	Cholesterol (mg)
Total	864.4	0.0	130.3	34.3	13.7	555.7
Per Serving	216.1	0.0	32.6	8.6	3.4	138.9

Pineapple Chicken

2 lbs. broiler-fryer   ³/₄ cup orange juice
   chicken pieces   ¹/₈ tsp. cinnamon
1 tsp. salt   ¹/₈ tsp. ground cloves
8 oz. can pineapple   1 tbsp. cornstarch
   chunks, juice-   1 tbsp. water
   packed

Before cooking: Drain the pineapple, reserving ¹/₄ cup of the juice.

Season the chicken with the salt. Heat a large non-stick skillet over moderate heat, add the chicken pieces, and brown them on both sides for about 20 minutes, turning them once. Pour off any fat that accumulates in the pan. Mix together the reserved pineapple juice and the orange juice, and add this mixture to the chicken. Stir in the cinnamon and ground cloves. Cover the skillet and simmer the chicken for about 30 minutes until it is tender. Remove the chicken from the skillet and place it on a platter in the oven to stay warm.

Add the pineapple chunks to the skillet. In a cup, blend the cornstarch with 1 tablespoon water, and add this mixture to the skillet, stirring rapidly. Cook the pineapple, stirring constantly, until the liquid has thickened and comes to a boil. To serve, spoon some of the sauce over the chicken on the platter and pass the remaining sauce.   *Makes 4 servings*

	Calories	Carbo-hydrate (gm)	Protein (gm)	Total Fat (gm)	Saturated Fat (gm)	Choles-terol (mg)
Total	1123.2	64.7	132.8	35.1	13.7	555.7
Per Serving	280.8	16.2	33.2	8.8	3.4	138.9

Spiced Chicken with Oranges

2 lbs. broiler-fryer
  chicken pieces
2 tbsp. flour
1 tsp. salt
  dash of pepper
$^1/_2$ tsp. cinnamon

$^1/_2$ tsp. ground cloves
4 oranges
1 tbsp. soy sauce
1 tbsp. brown sugar
  substitute
water

Before cooking: Combine the flour, salt, pepper, cinnamon, and cloves in a paper bag. Add the chicken, a few pieces at a time and shake the bag until the chicken is coated with the flour mixture. Peel the oranges and cut them into wedges. Save any juice that accumulates. Add enough water to the juice to make $^1/_2$ cup liquid.

Place the chicken, skin side up, in a non-stick baking pan. Bake it at 450° just until the chicken is brown. Before going any further, pour off all the fat that has accumulated in the pan. Mix the orange and water mixture with the soy sauce, orange wedges, and brown sugar, and pour the entire mixture over the chicken. Cover the baking pan with foil and continue to bake the chicken for 20 or 30 minutes longer — until the fleshiest part of the chicken is fork-tender.

Makes 4 servings

	Calories	Carbo-hydrate (gm)	Protein (gm)	Total Fat (gm)	Saturated Fat (gm)	Choles-terol (mg)
Total	1270.1	95.8	137.8	34.5	13.7	555.7
Per Serving	317.5	24.0	34.5	8.6	3.4	138.9

gm=grams; mg=milligrams. Nutritional figures are approximate. Figures are based on findings of U.S. Department of Agriculture.

Crispy Chicken

2 lbs. broiler-fryer
 chicken pieces
2 tsp. salt
1/4 tsp. pepper

1 cup crushed
 protein cereal,
 unsweetened
1/2 cup evaporated
 skim milk

Mix the crushed cereal, salt, and pepper together on a flat plate. Pour the evaporated skim milk into another plate. Dip the chicken pieces into the milk, and then roll them in the cereal mixture. Place them, skin side down, on a non-stick cookie sheet and bake them for 30 minutes at 350°. Turn the chicken pieces over and bake them on the other side for another 30 minutes.

Makes 4 servings

	Calories	Carbohydrate (gm)	Protein (gm)	Total Fat (gm)	Saturated Fat (gm)	Cholesterol (mg)
Total	1124.1	28.6	143.9	44.5	19.2	594.7
Per Serving	281.0	7.2	36.0	11.1	4.8	148.7

Easy Baked Chicken

2 (2 lbs. each) broiler-
 fryer chickens,
 quartered
1 1/2 tsp. salt
1 tsp. celery seed

1/2 tsp. dried
 marjoram
8 oz. can
 mushrooms,
 undrained

Before cooking: Drain the mushrooms, saving the liquid.

Sprinkle the chicken quarters with salt, and place them, skin side up, in a shallow baking dish. Season them with the celery seed and marjoram. Add the liquid from the mushrooms to the pan and bake the chicken at 350° for 30 minutes, occasionally spooning the liquid in the pan over the meat. Then add the mushrooms to the pan and continue to bake the chicken for 20 or 30 minutes longer until it is tender. Drain the liquid from the pan. Using a bulb-type baster, skim the fat from the liquid so the liquid can be used as a gravy.

Makes 8 servings

	Calories	Carbo-hydrate (gm)	Protein (gm)	Total Fat (gm)	Saturated Fat (gm)	Choles-terol (mg)
Total	1767.5	6.0	265.5	68.6	27.4	1110.5
Per Serving	220.9	0.8	33.2	8.6	3.4	138.8

Mushroom Stuffing

$^1/_2$ lb. fresh mushrooms
1 cup shredded carrots
1 cup diced celery
$^3/_4$ cup diced onion
$^1/_2$ cup nonfat dry milk

1 tbsp. chopped parsley
1 tsp. salt
$^1/_4$ tsp. ground sage
$^1/_8$ tsp. ground marjoram
dash ground red pepper

Before cooking: Rinse the mushrooms, and pat them dry. Then chop them into fine pieces.

Combine the mushrooms with the rest of the ingredients in a medium saucepan. Place the pan over low heat, and cook the stuffing for about 5 minutes — until liquid appears in the pan. Then cover the pan, and simmer the mixture for 30 minutes, stirring occasionally. The stuffing may be served hot, as is, or placed in the cavity of a chicken before roasting. This recipe makes about 2 cups of stuffing, which is enough for a 4-pound chicken.

Makes 8 servings

	Calories	Carbo-hydrate (gm)	Protein (gm)	Total Fat (gm)	Saturated Fat (gm)	Choles-terol (mg)
Total	378.5	68.5	33.0	2.5	0.0	7.5
Per Serving	47.3	8.6	4.1	0.3	0.0	0.9

---

gm=grams; mg=milligrams. Nutritional figures are approximate. Figures are based on findings of U.S. Department of Agriculture.

Oven-Baked Chicken Kiev

4 whole chicken
    breasts (about 1 lb.
    each)
4 oz. Neufchatel cheese
1 tbsp. freeze-dried
    chives
1 tsp. butter-flavored
    salt

$1/2$ tsp. thyme
$1/2$ tsp. marjoram
$1/4$ tsp. ground black
    pepper
2 eggs
2 tbsp. safflower oil
8 tbsp. seasoned
    bread crumbs

Before cooking: Skin and bone the chicken breasts carefully and cut them in half. Cut the cheese into 8 slices and chill them in the freezer.

Pound the chicken breast halves with a rolling pin until they are about $1/4$ inch thin. Sprinkle the chives and seasonings over the pounded chicken. Place a cheese slice on the edge of each piece of chicken and roll the chicken up tightly, tucking in the sides to enclose the cheese completely. Secure the rolls with toothpicks. Beat the eggs with the oil in a shallow dish. Place the bread crumbs in another shallow dish. Dip the chicken rolls in the egg mixture, and then roll them in the bread crumbs. Arrange the chicken in a single layer in a baking pan. Bake the chicken at 450° for 20 minutes. *Makes 8 servings*

	Calories	Carbo-hydrate (gm)	Protein (gm)	Total Fat (gm)	Saturated Fat (gm)	Choles-terol (mg)
Total	2381.2	41.3	311.1	102.0	40.3	1496.8
Per Serving	297.7	5.2	38.9	12.8	5.0	187.1

Chicken Cacciatore

2 lbs. broiler-fryer
    chicken pieces
2 tsp. salt
$1/4$ tsp. pepper
1 tbsp. parsley

1 tsp. oregano
1 tsp. garlic salt
4 cups canned
    tomatoes

Place the chicken in a non-stick skillet. Beginning with skin side down, brown the chicken over medium heat for about 15 minutes on each side. Do not add any oil to the pan because the chicken will release enough of its own fat for frying. When the chicken is brown, add the remaining ingredients to the pan. Cover the skillet, and simmer the contents for about 30 minutes until the chicken is tender. *Makes 4 servings*

	Calories	Carbo-hydrate (gm)	Protein (gm)	Total Fat (gm)	Saturated Fat (gm)	Choles-terol (mg)
Total	1065.4	40.0	138.3	38.3	13.7	555.7
Per Serving	266.4	10.0	34.6	9.6	3.4	138.9

Chicken Parmigiana

3 whole chicken
   breasts
1 egg
2 tbsp. safflower oil

$^1/_2$ cup Italian-flavored bread crumbs
3 oz. part-skim mozzarella cheese

Before cooking: Bone and skin the chicken breasts. Split them in half. Divide the cheese into 6 slices.

Whip the egg and oil together in a shallow dish. Place the bread crumbs in another shallow dish. Dip the chicken first into the egg mixture, then into the bread crumbs, to coat them lightly. Place the coated chicken in a single layer on a shallow non-stick baking tray or cookie sheet. Bake the chicken at 450° for 10 minutes, turning the pieces once. Then top each piece with a slice of cheese and return the chicken to the oven just until the cheese begins to melt. Serve the chicken as it is or with Quick Tomato Sauce (the recipe is in "The Flavor-Uppers"). *Makes 6 servings*

	Calories	Carbo-hydrate (gm)	Protein (gm)	Total Fat (gm)	Saturated Fat (gm)	Choles-terol (mg)
Total	1260.0	38.1	153.5	63.5	13.5	614.0
Per Serving	210.0	6.4	25.6	10.6	2.3	102.3

gm=grams; mg=milligrams. Nutritional figures are approximate. Figures are based on findings of U.S. Department of Agriculture.

Chicken Chili

2 lbs. broiler-fryer chicken pieces	1 green pepper
2 tsp. salt	3 cups canned tomatoes
1/4 tsp. pepper	2 cups canned kidney beans
1 onion	1 1/2 tsp. chili powder

Before cooking: Drain the kidney beans. Chop the onion and green pepper.

Arrange the chicken, skin side up, in a baking pan, and season it with the salt and pepper. Brown it in a 350° oven for about 30 minutes. Pour off the fat that has accumulated in the pan before going any further. Then add the rest of the ingredients. Cover the pan and continue to bake the chicken for 30 minutes longer until it is tender. *Makes 6 servings*

	Calories	Carbo-hydrate (gm)	Protein (gm)	Total Fat (gm)	Saturated Fat (gm)	Choles-terol (mg)
Total	1529.4	128.0	169.3	39.3	13.7	555.7
Per Serving	254.9	21.3	28.2	6.6	2.3	92.6

Chicken Pizza

2 lbs. chicken breasts, boned and skinned (2 1/2 lbs. with bone will yield 2 lbs. boned)	1/2 tsp. oregano
	4 oz. can mushrooms, undrained
1 tsp. onion salt	1 cup shredded part-skim mozzarella cheese (4 oz.)
1/2 tsp. pepper	
8 oz. can tomato sauce	

Season the chicken breasts with the onion salt and pepper, and arrange them in a shallow baking dish. Combine the tomato sauce, mushrooms, liquid, and oregano in a bowl; then pour this over the chicken. Bake the chicken, uncovered at 350° for 35 minutes or more until it is tender. Sprinkle the cheese over the top of the chicken, and return it to the oven for about 5 minutes, until the cheese is melted and bubbly.

Makes 8 servings

	Calories	Carbo-hydrate (gm)	Protein (gm)	Total Fat (gm)	Saturated Fat (gm)	Choles-terol (mg)
Total	1625.4	18.6	278.9	52.4	14.7	786.2
Per Serving	203.2	2.3	34.9	6.6	1.8	98.3

Chicken Scallopini

2 whole chicken
    breasts
4 tbsp. lemon juice
¼ cup chicken broth
1 tbsp. diet margarine

garlic salt
pepper
fresh parsley
1 fresh lemon

Before cooking: Bone and skin the chicken breasts. Split them in half. Cut the lemon into slices. Skim the fat from the broth by chilling it until the fat rises to the top and can be whisked away.

Combine the lemon juice, broth, and margarine in a large, non-stick skillet. Heat the mixture until the margarine has melted. Arrange the chicken in the skillet in a single layer. Season it with the garlic salt and pepper. Cook the chicken over high heat, un-covered, turning it occasionally When the liquid evaporates, the chicken is cooked through, and it will begin to brown in the remaining fat. Turn the chicken so it browns on both sides. Remove the chicken to a heated platter and garnish it with the parsley and lemon slices.

Makes 4 servings

Special note: If you do not have chicken broth, you may use canned broth, undiluted, or a bouillon cube mixed with ¼ cup water.

	Calories	Carbo-hydrate (gm)	Protein (gm)	Total Fat (gm)	Saturated Fat (gm)	Choles-terol (mg)
Total	406.5	5.5	65.0	14.0	5.0	207.5
Per Serving	101.6	1.4	16.3	3.5	1.3	51.9

gm=grams; mg=milligrams. Nutritional figures are approximate. Figures are based on findings of U.S. Department of Agriculture.

Chicken Pago-Pago

4 lbs. broiler-fryer
   chicken pieces
6 oz. can frozen
   pineapple juice
1 tsp. ground ginger

1 tsp. soy sauce
¼ cup flaked or
   grated coconut

Before cooking: Allow the pineapple juice to thaw, but
do not dilute it.

Arrange the chicken, skin side up, in a single layer in
a baking pan. In a bowl, mix together the melted
pineapple juice, ginger, and soy sauce. Pour this mixture over the chicken. Bake the chicken at 350° for
about 1 hour until it is tender, basting it as needed.
With a bulb-type baster, skim the fat from the pan liquid. Then sprinkle the coconut over the chicken, and
bake for 5 minutes longer until the coconut is brown.
Makes 8 servings

	Calories	Carbo-hydrate (gm)	Protein (gm)	Total Fat (gm)	Saturated Fat (gm)	Choles-terol (mg)
Total	2224.3	37.3	4388.8	80.1	37.2	1110.5
Per Serving	278.0	4.7	48.6	10.0	4.7	138.9

Italian Oven-Fried Chicken Breasts

3 whole chicken
   breasts
1½ oz. envelope
   spaghetti sauce mix

2 tbsp. fine dry bread
   crumbs

Before cooking: Split the chicken breasts in half.

Mix the spaghetti sauce mix and bread crumbs together in a paper bag. Dip the chicken in water, one
piece at a time, and then shake it in the bag to coat it
evenly with the bread crumbs. Place the chicken skin
side down in a baking pan and cover it with foil. Bake
the chicken at 350° for 30 minutes. Uncover the pan,
turn the chicken over and continue baking for another

30 minutes until it is tender and golden brown. Turn the chicken a few times during the last 30 minutes.

Makes 6 servings

	Calories	Carbo-hydrate (gm)	Protein (gm)	Total Fat (gm)	Saturated Fat (gm)	Choles-terol (mg)
Total	554.7	9.5	97.7	12.7	6.1	306.7
Per Serving	92.5	1.6	16.3	2.1	1.0	51.1

Chicken Breast Creole

2 lbs. chicken breasts,
    boned and skinned
    (2¹/₂ lbs. with bones
    will yield 2 lbs.
    when boned)
2 tbsp. diet margarine
1 large onion
1 cup mushrooms
2 green peppers

salt
pepper
oregano
thyme
garlic powder
onion powder
3 cups canned
    tomatoes
1¹/₂ cups dry white
    wine

Before cooking: Chop the onion and green peppers.

Melt the margarine in a heavy, non-stick skillet. Add the boned chicken breasts and brown them quickly on both sides. Remove them to a platter. Add the onions, green peppers, and mushrooms to the pan, and saute them until they are soft and golden brown. Then return the chicken to the pan. Season the chicken and vegetables with onion powder, garlic powder, salt, pepper, oregano, and thyme according to your own taste. Add the wine and tomatoes (with the liquid). Cover the pan, and simmer the chicken slowly for 1 hour.

Makes 8 servings

	Calories	Carbo-hydrate (gm)	Protein (gm)	Total Fat (gm)	Saturated Fat (gm)	Choles-terol (mg)
Total	1945.5	82.7	232.2	48.0	12.7	714.2
Per Serving	243.2	10.3	29.0	6.0	1.6	89.3

gm=grams; mg=milligrams. Nutritional figures are approximate. Figures are based on findings of U.S. Department of Agriculture.

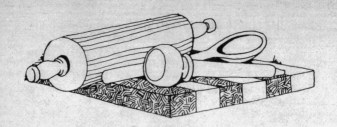

Passover Stuffed Chicken Breasts

3 chicken breasts
4 squares of matzos
½ cup orange juice
1 medium onion
2 eggs, beaten

1 tsp. grated orange
  peel
½ tsp. salt
2 seedless oranges
  parsley

Before cooking: Split the chicken breasts in half. Break the matzos into small pieces. Chop the onion. Section the oranges.

Mix the broken matzos, orange juice, onion, beaten eggs, grated orange peel, and salt in a bowl. Place the chicken breast halves, skin side down, in a foil-lined baking pan. Mound the matzos mixture on top of the breasts. Cover the pan with aluminum foil, and bake the chicken at 350° for about 1½ hours, until it is tender. For the last 20 minutes of baking, remove the foil and place the orange sections on top of the stuffing. Serve the chicken garnished with parsley.

Makes 6 servings

Diet hint: The calorie careful cook can save a giant 100 calories (almost 17 calories a serving) by using 4 egg whites instead of 2 whole eggs. The taste and texture will be the same, so only you will know what a clever calorie-wise trick you used. An extra bonus: you will also save 4 grams of saturated fat — what a nice thing to do for your heart.

	Calories	Carbo-hydrate (gm)	Protein (gm)	Total Fat (gm)	Saturated Fat (gm)	Choles-terol (mg)
Total	1411.0	159.5	121.0	28.5	10.0	810.0
Per Serving	235.2	26.6	20.2	4.8	1.7	135.0

CONSUMER GUIDE

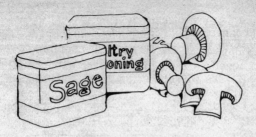

Chicken Stroganoff

2¹/₂ lbs. broiler-fryer
    chicken pieces
1 tsp. salt
¹/₈ tsp. pepper
¹/₈ tsp. garlic powder

8 oz. can tomato
    sauce
8 oz. can whole or
    sliced
    mushrooms
¹/₂ cup yogurt

Before cooking: Drain the mushrooms.

Place the chicken in a non-stick skillet and season it with the salt and pepper. Brown the chicken over medium heat for approximately 15 minutes on each side. Do not add any oil to the pan because the chicken will release enough of its own fat for frying. Mix together the tomato sauce and mushrooms, and pour this mixture over the chicken. Cover the pan and simmer the chicken for 30 minutes until it is tender. With a bulb-type baster skim off the fat from the sauce. Then stir in the yogurt and continue cooking until it is heated through. *Makes 6 servings*

Special note: If you like, you may serve Chicken Stroganoff over noodles. Plan 1 oz. of uncooked noodles per serving. The noodles should be cooked in boiling, salted water according to the package directions. The noodles will add 110 calories per serving.

	Calories	Carbo-hydrate (gm)	Protein (gm)	Total Fat (gm)	Saturated Fat (gm)	Choles-terol (mg)
Total	1550.3	84.9	184.7	48.9	20.2	804.0
Per Serving	258.4	14.2	30.8	8.1	3.4	134.0

gm=grams; mg=milligrams. Nutritional figures are approximate. Figures are based on findings of U.S. Department of Agriculture.

Chicken Goulash

1 lb. chicken breasts,
  boned and skinned
  (1¼ lbs. with bone
  will yield 1 lb.
  boned)
2 tsp. safflower or corn
  oil
2 onions
1 tbsp. paprika
3 tbsp. catsup

½ cup water
1½ tsp. salt
⅛ tsp. black pepper
⅛ tsp. red pepper
1 tsp. grated lemon
  peel
2 tbsp. flour
1 tbsp. nonfat dry
  milk

Before cooking: Cut the chicken into cubes. Slice the onions.

Heat the oil in a large, non-stick skillet, and sauté the onions until they are brown. Add the paprika and catsup, mixing well, and then add ½ cup water. Season the chicken cubes with salt and black pepper, and add them to the onions. At the same time, add the red pepper and lemon peel. Cover the pan and simmer the chicken for 20 minutes. Blend together the flour and dry milk and stir this into the chicken mixture. Continue to cook the chicken for another 5 minutes.

Makes 4 servings

	Calories	Carbo-hydrate (gm)	Protein (gm)	Total Fat (gm)	Saturated Fat (gm)	Choles-terol (mg)
Total	891.1	45.8	113.6	25.3	6.0	358.0
Per Serving	222.8	11.5	28.4	6.3	1.5	89.5

Arroz Con Pollo

2 lbs. broiler-fryer
  chicken pieces
1 medium onion
1 green pepper
4 cups stewed tomatoes

1 tsp. salt
1 cup uncooked rice
  pinch of saffron

Before cooking: Chop the onion, and chop the green pepper.

Place the chicken in a baking pan and bake it uncovered at 450° for 30 minutes. Pour off all the fat that accumulates in the pan. Then arrange the chicken with the onion in a 3-quart casserole. Sprinkle the rice and saffron around the chicken. Then add the tomatoes, green pepper, and salt. Cover the casserole tightly and bake it at 350° for 1 hour.   *Makes 6 servings*

	Calories	Carbo-hydrate (gm)	Protein (gm)	Total Fat (gm)	Saturated Fat (gm)	Choles-terol (mg)
Total	1789.4	203.0	153.3	39.3	13.7	555.7
Per Serving	298.2	33.8	25.6	6.6	2.3	92.6

Cornish Hens with Rice Dressing

2 small Cornish hens (2 lbs. total)
1 cup shredded carrots
½ cup sliced green onion
4 Tbsp. snipped parsley

½ cup uncooked long-grain rice
1½ cups chicken broth
½ tsp. salt
dash of pepper

Before cooking: Split the hens in half, lengthwise. Chill the broth until the fat rises to the top; skim off the fat.

Place the hens on a rack in a broiler pan, skin side up. Broil them just until the skin is crisp. Place the hens in a large oven-safe casserole, and add all the remaining ingredients. Cover the casserole and bake the contents at 350° for 30 minutes.   *Makes 4 servings*

	Calories	Carbo-hydrate (gm)	Protein (gm)	Total Fat (gm)	Saturated Fat (gm)	Choles-terol (mg)
Total	1624.8	94.0	191.9	48.5	24.0	763.5
Per Serving	406.2	23.5	47.9	12.1	6.0	190.9

---

gm=grams; mg=milligrams. Nutritional figures are approximate. Figures are based on findings of U.S. Department of Agriculture.

Turkey

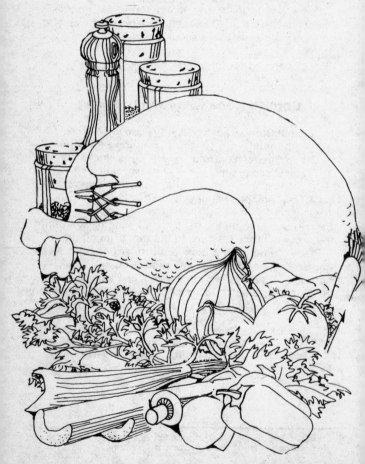

If the turkey is only a holiday visitor at your house, you are missing out on one of America's best buys in cost, calories, and nutrition. Like chicken, turkey is a lean and low-cal choice for figure-watchers and heart-smart cooks. With the increasing availability of smaller birds, boneless roasts, turkey-in-parts, and such recent innovations as turkey steaks, turkey cutlets, ground turkey meat, and even turkey sausage, there's no reason why turkey can't make a frequent appearance at the family dinner table.

Nowadays, most turkey comes to market relatively young, and that's good news. It's not only more convenient to cook and store a smaller bird, but the calorie-protein-fat ratio is more in keeping with the dieter's aims. Moreover, the old idea that big old birds offer more meat and less waste just isn't true, as the following chart shows.

TURKEY COMPARISON CHART

per pound*	waste	fat	protein	calories
Young under 24 weeks	27%	20 gm.	71 gm.	480
Medium up to 32 weeks	27%	52 gm.	66 gm.	752
Mature over 32 weeks	27%	97 gm.	61 gm.	1136

*Ready to cook. Source: USDA

How to Roast a Turkey

1. Most turkeys are bought frozen, so the first thing you must do is defrost it. When defrosting, leave the turkey in its original wrapper and use one of the following methods:

- **No Hurry.** Place the turkey on a tray and keep it in the refrigerator for 3 to 4 days.
- **Faster.** Place the turkey on a tray and leave it out at room temperature. This will take 1 hour per pound of turkey.
- **Fastest.** Place the turkey in the sink and cover it with cold water. Change the water occasionally. This will take ½ hour per pound of turkey.

2. The turkey should be refrigerated or roasted as soon as it has thawed. If you plan to stuff the turkey, don't do it until just before you are ready to roast it. If the turkey has been commercially-stuffed, follow the directions on the turkey wrapper, but omit the fat.

3. When you are ready to roast the turkey, remove the plastic wrapper; remove the neck and giblets from the bird's cavity.

4. Rinse the turkey, and wipe it dry.

5. Simmer the neck and giblets to make a broth for flavoring the stuffing or as a base for giblet gravy.

6. If you wish to stuff your turkey, follow your favorite stuffing recipe. (Several stuffing recipes are suggested in this chapter.) To stuff the turkey loosely, you will need $3/4$ cup stuffing per pound of oven-ready weight.

7. If you do not stuff the turkey, rub the cavity generously with salt. If you like, insert pieces of celery, carrot, onion, and parsley for added flavor. Unstuffed turkeys require about $1/2$ hour less roasting time.

8. Fasten down the bird's legs either by tying them together or by sticking them under the skin band. The neck skin should be skewered to the bird's back, and the wings should be twisted akimbo.

9. Place the turkey right-side-up on a rack in a shallow roasting pan. Don't brush it with any butter or oil.

10. If you like, insert a meat thermometer into the thickest part of the thigh. Make certain that the tip of the thermometer (the bulb) doesn't touch the bone.

11. A "tent" of foil placed loosely over the turkey will eliminate the need for basting, although the turkey may be basted if you like. If you use foil, remove it for the last $1/2$ hour of roasting so the bird gets nicely browned.

12. Or, if the turkey isn't too heavy for convenient handling, it can be roasted upside-down (using a V rack) for the first half of roasting time. In that case, don't insert the thermometer until the turkey has been turned over. This upside-down method results in juicier white meat.

13. Roast the turkey in a preheated 325° oven according to the following time chart, or until the meat

thermometer registers 180° to 185°. If you're not using a thermometer, you can tell that the turkey is done by pressing the drumstick. The turkey is done if the drumstick feels soft when pressed with your thumb and forefinger and when the drumstick and thigh move easily.

TIME CHART:
ROASTING UNSTUFFED TURKEY AT 325°

Ready-to-Cook Weight	Approximate Cooking Time
6 to 8 lbs.	3 - 3$^1/_2$ hours
8 to 12 lbs.	3$^1/_2$ - 4$^1/_2$ hours
12 to 16 lbs.	4$^1/_2$ - 5$^1/_2$ hours
16 to 20 lbs.	5$^1/_2$ - 6$^1/_2$ hours
20 to 24 lbs.	6$^1/_2$ - 7 hours

* If the turkey is stuffed, add $^1/_2$ hour to the total cooking time.

How to Roast a Boneless Turkey Breast Roast

The boneless turkey breast roast offers the same economical goodness and high nutritive value of a whole turkey, but it has the added advantage of coming in smaller sizes. A turkey roast is just the right size for the family's dinner or as an entree for a small dinner party.

The breast roast is particularly good for the weight-conscious person. Each average serving of white meat (3$^1/_2$ ounces) costs only 176 calories. It also has the least cholesterol of all the popular meats, yet it provides high-quality protein and generous amounts of the B vitamins, riboflavin, and niacin.

1. To thaw a turkey roast, leave it sealed in its plastic wrap, and place it on a tray in the refrigerator overnight. For quicker thawing, submerge the wrapped roast in cold water, changing the water occasionally. This will take $^1/_2$ hour per pound of turkey.

2. After the roast has thawed, unwrap it, rinse it in cool water, drain it, and pat it dry.

3. Skewer the turkey's skin to the meat along the cut

edges of the roast. This will prevent the skin from shrinking during the roasting time.

4. Rub the cavity of the roast lightly with salt.

5. If the wings are still attached, lay them flat over the breast and tie a string around the breast end to hold the wings down.

6. Insert a meat thermometer into the roast so that the tip of the thermometer (the bulb) is in the center of the meat.

7. Place the roast on a rack, skin side up, in a shallow roasting pan.

8. If you like, you may place a "tent" of foil loosely over the turkey. This will eliminate the need for basting, although the turkey may be basted if you wish. If you use foil, remove it for the last $1/2$ hour of roasting, so that the turkey gets nicely browned.

9. Roast the turkey in a 325° oven according to the following timetable. The meat is done when the thermometer reads 180° to 185°.

10. Let the roast stand for 15 minutes before carving it.

TIMETABLE FOR COOKING TURKEY BREAST ROAST

Ready-to-Cook Weight	Total Roasting Time
5 to 8 lbs.	$2^{1}/_{2}$ - $3^{1}/_{2}$ hours
8 to 10 lbs.	$3^{1}/_{2}$ - 4 hours
10 to 12 lbs.	4 - $4^{1}/_{2}$ hours

How to Make Low-Fat Turkey Gravy

What's turkey without gravy? It is like a beach without sand.

Gravy need not be the high-caloried no-no we fight to stay away from. All you have to do is remove the fat, and you have yourself a tasty sauce that adds enjoyment to your meal without adding inches to your hips. Low-fat turkey gravy has only about 75 calories in a cupful, or 5 calories per tablespoon.

For a de-calorized gravy:

1. Pour all the turkey drippings into a shallow metal saucepan, and set it in the freezer.

2. In 10 minutes, the fat will congeal on the surface of the drippings, making it easy to whisk away every last unnecessary calorie.

3. After the fat has been discarded, heat your fat-free broth, and season it with garlic salt and pepper.

4. To thicken the gravy, add $1/2$ cup cold water and 2 tablespoons flour for every cup of broth.

5. For a rich brown gravy, pour the heated gravy into your drained roasting pan, and scrape up the delectable residue.

Recipes

Savory Stuffing

2 cups minced celery	1 cup chicken broth
2 cups minced onion	10 cups dry whole
2 tsp. poultry seasoning	wheat or protein bread, cubed

Before cooking: Skim the fat from the broth by using a bulb-type baster or by chilling it until the fat floats to the top and can be lifted off.

Add the rest of the ingredients to the skimmed broth and mix them lightly. Loosely fill the cavity of a large turkey with the stuffing, or spoon it into a $1 1/2$-quart casserole. If you use a casserole, bake the stuffing at 350° for 45 minutes.   *Makes 12 servings*

	Calories	Carbo-hydrate (gm)	Protein (gm)	Total Fat (gm)	Saturated Fat (gm)	Choles-terol (mg)
Total	869.0	178.7	39.2	9.4	2.0	26.1
Per Serving	72.4	14.9	3.3	0.8	0.2	2.2

gm=grams; mg=milligrams. Nutritional figures are approximate. Figures are based on findings of U.S. Department of Agriculture.

Oven "Fried" Turkey

4 lbs. young turkey	2 tsp. salt
1/2 cup flour	1/4 tsp. pepper
2 tsp. paprika	1/4 tsp. poultry seasoning (optional)

Before cooking: Cut the turkey into serving pieces.

Combine the flour and seasonings in a paper bag. Add the turkey, a few pieces at a time, and shake the bag until they are coated with the flour mixture. Place the turkey pieces, skin side down, in a roasting pan and bake them uncovered at 450° for 15 to 20 minutes — just until they are brown. Using tongs or 2 spoons, turn the turkey pieces over. Turn down the oven to 350°, cover the roasting pan, and continue to cook the turkey for 1 hour or more. The turkey is done when the thickest pieces are fork-tender. During the last 10 minutes of baking, uncover the pan so the skin recrisps. *Makes 12 servings*

	Calories	Carbo-hydrate (gm)	Protein (gm)	Total Fat (gm)	Saturated Fat (gm)	Choles-terol (mg)
Total	3835.2	47.5	376.9	220.0	54.9	1440.4
Per Serving	319.6	4.0	31.4	18.3	4.6	120.0

Spanish Turkey

2 turkey drumsticks (about 3 lbs.)	1 small green pepper
2 tbsp. safflower oil	1 cup water
1 cup chopped celery	1 bay leaf
1/2 cup chopped onion	1 tsp. salt
1 cup fresh tomatoes, chopped or canned tomatoes, drained	6 stuffed green olives
	2 cups uncooked noodles

Before cooking: Cut the green pepper into slivers. Slice the olives. Wash the drumsticks and pat them dry with paper towel.

Place the drumsticks in a baking pan and bake them uncovered at 450° for 20 minutes. Then lower the oven to 350°. Add the celery, onion, tomatoes, green pepper, water, bay leaf, and salt. Cover the pan, and bake the mixture for about 2 hours until the turkey is tender. Add the olives and noodles, cover, and bake for an additional 20 minutes until the noodles are tender, adding more water if necessary. Cut the meat from the turkey legs, discarding the bones, and serve at once.

Makes 8 servings

	Calories	Carbo-hydrate (gm)	Protein (gm)	Total Fat (gm)	Saturated Fat (gm)	Choles-terol (mg)
Total	2948.6	160.2	304.2	111.1	32.9	1098.1
Per Serving	368.6	20.0	38.0	13.9	4.1	137.3

Apple Stuffing for Poultry

6 apples
2 cups cubed protein bread, stale or lightly toasted
$1/2$ cup chopped onion
$1/2$ cup cubed Canadian bacon
1 cup minced celery
$1/4$ cup chopped parsley
1 tsp. salt
$1/4$ tsp. pepper
1 tsp. poultry seasoning
$1/2$ cup hot giblet stock or boiling water

Before cooking: Peel and chop the apples.

Combine all of the ingredients and mix them lightly. Loosely fill the cavity of a turkey, chicken, or Rock Cornish hen. This recipe makes 4 cups of stuffing.

Makes 12 servings

	Calories	Carbo-hydrate (gm)	Protein (gm)	Total Fat (gm)	Saturated Fat (gm)	Choles-terol (mg)
Total	797.1	147.1	26.3	14.3	3.7	61.2
Per Serving	66.4	12.3	2.2	1.2	0.3	5.1

gm=grams; mg=milligrams. Nutritional figures are approximate. Figures are based on findings of U.S. Department of Agriculture.

Turkey Goulash

1¹/₄ lbs. turkey thigh
2 cups onion, cut in
   strips
2 green peppers
1 red pepper
4 tomatoes

1 cup water
1¹/₂ tsp. salt
¹/₄ tsp. black pepper
¹/₄ tsp. red pepper

Before cooking: Slice the onions, peppers, and tomatoes into strips. Discard the tomato seeds. Remove the turkey from the bone and cut the meat into ¹/₃-inch cubes.

Combine all the ingredients in a heavy non-stick skillet. Cover the skillet, and simmer the contents for about 35 minutes, until the turkey is tender.

Makes 4 servings

Serving note: This dish goes well with boiled potatoes.

	Calories	Carbo-hydrate (gm)	Protein (gm)	Total Fat (gm)	Saturated Fat (gm)	Choles-terol (mg)
Total	1452.1	69.0	186.3	45.7	17.1	576.7
Per Serving	363.0	17.3	46.6	11.4	4.3	144.2

Budget Marengo

3 lbs. turkey wings, tips
   removed
1 cup sliced onions
4 oz. can sliced
   mushrooms,
   undrained
1 lb. can tomatoes

¹/₂ cup dry white wine
2 cups water
1 tsp. salt
¹/₂ tsp. pepper
   dash of oregano

Before cooking: Separate the wing sections.

Place the wings in a non-stick Dutch oven and brown them. Don't add any oil to the pot. After the turkey has browned, add all of the remaining ingredients. Cover the pot and simmer the contents over low heat for 2 hours. Place the pot in the refrigerator until serving time.

Just before serving, remove the pot from the refrigerator. The fat will have floated to the top and congealed. Lift off the fat and discard it. Then reheat the turkey, uncovered, simmering it for 10 or 15 minutes, until most of the liquid has evaporated.

Makes 6 servings

	Calories	Carbo-hydrate (gm)	Protein (gm)	Total Fat (gm)	Saturated Fat (gm)	Choles-terol (mg)
Total	2059.8	37.6	193.6	111.7	27.4	719.8
Per Serving	343.2	6.3	32.3	18.6	4.6	120.0

Creole Turkey Cutlets

2 lbs. boned, skinless turkey white meat cut from breasts
2 tbsp. diet margarine
1 large onion
1 cup sliced mushrooms
2 green peppers

¹/₄ tsp. garlic powder
¹/₄ tsp. thyme
1 tsp. salt
¹/₄ tsp. pepper
2¹/₂ cups canned whole tomatoes, undrained
1 cup dry white wine (optional)

Before cooking: Chop the onion and green peppers.

Melt 1 tablespoon margarine in a large non-stick skillet. Add the cutlets, and brown them. Remove them to a platter. Then add the other tablespoon margarine and melt it. Sauté the onion, mushrooms, and green peppers until the mushrooms are brown. Return the cutlets to the skillet and add the seasonings. Add the tomatoes (with the liquid from the can) and the wine. Cover the skillet and simmer the turkey over low heat for 1 hour.

Makes 8 servings

	Calories	Carbo-hydrate (gm)	Protein (gm)	Total Fat (gm)	Saturated Fat (gm)	Choles-terol (mg)
Total	2206.3	73.2	319.6	52.1	11.1	703.8
Per Serving	275.8	9.2	40.0	6.5	1.4	88.0

---

gm=grams; mg=milligrams. Nutritional figures are approximate. Figures are based on findings of U.S. Department of Agriculture.

Turkey Ragout

1¼ lbs. turkey thigh
2 medium white
  potatoes
2 tbsp. water
2¼ cups water
1 cup tomato juice
2 onions

1 garlic clove
1 bay leaf
1 lb. small carrots,
  fresh or frozen
2 tbsp. flour
½ tsp. salt
¼ tsp. pepper

Before cooking: With a sharp knife, strip the turkey meat from the bone, and cut it into 1½-inch cubes. Peel the potatoes and cut them in half. Chop the onions and mince the garlic.

Put the turkey, skin side down, in a heavy non-stick Dutch oven and add 2 tablespoons water. Cover the pot, and cook the turkey over high heat until the water evaporates and the turkey cubes begin to brown in their own melted fat. Then lower the heat, uncover the pot, and continue to cook the turkey until it is brown on all sides. Before going any further, drain the accumulated fat from the pot. Then add 2 cups water and all the remaining ingredients, except the flour. Cover the pot and simmer the contents over low heat for 35 to 45 minutes — until the turkey is tender. Then combine the flour with ¼ cup cold water and stir this mixture into the pot. Continue to cook and stir until the gravy has thickened. *Makes 4 servings*

	Calories	Carbo-hydrate (gm)	Protein (gm)	Total Fat (gm)	Saturated Fat (gm)	Choles-terol (mg)
Total	1407.3	112.4	155.7	36.7	13.7	461.6
Per Serving	351.8	28.1	38.9	9.2	3.4	115.4

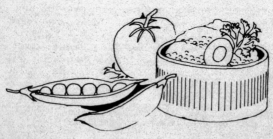

Turkey Chowder

1 lb. fresh ground turkey
2 tbsp. flour
1 tsp. salt
$^1/_8$ tsp. pepper
2 raw eggs
1 tbsp. grated onion
$^1/_2$ cup skim milk

8 cups turkey or chicken broth
6 medium-sized carrots
$^1/_2$ cup water
$^1/_4$ cup flour
2 tbsp. fresh lemon juice
2 tbsp. chopped parsley

Before cooking: Skim the fat from the broth by chilling it until the fat floats to the top and can be whisked away. Pare and slice the carrots.

Combine the turkey with the flour, salt, pepper, eggs, onion, and milk in a bowl. Shape the mixture into 36 small balls. In a stock pot, bring the broth to a boil. Add the meatballs, cover the pot and simmer them for 10 minutes. Remove the meatballs from the broth and set them aside. Then add the carrots to the broth and cook them in the same way for 20 minutes. In a cup combine the water and flour, and mix them well. Add the mixture to the broth and carrots, and continue cooking for abut 2 minutes until it is bubbly. Then add the lemon juice and meatballs. Serve the chowder garnished with chopped parsley.   *Makes 10 servings*

	Calories	Carbo-hydrate (gm)	Protein (gm)	Total Fat (gm)	Saturated Fat (gm)	Choles-terol (mg)
Total	1577.2	96.1	198.5	39.8	13.1	1025.2
Per Serving	157.7	9.6	19.9	4.0	1.3	102.5

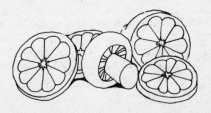

gm=grams; mg=milligrams. Nutritional figures are approximate. Figures are based on findings of U.S. Department of Agriculture.

Turkey Dressing Casserole

2 cups skim milk
3 medium eggs
2 onions
2 celery stalks

1 garlic clove
2 cups seasoned
   stuffing mix
salt
pepper

Before cooking: Scald the milk, and allow it to cool. Mince the onion, celery, and garlic.

Add the eggs to the cooled milk and whip the mixture lightly with a fork. Stir in the minced onion, celery, and garlic. Then add in the seasoned stuffing mix. Spoon the mixture into a non-stick loaf pan or oven-safe casserole and bake it at 325° for 50 minutes, until it sets. For individual servings, pile the mixture into a non-stick muffin pan and bake for only 30 minutes.
Makes 8 servings

For variety: Add ¹/₂ cup drained canned mushrooms (10 calories). Or stir in the contents of a 2¹/₂-ounce can of deviled ham (200 calories).

For extra protein: Use 2 cups cubed high-protein bread instead of the stuffing mix. Add 1 teaspoon poultry seasoning. If the bread is fresh, toast it lightly before cutting it into cubes.

If you're in a hurry: Use 1 cup evaporated skim milk and 1 cup water instead of 2 cups skim milk scalded. The minced vegetables can be replaced with 2 tablespoons dried onion flakes and 1 tablespoon dried celery. Season with garlic salt instead of using minced garlic.

	Calories	Carbo-hydrate (gm)	Protein (gm)	Total Fat (gm)	Saturated Fat (gm)	Choles-terol (mg)
Total	1252.0	192.0	66.0	26.0	8.0	774.0
Per Serving	156.5	24.0	8.3	3.3	1.0	96.8

---

gm=grams; mg=milligrams. Nutritional figures are approximate. Figures are based on findings of U.S. Department of Agriculture.

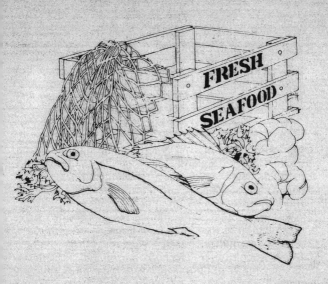

Seafood

I f you are a seafood fan, this section is for you. If you are *not* . . . then this section is *especially* for you. We suspect that most overweights who claim to dislike fish have never really had it — good fish, we mean!

If your seafood sampling history is limited to frozen fish sticks, diner-fried "fish" fillets of indeterminate species, or the Friday fish special dished up in the company or school cafeteria, then you should count yourself among the vast number of Americans who have never had really good fish.

What is good fish? To begin with, it must be absolutely fresh. Fish that "smells like fish" isn't fresh — because really fresh fish has no odor. The admonition that fish must be fresh doesn't mean you have to catch your own or barter with a charterboat operator down at the docks. And it doesn't mean that you must limit your marketing to fancy fish stores; perfectly good fresh fish is available bargain-priced in your supermarket freezer case. Yes, frozen fish can be the freshest of all — if it has been properly handled. Frozen fish is frequently processed right on the commercial vessel on which it is caught. However, partial thawing or careless handling anywhere along the distribution route can result in sub-quality seafood when you thaw it out at home. If frozen seafood shows signs of mishandling when you thaw it out, simply wrap it in plastic and return it to the store for a refund.

Good seafood is also properly cooked. And here's where lots of perfectly fine fish wind up a culinary casualty.

Unlike meat, fish doesn't need cooking to make it tender. The purpose of cooking fish is to develop its fine flavor. Overcooking — either too much or for too long — only results in toughness, dryness, and unpleasant flavor. Fish that has been overfloured and carelessly tossed into a skillet full of fat is not only fattening, it is unappetizing in taste, texture, and appearance. If that's the sort of seafood you've been exposed to, it is time to give fish a fighting chance.

Why the Emphasis on Fish for Slimming?

Anyone who has a nodding acquaintance with diets and dieting knows that seafood turns up with sometimes monotonous frequency on most lose-weight plans. The reason is that seafood is the slimmest of all main course choices — the one that's highest in protein and lowest in fat.

All fish is low-calorie when compared with most meat — even so-called "fatty" fish. Flounder, a lean fish, is only 308 calories a pound compared with 1,818 calories for rib roast — both have a comparable protein content. Mackerel, which is a "fat" fish, has only

866 calories a pound and *more* protein than rib roast. To see how other popular species of seafood compare, check the following list.

One pound*	Calories
Beef, rib	1,818
Bass, striped	476
Bluefish	530
Butterfish	522
Carp	522
Catfish	467
Clam meat	363
Cod	354
Crab meat	422
Flounder	308
Haddock	358
Halibut	453
Lake Trout	1,093
Lobster	413
Mackerel	866
Oyster meat	299
Perch	431
Pompano	753
Porgy	508
Pike	408
Red Snapper	422
Rockfish	440
Salmon	939
Sole	308
Sardines canned in tomato sauce	893
Scallops	367
Smelt	445
Shrimp	412
Swordfish	535
Tuna canned in oil	1,306
Tuna canned in water	576
Whitefish	703

*meat only, raw; except for canned seafood

Buying Fresh Fish

Here is the advice of the National Marine Fisheries Service on selecting the freshest fish*. Look for these qualities:

Flesh: Firm flesh, not separating from the bones, indicates fish are fresh and have been handled carefully.

Odor: Fresh and mild. A fish just taken from the water has practically no "fish" odor. The fishy odor becomes more pronounced with passage of time, but it should not be disagreeably strong when the fish are bought.

Eyes: Bright, clear, and full. The eyes of fresh fish are bright and transparent; as the fish becomes stale, the eyes become cloudy and often turn pink. When fish are fresh, the eyes often protrude; but with increasing staleness, the eyes tend to become sunken.

Gills: Red and free from slime. The color gradually fades with age to a light pink, then gray, and finally brownish or greenish.

Skin: Shiny, with color unfaded. When first taken from the water, most fish have an irridescent appearance. Each species has its characteristic markings and colors which fade and become less pronounced as the fish loses freshness.

Fresh fillets, steaks, and chunks have the following characteristics:

Flesh: Fresh-cut in appearance. It should be firm in texture without traces of browning or drying around the edges.

Odor: Fresh and mild.

Wrapping: If the fillets, steaks, or chunks are wrapped, the wrapping should be a moisture-vapor-proof material. There should be little or no air space between the fish and the wrapping.

Buying Frozen Fish

High quality frozen fish that are properly processed,

---

* "Let's Cook Fish: A Complete Guide to Fish Cookery." *Fishery Market Development Series No. 8.* U.S. Department of Interior, Fish and Wildlife Service, Bureau of Commercial Fisheries, U.S. Govt. Printing Office, 60 cents.

TIMETABLE FOR COOKING FISH

Method of Cooking	Market Form	Cooking Temp.	Approximate Cooking Time (Minutes)
Baking	Dressed	350°	45 to 60
	Pan-dressed	350°	25 to 30
	Fillets or steaks	350°	20 to 25
Broiling	Pan-dressed	3 to 4 inches from heat	10 to 16 turning once
	Fillets or steaks		10 to 15
	Frozen fried fish		10 to 15
	Frozen fried fish sticks		10 to 15
Charcoal Broiling	Pan-dressed	Moderate	10 to 16 turning once
	Fillets or steaks	Moderate	10 to 16
Oven-Frying	Pan-dressed	500°	15 to 20
	Fillets or steaks	500°	10 to 12
Pan-Frying	Pan-dressed	Moderate	8 to 10 turning once
	Fillets or steaks	Moderate	8 to 10
Poaching	Fillets or steaks	Simmer	5 to 10
Steaming	Fillets or steaks	Boil	5 to 10

packaged, and held at 0° or below, will remain in good condition for relatively long periods of time. Frozen fish of good quality have the following characteristics:

Flesh: Should be solidly frozen when bought. The flesh should have no discoloration or freezer burn. Virtually all deterioration in quality is prevented when fish are properly held in the frozen state. Frozen fish which have been thawed and then re-frozen are poorer in quality.

Odor: Frozen fish should have little or no odor. A strong fish odor means poor quality.

Wrapping: Most frozen fillets, steaks, chunks, portions, and sticks are wrapped either individually or in packages of various weights. The wrapping should be of moisture-vapor-proof material. There should be little or no air space between the fish and the wrapping.

How Much Fish Should You Buy?

Whole: This is fish as it comes from the water. Before cooking, the fish must be scaled and gutted. Usually the head, tail and fins are removed. The fish may then be cooked, filleted, or cut into steaks or chunks. Allow $2/3$ to $3/4$ pound per serving.

Dressed: This is fish with scales and entrails removed. Usually the head, tail, and fins are also removed. The fish may then be cooked, filleted, or cut into steaks or chunks. (The smaller size fish are called pan-dressed and are ready to cook as purchased.) About $1/3$ to $1/2$ pound equals one serving.

Fillets: These are boneless, usually skinless — the sides of the fish cut lengthwise away from the backbone. They are ready to cook as purchased. Allow $1/4$ pound per serving.

Steaks: These are cross section slices from large dressed fish cut $1/2$ to 1 inch thick. A cross section of the backbone is the only bone in a steak. They are ready to cook as purchased. Allow $1/4$ to $1/3$ pound per serving.

Chunks: These are cross-sections of large dressed fish. A cross section of the backbone is the only bone in a chunk. They are ready to cook as purchased. Allow $1/3$ to $1/4$ pound per serving.

What Dieters Should Avoid

Although fish is the best calorie and nutrition bargain you can buy, there are some types of frozen fish that dieters should stay away from. Fish is often frozen already breaded as a "convenience" to busy home-makers. What you get when you pay for already-breaded fish is a lot of breading and not much fish. You also get a lot of extra calories.

Raw breaded fish portions: These are portions cut from frozen fish blocks, coated with a batter, breaded, packaged, and frozen. Raw breaded fish portions generally contain only 75 percent fish.

Fried fish sticks: These are cut from frozen fish blocks. They are coated with a batter, then fried in fat, and frozen. Fried fish sticks are only 60 percent fish.

Recipes

Cheese Chowder

1 tbsp. finely chopped onion
1 can condensed cheddar cheese soup
½ cup skim milk
16 oz. can tomatoes, undrained

7 oz. can minced clams, undrained
parsley sprigs
coarse freshly ground pepper

Before cooking: Break the tomatoes into small pieces.

Combine all the ingredients (including the liquid from the cans of tomatoes and clams) in a large saucepan. Simmer the mixture, covered, for 10 to 12 minutes.   *Makes 4 servings*

	Calories	Carbo-hydrate (gm)	Protein (gm)	Total Fat (gm)	Saturated Fat (gm)	Choles-terol (mg)
Total	630.3	56.5	37.5	29.5	12.6	128.4
Per Serving	157.6	14.1	9.4	7.4	3.2	32.1

gm=grams; mg=milligrams. Nutritional figures are approximate. Figures are based on findings of U.S. Department of Agriculture.

Egg Sauce for Fish

2 tbsp. flour
1/2 tsp. butter salt
dash white pepper
13 oz. can evaporated
skim milk

1 tbsp. fresh lemon
juice
2 eggs
2 tbsp. diced
pimiento
(optional)

Before cooking: Hard boil the eggs, peel them and chop them coarsely.

Place the flour, salt, and pepper in a saucepan. Stir in the milk. Cook this mixture slowly, stirring constantly, until it has become thick and smooth. Then fold in the lemon juice, chopped eggs, and pimiento. Continue to cook the sauce just until it is heated through. Serve it with baked fish.   *Makes 6 servings*

	Calories	Carbo-hydrate (gm)	Protein (gm)	Total Fat (gm)	Saturated Fat (gm)	Choles-terol (mg)
Total	777.1	51.5	42.9	44.5	21.8	630.4
Per Serving	129.5	8.6	7.2	7.4	3.6	105.1

Stuffed Salmon with Egg Sauce

3 1/2 lbs. dressed salmon,
fresh or frozen
1 1/2 tsp. salt
2 cups diced celery
2 cups chopped onion
1 finely minced garlic
clove

1 small crumbled
bay leaf
1/4 cup water
3 cups soft bread
crumbs
2 tbsp. chopped
parsley
1/2 tsp. rosemary
dash pepper

Before cooking: If the fish is frozen, let it thaw in the refrigerator or at room temperature. Rinse the fish, and pat it dry.

Sprinkle 1 teaspoon salt over the inside of the fish, and place it in a non-stick baking pan. In a covered saucepan, simmer the celery, onion, garlic, and bay leaf in 1/4 cup water until the vegetables are tender.

Then add the remaining ¹/₂ tsp. salt, bread crumbs, parsley, rosemary, and pepper to the pan; and toss the mixture together lightly. Stuff the cavity of the fish loosely with this mixture. Cover the fins and tail of the fish loosely with foil. Bake the stuffed fish at 350° for 45 to 60 minutes or until it flakes easily when tested with a fork. Serve the salmon plain or with Egg Sauce.

Makes 10 servings

	Calories	Carbo-hydrate (gm)	Protein (gm)	Total Fat (gm)	Saturated Fat (gm)	Choles-terol (mg)
Total	3250.9	77.8	441.2	115.0	37.9	749.6
Per Serving	325.1	7.8	44.1	11.5	3.8	75.0

Broiled Cheddar Cod

2 lbs. cod or other white fish fillets, fresh or frozen	8 oz. can tomato sauce
1 tbsp. fresh lemon juice	1 medium onion
2 tsp. salt	5 tbsp. grated extra-sharp cheddar cheese

Before cooking: If the fish is frozen, let it thaw in the refrigerator or at room temperature. Cut the thawed fish into 8 portions. Chop the onion.

Spray a non-stick baking pan with spray-on vegetable coating for no-fat cooking. Arrange the fish in a single layer in the pan and brush it with lemon juice. Season it with salt. Broil the fish about 3 inches from the heat source for about 8 minutes. Then pour the tomato sauce over the fish and sprinkle on the onion and cheese. Continue broiling for about 4 minutes until the cheese melts and the fish flakes easily when tested with a fork.

Makes 8 servings

	Calories	Carbo-hydrate (gm)	Protein (gm)	Total Fat (gm)	Saturated Fat (gm)	Choles-terol (mg)
Total	2017.1	28.9	282.8	82.1	26.5	824.0
Per Serving	252.1	3.6	35.4	10.3	3.3	103.0

gm = grams; mg = milligrams. Nutritional figures are approximate. Figures are based on findings of U.S. Department of Agriculture.

Cod Steaks Amandine

1 1/2 lbs. cod steaks
2 tbsp. flour
1/2 tsp. salt
    dash pepper

1/2 cup cold skim milk
2 tbsp. lemon juice
2 beaten egg yolks
2 tbsp. sliced
    almonds

Before cooking: Toast the almonds by spreading them out on a cookie sheet and baking them at 350° until they are lightly browned.

Place the fish steaks in a small skillet or saucepan and add just enough water to cover them. Cover the pot and simmer the fish for 8 to 10 minutes — until it flakes easily. Drain the liquid from the pan, but reserve 1 cup. In another saucepan, stir the cold milk and flour together over low heat until the mixture thickens. Then add the reserved liquid from cooking the fish, and the salt and pepper. Cook and stir the mixture until it is bubbly. Then stir in the lemon juice. Stir a small amount of this hot mixture into the beaten egg yolks; then stir the egg yolk mixture back into the saucepan. Cook the sauce over low heat, stirring constantly, for about 1 minute until it has thickened. (If you accidentally overcook it and the egg curdles, simply beat it smooth again in your blender.) Pour the hot sauce over the poached fish steaks, and sprinkle them with the toasted almonds. *Makes 6 servings*

	Calories	Carbo-hydrate (gm)	Protein (gm)	Total Fat (gm)	Saturated Fat (gm)	Choles-terol (mg)
Total	1488.0	23.2	207.1	59.3	12.7	1058.1
Per Serving	248.0	3.9	34.5	9.9	2.1	176.4

Swordfish Teriyaki

1 1/2 lbs. swordfish steaks
2 tbsp. fresh lemon
    juice
2 tbsp. soy sauce

1/2 tsp. dry mustard
1/2 tsp. ground ginger
1/8 tsp. garlic powder

Before cooking: Place the fish in a shallow pan. Combine the lemon juice, soy sauce, mustard, ginger, and garlic powder. Pour this over the fish and let it stand at room temperature for 1 hour, turning it once.

Remove the fish steaks from the marinade and place them on a broiler pan. Broil them 3 inches from the heat source for 5 minutes. Then turn them over, brush them with the marinade, and broil them for another 5 to 10 minutes — until the fish flakes easily when tested with a fork. *Makes 6 servings*

	Calories	Carbo-hydrate (gm)	Protein (gm)	Total Fat (gm)	Saturated Fat (gm)	Choles-terol (mg)
Total	1227.2	4.4	194.1	40.0	0.0	544.0
Per Serving	204.5	0.7	32.4	6.7	0.0	90.7

Curried Fish

1 lb. fish fillets
¾ tsp. salt
¾ cup water
2 tbsp. flour

1 tsp. curry powder
1 tbsp. onion flakes
dash ground ginger
¾ cup skim milk

Pour the water and ½ teaspoon salt into a skillet, and bring them to a boil. Lower the heat, add the fish, and cover the pan. Simmer the fish for 6 to 10 minutes or until it flakes easily when tested with a fork. Drain the liquid from the pan, reserving ¼ cup. Remove the fillets, and break them into 2-inch pieces. Combine the flour, curry powder, onion flakes, ¼ tsp. salt, ginger, milk, and reserved liquid in the now-empty skillet. Heat this mixture to boiling, stirring constantly, and boil and stir it for 1 minute. Then stir in the fish and heat it through. Serve Curried Fish with Skinny Rice (the recipe is in "Potatoes, Pasta, and Rice").

Makes 4 servings

	Calories	Carbo-hydrate (gm)	Protein (gm)	Total Fat (gm)	Saturated Fat (gm)	Choles-terol (mg)
Total	1049.4	22.9	147.3	37.4	10.7	414.2
Per Serving	262.4	5.7	36.8	9.4	2.7	103.6

---

gm=grams; mg=milligrams. Nutritional figures are approximate. Figures are based on findings of U.S. Department of Agriculture.

Bluefish Curry

1½ lbs. bluefish fillets
1½ tbsp. fresh lemon
  juice
½ tsp. butter-flavored
  salt
¼ tsp. pepper

1 can condensed
  cream of celery
  soup
¼ cup skim milk
1 tsp. curry powder
  (or more to taste)

Before cooking: Cut the fillets into 6 serving pieces.
  Arrange the fish in a single layer in a baking dish. Season them with the lemon juice, salt, and pepper, and bake them uncovered at 425° for 12 minutes. While the fish is baking, heat the condensed soup in a saucepan. Stir in the milk, a little at a time. When the sauce is smooth, add the curry powder. To serve, place the baked fillets on a platter and spoon the sauce over the fish.   *Makes 6 servings*

	Calories	Carbo-hydrate (gm)	Protein (gm)	Total Fat (gm)	Saturated Fat (gm)	Choles-terol (mg)
Total	1328.7	26.7	183.6	45.2	0.0	499.7
Per Serving	221.5	4.5	30.6	7.5	0.0	83.3

Flounder Parmesan

2 lbs. skinless flounder
  fillets or other fish
  fillets, fresh or
  frozen
2 tbsp. fresh lemon
  juice
5 tbsp. grated
  Parmesan cheese

4 tbsp. diet
  mayonnaise
3 tbsp. chopped
  green onion
¼ tsp. salt
  dash hot pepper
  sauce

Before cooking: If the fish is frozen, let it thaw in the refrigerator or at room temperature. Spray a bake-and-serve platter with spray-on vegetable coating. Arrange the fillets in a single layer on the platter and brush them with lemon juice. Let them stand for 10 minutes.
  Combine the remaining ingredients in a bowl. Broil the fillets about 4 inches from the heat source for 5 to 6

minutes. Remove them from the broiler and spread the cheese mixture over them. Return the fillets to the broiler, and continue to broil them for 3 to 4 minutes longer — until they are lightly browned.

Makes 8 servings

	Calories	Carbo-hydrate (gm)	Protein (gm)	Total Fat (gm)	Saturated Fat (gm)	Choles-terol (mg)
Total	2318.3	11.3	313.7	109.6	36.3	933.8
Per Serving	289.8	1.4	39.2	13.7	4.5	116.7

Flounder Mozzarella

2 lbs. skinless flounder
fillets or other fish
fillets, fresh or
frozen
2 tbsp. grated onion
1¹/₂ tsp. garlic salt

¹/₈ tsp. pepper
2 large tomatoes
1 cup shredded part-
skim mozzarella
cheese
¹/₂ tsp. oregano

Before cooking: If the fish is frozen, let it thaw in the refrigerator or at room temperature. Cut the tomatoes into small pieces.

Spray a bake-and-serve platter with spray-on vegetable coating for no-fat, no-stick cooking. Arrange the fillets in a single layer on the platter and sprinkle over them the grated onion, oregano, salt, and pepper. Then cover the fillets with the tomato pieces. Broil the fish about 4 inches from the heat source for 10 to 12 minutes or until the fillets flake easily when tested with a fork. Sprinkle the cheese over the fish, and continue to broil for 2 to 3 minutes longer — until the cheese melts.

Makes 8 servings

	Calories	Carbo-hydrate (gm)	Protein (gm)	Total Fat (gm)	Saturated Fat (gm)	Choles-terol (mg)
Total	2226.7	21.5	341.5	94.6	25.3	892.8
Per Serving	278.3	2.7	42.7	11.8	3.2	111.6

gm = grams; mg = milligrams. Nutritional figures are approximate. Figures are based on findings of U.S. Department of Agriculture.

Basic Steamed Fish

1½ lbs. fish fillets, steaks,   1½ tsp. salt
   or pan-dressed fish,
   fresh or frozen

Before cooking: If the fish is frozen, let it defrost in the refrigerator or at room temperature.

Fill the bottom of a fish steamer with just enough water so it does not rise above the insert basket. Bring the water and salt to a boil. Grease the insert basket and place the fish inside. Cover the steamer, and cook the fish over the boiling water for 5 to 10 minutes or until the fish flakes easily when tested with a fork. Let the fish cool, then remove the skin and bones.

Makes 6 servings

Special note: Steamed fish that has been chilled is a perfect beginning for a beautiful luncheon salad.

	Calories	Carbo-hydrate (gm)	Protein (gm)	Total Fat (gm)	Saturated Fat (gm)	Choles-terol (mg)
Total	1386.1	0.0	209.6	56.4	16.1	620.5
Per Serving	231.0	0.0	34.9	9.4	2.7	103.4

Basic Barbecued Fillets or Steaks

2 lbs. fish fillets or
   steaks, fresh or
   frozen
Barbecue Sauce:
¼ cup chopped onion
2 tbsp. chopped green
   pepper
1 finely chopped garlic
   clove

8 oz. can tomato
   sauce
2 tbsp. fresh lemon
   juice
1 tbsp.
   Worcestershire
   sauce
1 tbsp. sugar
2 tsp. salt
¼ tsp. pepper

Before cooking: If the fish is frozen, let it thaw in the refrigerator or at room temperature. Cut the fish into 8 portions.

Combine all of the ingredients except the fish in a

saucepan and cook them over moderate heat for 5 minutes, stirring occasionally. Allow this sauce to cool. Arrange the fish in a single layer in a shallow baking dish. Pour the sauce over the fish and let it stand at room temperature for 30 minutes, turning the fish once. Then remove the fish from the baking dish and save the sauce for basting. Place the fish in a well-oiled, hinged wire grill. Place the grill about 4 inches from moderately hot coals and cook the fish for 5 to 8 minutes. Baste it with the sauce; turn the fish over and cook it for 5 to 8 minutes longer or until the fish flakes easily when tested with a fork.   *Makes 8 servings*

	Calories	Carbo-hydrate (gm)	Protein (gm)	Total Fat (gm)	Saturated Fat (gm)	Choles-terol (mg)
Total	1683.5	33.8	227.8	64.4	21.3	543.7
Per Serving	210.4	4.2	28.5	8.1	2.7	68.0

"Deep-Fried" Fish Fillets

1 lb. fish fillets
1 egg

2 tbsp. corn or safflower oil
1/2 cup seasoned bread crumbs

Combine the egg and oil and whip them together with a fork. Pour this mixture onto a plate. Place the bread crumbs on another plate. Dip the fillets first into the egg mixture and then into the bread crumbs so they are lightly coated. Place the breaded fillets on a non-stick cookie sheet or other shallow pan with no-stick coating and bake them at 450° for 10 to 12 minutes, until they are golden and cooked through.

Makes 4 servings

	Calories	Carbo-hydrate (gm)	Protein (gm)	Total Fat (gm)	Saturated Fat (gm)	Choles-terol (mg)
Total	1441.8	36.5	151.1	73.8	15.2	664.9
Per Serving	360.5	9.1	37.7	18.5	3.8	166.2

---

gm=grams; mg=milligrams. Nutritional figures are approximate. Figures are based on findings of U.S. Department of Agriculture.

Oriental Fish Broil

2 lbs. skinless fish
    fillets, fresh or
    frozen
1/4 cup low-calorie
    French dressing

3 tbsp. soy sauce
3/4 tsp. ground ginger
    lemon slices

Before cooking: If the fish is frozen, let it thaw in the refrigerator or at room temperature. Spray a bake-and-serve platter with spray-on vegetable coating, and arrange the fillets on it in a single layer. Combine the French dressing, soy sauce, and ginger and pour this mixture over the fish. Let the fish stand for 10 minutes.

Broil the fillets about 4 inches from the heat source for 10 to 15 minutes or until they flake easily when tested with a fork. Baste them once during the broiling time with the sauce in the platter. To serve, garnish the fish with lemon slices.   *Makes 8 servings*

	Calories	Carbo-hydrate (gm)	Protein (gm)	Total Fat (gm)	Saturated Fat (gm)	Choles-terol (mg)
Total	1867.5	3.0	280.2	74.6	21.3	820.8
Per Serving	233.4	0.4	35.0	9.3	2.7	102.6

Broiled Fillets or Steaks

2 lbs. fish fillets or
    steaks, fresh or
    frozen
1 tbsp. diet margarine
2 tbsp. fresh lemon
    juice

1 tsp. salt
1/2 tsp. paprika
    dash pepper

Before cooking: If the fish is frozen, let it thaw in the refrigerator or at room temperature. Cut the fish into 8 portions.

Place the fish portions in a single layer, skin side down, on a non-stick baking pan. Dot them with diet margarine, and sprinkle them with lemon juice, salt, paprika, and a dash of pepper. Broil the fish about 4 inches from the heat source for 10 to 15 minutes or un-

til it flakes easily when tested with a fork. Baste the fish
during the broiling with the liquid in the pan, but don't
turn the fish over. *Makes 8 servings*

	Calories	Carbo-hydrate (gm)	Protein (gm)	Total Fat (gm)	Saturated Fat (gm)	Choles-terol (mg)
Total	856.7	2.4	170.7	16.7	1.0	501.0
Per Serving	107.1	0.3	21.3	2.1	0.1	62.6

Fish Steaks in Mushroom Sauce

8 oz. can sliced
    mushrooms
2 lbs. fish steaks
1 lb. can tomatoes
¼ cup finely chopped
    onion
1 small minced garlic
    clove

¼ cup water
2 tbsp. flour
¾ tsp. salt
⅛ tsp. coarse freshly
    ground black
    pepper

Before cooking: Drain the mushrooms, reserving the
liquid, and do the same with the tomatoes.

Arrange the fish in a shallow baking dish. Break the
tomatoes into pieces and spoon them over the fish
along with the mushrooms, chopped onion, and
minced garlic. In a bowl, combine the reserved liquid
from the mushrooms and tomatoes with ¼ cup water.
Mix in the flour, salt, and pepper. Pour this mixture
over the fish. Cover the baking dish, and bake the fish
in a preheated 375° oven for 15 minutes. Then remove
the cover and bake the fish for 15 to 20 minutes longer
or until the fish flakes when tested with a fork.

Makes 6 servings

	Calories	Carbo-hydrate (gm)	Protein (gm)	Total Fat (gm)	Saturated Fat (gm)	Choles-terol (mg)
Total	1750.3	39.9	235.0	66.1	21.3	543.7
Per Serving	291.7	6.7	39.2	11.0	3.6	90.6

---

*gm=grams; mg=milligrams. Nutritional figures are approximate. Figures
are based on findings of U.S. Department of Agriculture.*

Stuffed Fish Fillets with Crab Meat

7¹/₂ oz. can crab meat
1 lb. sole or flounder fillet
3 tbsp. soft bread crumbs
¹/₂ cup minced celery
¹/₄ tsp. onion powder
¹/₂ tsp. butter-flavored salt
pinch of pepper
pinch of tarragon
2 tbsp. diet margarine
1¹/₂ tbsp. fresh lemon juice
¹/₄ cup dry white wine
paprika

Before cooking: Drain the crab meat; bone it and flake it. Cut the fillet into 6 pieces.

Combine the crab meat, bread crumbs, celery, onion powder, salt, pepper, and tarragon in a bowl. Lay the pieces of fillet out flat and place an equal portion of the crab meat filling at one end of each piece. Roll up the fillets and fasten them closed with wooden picks. Place the rolls in a shallow baking dish. Pour the lemon juice and wine over them and pat them with the diet margarine. Bake the fish rolls at 350° — basting occasionally — for about 20 minutes or until the fish flakes easily when tested with a fork. Sprinkle them with paprika before serving.   *Makes 6 servings*

	Calories	Carbo-hydrate (gm)	Protein (gm)	Total Fat (gm)	Saturated Fat (gm)	Choles-terol (mg)
Total	1337.6	12.0	176.2	54.3	12.7	622.9
Per Serving	222.9	2.0	29.4	9.1	2.1	103.8

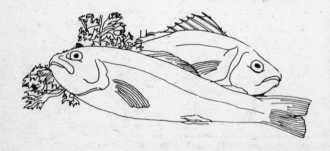

Green Peppers Stuffed with Crab Meat

4 medium green
   peppers
8 oz. crab meat (fresh,
   frozen, or canned)
1 cup cooked rice
2 eggs, slightly beaten
2 tbsp. lemon juice

1 tbsp. chopped
   onion
1/2 tsp. curry
1/4 tsp. salt
   dash of cayenne
1/2 cup crushed rice
   cereal
1 tbsp. diet
   margarine

Before cooking: Cook the rice according to the directions on the package to yield 1 cup. Cut the green peppers in half lengthwise and remove the seeds. Cook the peppers in boiling salted water for 5 minutes and then drain them. Flake the crab meat and remove any pieces of shell that may be present.

Combine the crab meat with the beaten eggs, rice, lemon juice, onion, curry, salt, and cayenne. Fill the pepper halves with the crab mixture. Then combine the crushed cereal with the margarine and sprinkle this over the crab mixture. Place the stuffed green peppers on a baking sheet and bake them at 400° for 15 minutes.   *Makes 4 servings*

	Calories	Carbo-hydrate (gm)	Protein (gm)	Total Fat (gm)	Saturated Fat (gm)	Choles-terol (mg)
Total	745.5	71.5	60.8	23.3	5.0	731.0
Per Serving	186.4	17.9	15.2	5.8	1.3	182.8

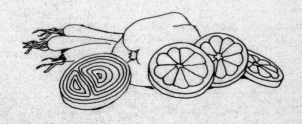

gm=grams; mg=milligrams. Nutritional figures are approximate. Figures are based on findings of U.S. Department of Agriculture.

Seafood Skillet

2 lbs. skinless fish
    fillets, fresh or
    frozen
2 cups chopped onion
2 tbsp. diet margarine
1½ tsp. salt

¼ tsp. pepper
2 tomatoes
1 lemon
1 large bay leaf
¼ cup water
1 tsp. cider vinegar

Before cooking: If the fish is frozen, let it thaw in the refrigerator or at room temperature. Cut the thawed fillets crosswise into strips about ½ inch wide. Slice the tomatoes and lemon.

Melt the margarine in a large non-stick skillet. Add the chopped onions and sauté them until they are tender. Arrange the fish strips over the onions and season them with salt and pepper. Then cover the fish with the tomato and lemon slices. Add the bay leaf. In a cup, combine the vinegar and water and pour this over the fish mixture. Cover the skillet, and simmer the fish for 10 to 15 minutes or until the fish flakes easily when tested with a fork. Before serving, remove the bay leaf.

Makes 8 servings

	Calories	Carbo-hydrate (gm)	Protein (gm)	Total Fat (gm)	Saturated Fat (gm)	Choles-terol (mg)
Total	1079.9	44.4	179.6	22.7	2.0	501.0
Per Serving	135.0	5.6	22.5	2.8	0.3	62.6

Snapper á l'Orange

2 lbs. skinless snapper
    fillets or other fish
    fillets, fresh or
    frozen
½ cup frozen orange
    juice concentrate
1 tbsp. corn or safflower
    oil

¼ cup soy sauce
¼ cup cider vinegar
½ tsp. salt
    chopped parsley
    orange slices
    (optional)

Before cooking: If the fish is frozen, let it thaw in the refrigerator or at room temperature. Let the orange juice thaw also. Cut the fillets into 8 portions.

Spray a 15"x10"x1" baking pan with spray-on vegetable coating for no-fat cooking. Arrange the fish, skinned side up, in a single layer. In a bowl, combine the orange juice, oil, soy sauce, vinegar, and salt. Brush the fish with this sauce. Broil the fish about 4 inches from the heat source for 5 minutes. Turn the fish carefully and brush it again with the sauce. Continue to broil it for another 5 to 7 minutes — until it has lightly browned and the fish flakes easily when tested with a fork. Sprinkle chopped parsley over the top. Garnish the platter with orange slices if you like.

Makes 8 servings

	Calories	Carbo-hydrate (gm)	Protein (gm)	Total Fat (gm)	Saturated Fat (gm)	Choles-terol (mg)
Total	1252.3	66.3	188.6	24.7	1.0	501.0
Per Serving	156.5	8.3	23.6	3.1	0.1	62.6

Broiled Rock Lobster Tails

4 rock lobster tails (5 oz. each)
1/4 cup chicken bouillon
2-3 drops butter flavoring

1 tbsp. fresh lemon juice
1/8 tsp. bitters
1/8 tsp. ground ginger
1/8 tsp. chili powder

Before cooking: Cut through the shells lengthwise to keep the lobster tails from curling during cooking.

Combine the bouillon, butter flavoring, lemon juice, bitters, ginger, and chili powder in a bowl. (For the bouillon, you may use canned bouillon undiluted or a bouillon cube mixed with 1/4 cup water.) Place the lobster tails on a broiler rack, meat side up, and brush the meat with the bouillon mixture. Broil the lobster about 4 inches from the heat source for 8 to 10 minutes.

Makes 4 servings

	Calories	Carbo-hydrate (gm)	Protein (gm)	Total Fat (gm)	Saturated Fat (gm)	Choles-terol (mg)
Total	554.9	2.2	108.3	6.7	0.0	487.2
Per Serving	138.7	0.6	27.1	1.7	0.0	121.8

gm=grams; mg=milligrams. Nutritional figures are approximate. Figures are based on findings of U.S. Department of Agriculture.

Happy Halibut

2 lbs. halibut steaks or other fish steaks, fresh or frozen

1/3 cup hickory-smoke-flavored barbecue sauce

1/4 cup juice-packed crushed pineapple, undrained

1 tbsp. fresh lemon juice

1 tbsp. instant minced onion

1/4 tsp. salt

Before cooking: If the fish is frozen, let it thaw in the refrigerator or at room temperature.

Spray a bake-and-serve platter with spray-on vegetable coating for no-fat, no-stick cooking. Arrange the steaks in a single layer on the platter. In a bowl, combine the rest of the ingredients. Brush the steaks generously with this sauce. Broil the fish about 4 inches from the heat source for 10 to 15 minutes or until the steaks flake easily when tested with a fork. Baste them once with the remaining sauce during the broiling period.   *Makes 8 servings*

	Calories	Carbo-hydrate (gm)	Protein (gm)	Total Fat (gm)	Saturated Fat (gm)	Choles-terol (mg)
Total	1673.5	20.1	225.9	69.6	22.0	543.7
Per Serving	209.2	2.5	28.2	8.7	2.8	68.0

Fruited Halibut

2 lbs. 3/4-inch halibut steaks, fresh or frozen

2 cups boiling water

2 tbsp. fresh lemon juice

1 tsp. salt

1 tbsp. cornstarch

1/2 cup orange juice

1/2 cup cold water

2 tsp. grated orange peel

1 tsp. lemon juice

sugar substitute to equal 1 tbsp.

11 oz. can mandarin orange segments

1 cup seeded green grape halves

Before cooking: If the fish is frozen, let it thaw in the refrigerator or at room temperature. Cut it into 8 portions. Drain the can of mandarin orange segments.

Place the fish in a large skillet. Add 2 cups boiling water, 2 tbsp. lemon juice and the salt. Cover the pan and simmer the fish for 8 to 10 minutes until it flakes easily when tested with a fork. While the fish is simmering, prepare the sauce.

Combine the cornstarch, orange juice and $\frac{1}{2}$ cup cold water in a saucepan. Cook this mixture slowly, stirring constantly, until it thickens. Then stir in the orange peel, and 1 teaspoon lemon juice. Add the orange segments and grape halves. Continue cooking the sauce just until it is heated through. Remove the pan from the heat and stir in the sugar substitute.

Transfer the cooked, drained fish carefully to a hot serving platter. Spoon the sauce over the halibut.

Makes 8 servings

	Calories	Carbo-hydrate (gm)	Protein (gm)	Total Fat (gm)	Saturated Fat (gm)	Choles-terol (mg)
Total	1818.2	67.2	227.7	64.8	21.3	543.7
Per Serving	227.3	8.4	28.5	8.1	2.7	68.0

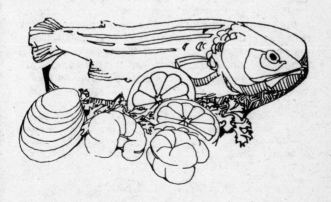

gm = grams; mg = milligrams. Nutritional figures are approximate. Figures are based on findings of U.S. Department of Agriculture.

Oven Paella

1 broiler-fryer chicken
(2 lbs.)
1 lb. medium shrimp
12 small clams (in shell)
10¹/₂ oz. can chicken broth
2 tbsp. instant minced
onion
1¹/₂ tsp. garlic salt

¹/₄ tsp. pepper
¹/₈ tsp. powdered
saffron
1¹/₂ cups uncooked
converted rice
10 oz. package frozen
peas
1 whole pimiento

Before cooking: Cut the chicken into small pieces.
Skim the broth of fat by chilling it until the fat rises to
the top and can be whisked away. Shell and devein the
shrimp. Cut the pimiento into strips. Allow the peas to
become partially thawed.

Arrange the chicken pieces, skin side up, in a large
non-stick baking pan. Bake them, uncovered, in a preheated 450° oven for about 20 minutes — until they are
brown. Remove the pan from the oven. Pour off all the
fat that accumulates in the pan. Lower the oven to
350°. Add enough water to the broth to make 3 cups.
Pour 1 cup of the broth mixture into the pan with the
chicken. Then stir in the onion, garlic salt, pepper, and
saffron. Cover the pan with foil and bake the contents
for 25 minutes. Sprinkle the rice into the pan and pour
in the remaining broth. Arrange the shrimp and clams
over this mixture and sprinkle the peas over all. Cover
the pan again, and return it to the oven for about 25
minutes — until the rice is cooked and the liquid is absorbed. Garnish the Paella with the pimiento and serve
it right from the pan.   *Makes 10 servings*

	Calories	Carbo-hydrate (gm)	Protein (gm)	Total Fat (gm)	Saturated Fat (gm)	Choles-terol (mg)
Total	2691.3	278.8	273.3	43.6	13.7	1360.7
Per Serving	269.1	27.9	27.3	4.4	1.4	136.1

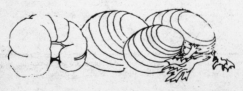

Angler's Spaghetti Stew

2 lbs. rockfish, ling,
    cod, ocean perch,
    salmon, halibut, or
    other firm fish, fresh
    or frozen
2 tbsp. diet margarine
2 cups sliced celery
1 cup chopped onion
1 minced garlic clove
1 lb. 12 oz. can
    tomatoes,
    undrained

8 oz. can tomato
    sauce
2 tsp. salt
1/2 tsp. paprika
1/2 tsp. chili powder
1/4 tsp. pepper
6 oz. uncooked
    spaghetti
2 cups boiling water
2 tbsp. grated
    Parmesan
    cheese

Before cooking: If the fish is frozen, let it thaw in the refrigerator or at room temperature. Cut the fish into 1-inch chunks.

Melt the diet margarine in a large, heavy non-stick skillet. Sauté the celery, onion, and garlic in the margarine until they are tender. Then add the tomatoes (with the liquid from the can), tomato sauce, and seasonings. Bring this mixture to a simmer, cover the pan, and cook it slowly for 15 to 20 minutes. Then add the uncooked spaghetti and the boiling water. Cover the pan and cook the contents slowly for about 10 minutes or until the spaghetti is almost tender. Then add the fish, cover the pan again, and continue to cook slowly for another 10 minutes or until the fish flakes easily when tested with a fork. Serve with Parmesan cheese sprinkled over the top.   *Makes 8 servings*

	Calories	Carbo-hydrate (gm)	Protein (gm)	Total Fat (gm)	Saturated Fat (gm)	Choles-terol (mg)
Total	2806.7	193.0	292.0	91.4	29.3	458.8
Per Serving	350.8	24.1	36.5	11.4	3.7	57.4

gm=grams; mg=milligrams. Nutritional figures are approximate. Figures are based on findings of U.S. Department of Agriculture.

Skillet Soy Scallops

2 lbs. scallops, fresh or frozen	¼ cup water
	2 tbsp. cornstarch
7 oz. package frozen pea pods	1 tbsp. soy sauce
	½ tsp. salt
2 tbsp. diet margarine	⅛ tsp. pepper
2 tomatoes	

Before cooking: If the scallops are frozen, allow them to thaw at room temperature. Also allow the pea pods to thaw. Rinse the scallops with cold water to remove any shell particles. Cut the large scallops in half crosswise. Drain the pea pods. Cut the tomatoes into eighths.

Melt the margarine in a 10-inch non-stick skillet. Add the scallops, and sauté them over low heat for 3 or 4 minutes, stirring frequently. Then add the pea pods and tomatoes. In a cup, combine the water, cornstarch, soy sauce, salt, and pepper. Add this mixture to the skillet and cook the whole mixture, stirring constantly, until the sauce is thick. Serve Skillet Soy Scallops with Skinny Rice (the receipe is in "Potatoes, Pasta, and Rice"). *Makes 6 servings*

	Calories	Carbo-hydrate (gm)	Protein (gm)	Total Fat (gm)	Saturated Fat (gm)	Choles-terol (mg)
Total	1357.4	89.3	218.2	22.7	2.0	479.7
Per Serving	226.2	14.9	36.4	3.8	0.3	80.0

Scallops on Skewers

1 lb. small scallops	1 tbsp. corn or safflower oil
½ lb. Canadian bacon	
1 large onion	2 tbsp. soy sauce
2 green peppers	garlic salt
½ lb. fresh mushrooms	dash of cayenne

Before cooking: Rinse the scallops and pat them dry. Cut the Canadian bacon into 1-inch cubes. Cut the onion and green peppers into chunks. If the mushrooms are large, cut in half; otherwise, leave whole.

CONSUMER GUIDE

Thread the scallops on 6 skewers, alternating them with the bacon cubes and vegetable chunks. Combine the oil, soy sauce, and seasonings in a shallow plate. Rotate the skewers in this mixture to coat the scallops and vegetables evenly. Place the skewers 3 or 4 inches over hot coals for 15 minutes, turning them frequently. Or place the skewers on a shallow non-stick roasting pan or cookie sheet. Pour on the remaining sauce. Bake them in a preheated 450° oven for 15 minutes, turning once or twice during cooking. *Makes 6 servings*

	Calories	Carbo-hydrate (gm)	Protein (gm)	Total Fat (gm)	Saturated Fat (gm)	Choles-terol (mg)
Total	1548.7	73.5	193.5	61.9	11.7	429.5
Per Serving	258.1	12.3	32.3	10.3	2.0	71.6

Shrimp Bisque

14 oz. shrimp
1/4 cup finely chopped onion
1/4 cup finely chopped celery
1/4 cup water
2 tbsp. flour

1 tsp. butter-flavored salt
1/4 tsp. paprika
dash white pepper
4 cups skim milk

Before cooking: For this recipe, you may use shrimp that is canned, frozen, cooked or boiled fresh. Chop the shrimp coarsely.

Place the onion, celery, and water in a non-stick skillet. Cook the vegetables in the water until they are tender. Then stir in the seasonings and the flour. Add the milk to the skillet, and cook the entire mixture over low heat, stirring constantly, until it is thick. Then fold in the shrimp. Continue cooking just until the shrimp is heated through, then serve it at once. *Makes 6 servings*

	Calories	Carbo-hydrate (gm)	Protein (gm)	Total Fat (gm)	Saturated Fat (gm)	Choles-terol (mg)
Total	787.2	63.4	108.0	4.8	0.0	616.5
Per Serving	131.2	10.6	18.0	0.8	0.0	102.7

gm=grams; mg=milligrams. Nutritional figures are approximate. Figures are based on findings of U.S. Department of Agriculture.

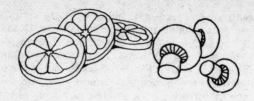

Crab Casserole

1 lb. crab meat, fresh or frozen
15 oz. can artichoke hearts
4 oz. can sliced mushrooms
2½ tbsp. flour
½ tsp. butter-flavored salt
dash cayenne

1 cup evaporated skim milk
2 tbsp. dry sherry
2 tbsp. crushed high-protein cereal, unsweetened
1 tbsp. grated Parmesan cheese
paprika

Before cooking: If the crab meat is frozen, let it thaw in the refrigerator or at room temperature; then drain it and remove any remaining shell or cartilage. Drain the can of artichoke hearts and the can of mushrooms. Cut the artichoke hearts in half.

Spray a shallow 1½-quart casserole with spray-on vegetable coating. Place the artichokes in the casserole and cover them with the mushrooms and crab meat. In a saucepan, combine the milk, flour and seasonings. Cook this mixture slowly, stirring constantly, until it is thick. Then stir in the sherry. Pour the sauce over the crab meat. Combine the cereal crumbs and cheese, and sprinkle them over the sauce. Sprinkle paprika over all. Bake the casserole at 450° for 12 to 15 minutes — until it is bubbly.

Makes 6 servings

	Calories	Carbo-hydrate (gm)	Protein (gm)	Total Fat (gm)	Saturated Fat (gm)	Choles-terol (mg)
Total	1098.4	79.8	123.1	36.4	14.0	547.3
Per Serving	183.1	13.3	20.5	6.1	2.3	91.2

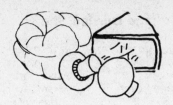

Crab and Shrimp Au Gratin

6 oz. package frozen
king crab meat
7 oz. cooked Pacific
pink shrimp
1 tbsp. diet margarine
1/3 cup sliced green
onions
1/4 cup flour
1 tsp. salt
1/8 tsp. white pepper

13 oz. can evaporated
skim milk
2 tbsp. fresh lemon
juice
6 oz. can sliced
water chestnuts
2 1/2 cups cooked rice
2 tbsp. diced
pimiento
1/2 cup shredded
cheddar cheese

Before cooking: Let the crab meat thaw at room temperature. Drain the water chestnuts. You may use shrimp that is canned, frozen, cooked or freshly boiled.

Melt the margarine in a small non-stick skillet. Sauté the green onions in the margarine until they are tender. In a large saucepan, blend together the flour, salt, and pepper; then add the milk. Cook this mixture over low heat, stirring constantly, until it is thick and smooth. Then stir in the lemon juice, crab meat, shrimp, water chestnuts, cooked rice, pimiento, and sautéed green onions. Spoon the entire mixture into 6 individual-size ramekins at 350° for about 25 minutes until the mixture is hot and bubbly. *Makes 6 servings*

	Calories	Carbo-hydrate (gm)	Protein (gm)	Total Fat (gm)	Saturated Fat (gm)	Choles-terol (mg)
Total	2364.6	234.6	145.4	90.6	44.1	735.8
Per Serving	394.1	39.1	24.2	15.1	7.4	122.6

gm=grams; mg=milligrams. Nutritional figures are approximate. Figures are based on findings of U.S. Department of Agriculture.

Cottage Curried Shrimp

1 lb. package frozen
    shelled deveined
    shrimp
10 oz. package frozen
    peas
1 tbsp. diet margarine
1/4 cup finely chopped
    peeled apple
2 tbsp. finely chopped
    onion

2 1/2 tbsp. flour
1 tbsp. curry powder
1/2 tsp. salt
1/4 tsp. savory
    dash of cayenne
1 cup skim milk
2 cups 99% fat free
    cottage cheese

Before cooking: Cook the peas according to package directions, and drain them. Cook and drain the shrimp also.

Melt the margarine in a saucepan. Add the apple and onion and sauté them until they are tender. Blend in the flour, curry, salt, savory, and cayenne pepper. Remove the pot from the heat and gradually add the milk and cottage cheese. Cook the entire mixture over medium heat, stirring constantly, until it has thickened. Then cook it for 2 more minutes. Stir in the peas and shrimp and continue to cook the mixture just until it is heated through.   *Makes 6 servings*

	Calories	Carbo-hydrate (gm)	Protein (gm)	Total Fat (gm)	Saturated Fat (gm)	Choles-terol (mg)
Total	1196.6	71.3	136.0	15.6	3.4	726.0
Per Serving	199.4	11.9	22.7	2.6	0.6	121.0

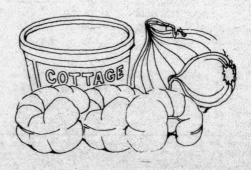

Tuna Stroganoff

2 (7 oz.) cans chunk
tuna, packed in
water
¹/₄ cup flour
13¹/₂ oz. can chicken broth
8 oz. can tomato sauce

¹/₄ cup instant
chopped onions
4 oz. can
mushrooms,
undrained
1 tsp. parsley flakes
1 cup plain yogurt

Before cooking: Skim the fat from the chicken broth. An easy way to do this is to chill the broth until the fat floats to the top and can be whisked away. Drain the tuna, reserving the liquid.

Combine the flour with the liquid from the tuna in a saucepan. Gradually stir in the broth and cook this mixture over low heat, stirring constantly, until it has thickened. Then stir in the tomato sauce, onions, mushrooms, parsley, and tuna. Cover the pot and simmer the contents until they are heated through. Stir in the yogurt, and continue cooking just until hot — do not boil. Serve the Tuna Stroganoff over Skinny Rice (the recipe is in "Potatoes, Pasta, and Rice").

Makes 8 servings

	Calories	Carbo-hydrate (gm)	Protein (gm)	Total Fat (gm)	Saturated Fat (gm)	Choles-terol (mg)
Total	930.2	72.9	134.6	8.6	2.0	306.7
Per Serving	116.3	9.1	16.8	1.1	0.3	38.3

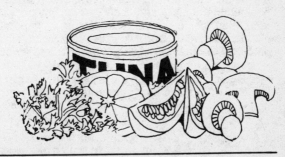

gm = grams; mg = milligrams. Nutritional figures are approximate. Figures are based on findings of U.S. Department of Agriculture.

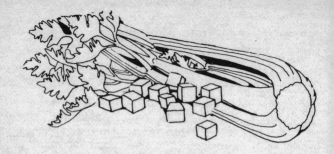

Tuna Veronique

7 oz. can water-packed
  tuna
²/₃ cup boiling water
¹/₂ cup instant rice
1 vegetable bouillon
  cube
¹/₄ cup finely chopped
  celery
2 tbsp. snipped parsley

2 tbsp. all-purpose
  flour
¹/₂ tsp. salt
1 cup evaporated
  skim milk
¹/₂ cup seedless
  green grapes,
  halved
2 tbsp. dry white
  wine
1 tbsp. lemon juice

Before cooking: Drain the tuna, and break it into chunks.

Bring the ²/₃ cup water to a boil in a saucepan. Add the rice, bouillon, celery, and parsley, and cook them for 2 minutes. Spray 4 individual casseroles with spray-on vegetable coating and spoon the rice mixture into them. Then, combine the flour, salt, and evaporated milk in a saucepan. Cook them over low heat, stirring constantly, until the mixture is thick and bubbly. Remove the pot from the heat and stir in the remaining ingredients. Spoon this mixture into the casseroles over the rice. Bake the casseroles at 350° for 20 minutes.   *Makes 4 servings*

	Calories	Carbo-hydrate (gm)	Protein (gm)	Total Fat (gm)	Saturated Fat (gm)	Choles-terol (mg)
Total	1076.3	134.2	94.9	30.3	13.2	204.0
Per Serving	269.1	33.6	23.7	7.6	3.3	51.0

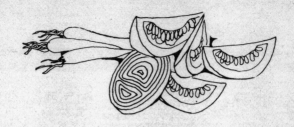

Cioppino

1½ lbs. halibut, ling, cod,
    rockfish, or sea
    bass, fresh or
    frozen
2 cups sliced onion
2 finely minced garlic
    cloves
1 lb. 12 oz. can Italian
    tomatoes,
    undrained
8 oz. can tomato sauce

1 cup water
¼ cup chopped
    parsley
2 tsp. salt
1 tsp. basil
½ tsp. oregano
¼ tsp. pepper
1 doz. clams in shell
1 cup cooked shrimp

Before cooking: If the fish is frozen, let it thaw in the refrigerator or at room temperature. Cut the thawed fish into 1½-inch chunks. Wash the clams. Boil the shrimp; then peel and devein them.

Combine all the ingredients except the fish, clams, and shrimp in a Dutch oven. Cover the pot and simmer the contents gently for 30 minutes. Add the fish chunks and continue to simmer, covered, for about 15 minutes. Then add the clams in their shells and the shrimp. Cover the pot and continue to simmer for about 10 minutes or until the fish chunks flake easily when tested with a fork. *Makes 8 servings*

	Calories	Carbo-hydrate (gm)	Protein (gm)	Total Fat (gm)	Saturated Fat (gm)	Choles-terol (mg)
Total	1723.8	76.8	224.2	55.2	16.0	664.2
Per Serving	215.5	9.6	28.0	6.9	2.0	83.0

gm = grams; mg = milligrams. Nutritional figures are approximate. Figures are based on findings of U.S. Department of Agriculture.

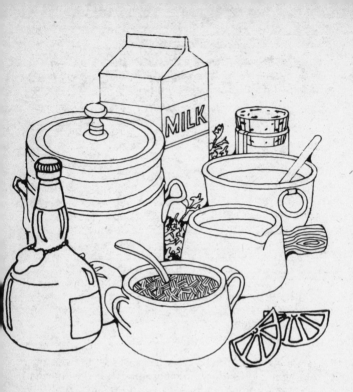

The Flavor-Uppers:

Sauces, Marinades, And Gravy

Most diet plans warn the would-be slimmer to stay away from sauces and gravies. And with good reason — most sauces are calorie-rich. But thickeners aren't the main source of a sauce's calories. The real culprit is hidden fat — in the form of butter, cream, margarine, oil, or meat fat. Without these unneeded fat calories, sauces and gravies can serve as savory toppings for lean meat, fish, and poultry — or a replacement for butter or margarine on top of vegetables.

How To Make Low-Fat Gravy

Fat is not a necessary ingredient in gravy. You can subtract 100 calories for every tablespoon of meat fat you skim from pan drippings.

1. The easy way to do this is to drain the drippings into a cup and quick-chill it in your freezer until the fat rises to the surface and hardens. Then, simply lift the fat off and discard it. If you're in a real rush, pour the hot drippings in a tall narrow heat-proof container and wait a minute or two until the fat reaches the surface. Then *zoop* it up with a bulb-type baster.

2. Measure the stock, and heat it to boiling.

3. For each cup of stock, combine 2 tablespoons flour and ¼ cup cold water in a small cup. Stir until smooth and lump-free, then stir the flour mixture into the simmering stock to thicken it. (Never add flour directly to a hot liquid or it will lump.)

4. Simmer the gravy over very low heat until it is the desired thickness. If it gets too thick, thin it with a little water.

5. For a darker gravy, stir in a little soy sauce or brown gravy coloring. Season the gravy to your taste with salt, pepper, onion powder, or herbs.

Canned beef broth or chicken broth can be used in place of meat drippings for gravy-making. When you open the can, be sure to remove any globules of grease floating on the surface. Use condensed products "straight," without diluting. But do not use canned cream-soups for sauces because these contain unneeded fat. (A can of Cream of Chicken soup is 245 calories.)

How to Make a Cream Sauce
(White Sauce)

Cream sauce doesn't need cream or butter for a dairy-rich flavor. Canned evaporated skim milk is an ideal stand-in for cream. It has only a fraction of the fat and calories and it's much higher in protein.

1. For a medium cream sauce (white sauce) combine one 13-ounce can of evaporated skim milk with 4 tablespoons flour in a non-stick saucepan over very low heat. Cook and stir until the sauce begins to bubble. Simmer two minutes.

2. Season to taste with chopped parsley, a pinch of nutmeg, white pepper and butter-flavored salt (or bottled butter flavoring).

3. Increase or decrease the amount of flour for a thick or thin white sauce.

This sauce can be used in any favorite recipe that calls for white sauce as a base:

Wine sauce Add 3 tablespoons dry white wine. Simmer 2 minutes.

Cheese Sauce Add 6 tablespoons shredded cheese. Stir until melted.

Curry Sauce Add 1 (or more) tsp. curry powder.

Bechamel Sauce Omit salt, add 2 cubes or teaspoon chicken bouillon.

Recipes

Applesauce Glaze

1 cup diet applesauce   ⅛ tsp. allspice

Combine the applesauce and allspice. Brush the glaze on meat during cooking.   *Makes 1 cup*
(4 servings)

	Calories	Carbo-hydrate (gm)	Protein (gm)	Total Fat (gm)	Saturated Fat (gm)	Choles-terol (mg)
Total	100.0	26.0	1.0	0.0	0.0	0.0
Per Serving	25.0	6.5	0.3	0.0	0.0	0.0

Orange Poultry Glaze

1 tsp. paprika   ³/₄ cup orange juice
1 tbsp. soy sauce

Combine all of the ingredients in a bowl. Use the mixture as a baste when barbecuing or roasting poultry.

Makes ³/₄ cup
(4 servings)

	Calories	Carbo-hydrate (gm)	Protein (gm)	Total Fat (gm)	Saturated Fat (gm)	Choles-terol (mg)
Total	92.5	20.5	2.5	0.8	0.0	0.0
Per Serving	23.1	5.1	0.6	0.2	0.0	0.0

Chunky Orange Sauce for Meat or Poultry

1 tbsp. cornstarch   1 orange
1 cup orange juice   2 tsp. grated orange
    sugar substitute to   peel
    equal 2 tsp.

Before cooking: Peel the orange. Section it, and then cut the sections into ¹/₂-inch pieces.

Combine the cornstarch and orange juice in a saucepan. Cook the mixture over moderate heat, stirring constantly, until it has thickened and is clear. Then stir in the sugar substitute, orange pieces and grated orange peel. This sauce is especially good with smoked ham slices.

Makes 1¹/₂ cups
(6 servings)

	Calories	Carbo-hydrate (gm)	Protein (gm)	Total Fat (gm)	Saturated Fat (gm)	Choles-terol (mg)
Total	229.7	55.3	3.1	1.0	0.0	0.0
Per Serving	38.3	9.2	0.5	0.2	0.0	0.0

---

gm=grams; mg=milligrams. Nutritional figures are approximate. Figures are based on findings of U.S. Department of Agriculture.

Soy Basting Sauce

¼ cup dry wine
¼ cup soy sauce
1 tsp. ground ginger

1 tsp. dry mustard
¼ tsp. pepper
1 garlic clove

Before cooking: Mince the garlic clove.
   Combine all of the ingredients in a bowl. Use the mixture to baste meat, chicken, or seafood while cooking over coals or in the oven. *Makes ½ cup*
(3 servings)

	Calories	Carbo-hydrate (gm)	Protein (gm)	Total Fat (gm)	Saturated Fat (gm)	Choles-terol (mg)
Total	88.5	6.3	4.0	0.0	0.0	0.0
Per Serving	29.5	2.1	1.3	0.0	0.0	0.0

Luau Sauce

1 jar (7¾ oz.) baby food
   peaches or apricots
⅓ cup catsup
¼ cup brown sugar
   substitute

⅓ cup cider vinegar
1 tbsp. soy sauce
1 tsp. ground ginger
⅛ tsp. garlic powder

Combine all of the ingredients in a small saucepan. Bring the mixture to a boil, stirring frequently. Serve with broiled pork or chicken. *Makes 1½ cups*
(5 servings)

	Calories	Carbo-hydrate (gm)	Protein (gm)	Total Fat (gm)	Saturated Fat (gm)	Choles-terol (mg)
Total	274.3	74.0	3.2	0.0	0.0	0.0
Per Serving	54.9	14.8	0.6	0.0	0.0	0.0

Mustard Sauce

½ cup plain yogurt
1½ tbsp. prepared
   mustard

½ tsp. parsley flakes
⅛ tsp. butter salt

Combine all of the ingredients in a saucepan. Heat the mixture slowly, stirring occasionally, but don't let it boil. Serve with fish and cooked vegetables.

Makes 10 tablespoons
(5 servings)

	Calories	Carbo-hydrate (gm)	Protein (gm)	Total Fat (gm)	Saturated Fat (gm)	Choles-terol (mg)
Total	236.5	50.0	4.0	2.0	1.0	10.0
Per Serving	47.3	10.0	0.8	0.4	0.2	2.0

Barbecue Sauce

1 cup tomato puree
1 cup water
1 small onion
1 tbsp. Worcestershire
    sauce
1/2 tsp. seasoned meat
    tenderizer
1/4 cup vinegar

2 tsp. dry mustard
1 tsp. paprika
1 tsp. chili powder
1 garlic clove
1 tbsp. brown sugar
    substitute

Before cooking: Chop the onion and garlic clove.

Combine all of the ingredients in a saucepan except the brown sugar substitute. Cover the pan and simmer the mixture slowly for 30 minutes. Then stir in the sugar substitute. (If you want a hotter sauce, add a dash of cayenne or more chili powder.)   *Makes 2¹/₂ cups*
(10 servings)

	Calories	Carbo-hydrate (gm)	Protein (gm)	Total Fat (gm)	Saturated Fat (gm)	Choles-terol (mg)
Total	138.0	35.0	6.0	0.0	0.0	0.0
Per Serving	13.8	3.5	0.6	0.0	0.0	0.0

---

gm=grams; mg=milligrams. Nutritional figures are approximate. Figures are based on findings of U.S. Department of Agriculture.

Barbecue Basting Sauce

6 oz. tomato juice
¼ cup chili sauce, or
catsup
2 tbsp. lemon juice

2 tsp. prepared
mustard
few drops hot
pepper sauce

Combine all of the ingredients in a bowl. Use this sauce to baste meat, fish, or poultry as it broils or barbecues.
*Makes 1⅛ cups
(5 servings)*

	Calories	Carbo-hydrate (gm)	Protein (gm)	Total Fat (gm)	Saturated Fat (gm)	Choles-terol (mg)
Total	180.0	45.8	1.6	0.0	0.0	0.0
Per Serving	36.0	9.2	0.3	0.0	0.0	0.0

Tomato Barbecue Sauce

1 cup catsup
⅔ cup tomato juice

1 tbsp. vinegar
3 tbsp. brown sugar
substitute

Combine all of the ingredients in a bowl. Brush the meat or chicken with the barbecue sauce during the last 30 minutes of cooking.
*Makes 1⅔ cups
(6 servings)*

	Calories	Carbo-hydrate (gm)	Protein (gm)	Total Fat (gm)	Saturated Fat (gm)	Choles-terol (mg)
Total	270.7	71.6	1.3	0.0	0.0	0.0
Per Serving	45.1	11.9	0.2	0.0	0.0	0.0

Quick Tomato Sauce

1 tsp. diet margarine
2 cups coarsely
chopped tomatoes
(1 lb. can)

¼ cup finely chopped
onion
2 tsp. instant
bouillon (or 2
bouillon cubes)

Melt the margarine in a non-stick skillet, and sauté

the onions until they are tender. Then stir in the tomatoes and bouillon. Simmer the mixture, uncovered, for about 15 minutes — until the sauce is thick and well blended. *Makes 1¹/₂ cups*
(6 servings)

	Calories	Carbo-hydrate (gm)	Protein (gm)	Total Fat (gm)	Saturated Fat (gm)	Choles-terol (mg)
Total	136.5	22.5	6.5	4.0	0.3	6.0
Per Serving	22.8	3.8	1.1	0.7	0.1	1.0

Quick Tartar Sauce

¹/₂ cup diet mayonnaise   ¹/₄ cup pickle relish

Drain the pickle relish and mix it with the mayonnaise. Serve with fish.
Special hint: If you like spice in your life, add ¹/₂ teaspoon horseradish and 1 teaspoon Worcestershire sauce. *Makes ³/₄ cup*
(6 servings)

	Calories	Carbo-hydrate (gm)	Protein (gm)	Total Fat (gm)	Saturated Fat (gm)	Choles-terol (mg)
Total	240.0	28.0	0.0	16.0	0.0	64.0
Per Serving	40.0	4.7	0.0	2.7	0.0	10.7

Cream Sauce for Vegetables

¹/₄ cup flour   ¹/₈ tsp. pepper
2 cups skim milk   dash of nutmeg
³/₄ tsp. butter salt   dash of cayenne

Blend the ingredients in a non-stick saucepan over moderate heat, stirring constantly until the sauce is thick and smooth. *Makes 2 cups*
(8 servings)

	Calories	Carbo-hydrate (gm)	Protein (gm)	Total Fat (gm)	Saturated Fat (gm)	Choles-terol (mg)
Total	293.8	47.8	21.3	0.3	0.0	10.0
Per Serving	36.7	6.0	2.7	0.0	0.0	1.3

gm=grams; mg=milligrams. *Nutritional figures are approximate. Figures are based on findings of U.S. Department of Agriculture.*

Quick Curry Sauce

2 tsp. instant chicken
    bouillon or 2
    chicken bouillon
    cubes
1 cup dry skim milk
    powder

1/4 cup all-purpose
    flour
3/4 tsp. curry powder
2 cups cold water

Combine all of the ingredients in a saucepan. Cook the mixture over moderate heat, stirring constantly, until it thickens and boils. Serve the sauce hot over cooked vegetables or fish.

*Makes 2 1/2 cups
(20 servings)*

	Calories	Carbo-hydrate (gm)	Protein (gm)	Total Fat (gm)	Saturated Fat (gm)	Choles-terol (mg)
Total	391.0	99.6	47.2	14.3	4.0	15.0
Per Serving	19.6	5.0	2.4	0.7	0.2	0.8

Hollandaise Sauce

3/4 cup diet mayonnaise
3 tbsp. skim milk
1/4 tsp. salt

dash white pepper
1 tbsp. lemon juice
1 tbsp. grated lemon
    peel

Combine the mayonnaise, milk, salt, and pepper in a saucepan. Heat this mixture very slowly, stirring constantly, until it is warm. Then stir in the lemon juice and grated lemon peel. Serve with cooked vegetables or fish.

*Makes 16 tablespoons
(8 servings)*

	Calories	Carbo-hydrate (gm)	Protein (gm)	Total Fat (gm)	Saturated Fat (gm)	Choles-terol (mg)
Total	261.1	13.7	1.7	20.0	0.0	10.0
Per Serving	32.6	1.7	0.2	2.5	0.0	1.3

Yogurt Marinade

¹/₂ cup plain yogurt	¹/₂ tsp. garlic salt
2 tbsp. lemon juice	¹/₂ tsp. salt
¹/₄ cup chopped onion	¹/₈ tsp. pepper
1 tsp. dry mustard	

Combine all of the ingredients in a bowl. Pour this mixture over meat and let it stand at room temperature, uncovered, for several hours — or in the refrigerator, covered, overnight. During cooking, brush the meat with the remaining marinade.

Makes ⁷/₈ cup
(4 servings)

	Calories	Carbo-hydrate (gm)	Protein (gm)	Total Fat (gm)	Saturated Fat (gm)	Choles-terol (mg)
Total	80.3	11.6	4.6	2.0	1.0	10.0
Per Serving	20.1	2.9	1.2	0.5	0.3	2.5

Mandarin Marinade

1 cup soy sauce	1 tsp. ground ginger
1 cup orange juice	¹/₄ tsp. pepper
2 cloves garlic	

Before cooking: Mince the garlic cloves.

Combine all of the ingredients in a bowl. Pour the mixture over meat and let it stand at room temperature, uncovered, for several hours — or in the refrigerator, covered, overnight. During cooking, brush the meat with the remaining marinade.

Makes 2 cups
(8 servings)

	Calories	Carbo-hydrate (gm)	Protein (gm)	Total Fat (gm)	Saturated Fat (gm)	Choles-terol (mg)
Total	270.0	42.0	18.0	1.0	0.0	0.0
Per Serving	33.8	5.3	2.3	0.1	0.0	0.0

---

gm=grams; mg=milligrams. Nutritional figures are approximate. Figures are based on findings of U.S. Department of Agriculture.

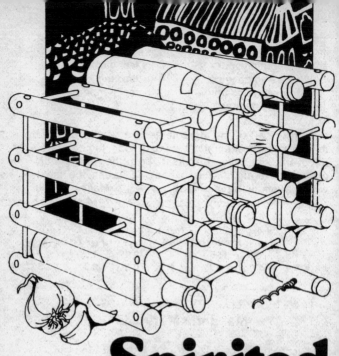

Spirited Cooking

Dieters are always cautioned against the overuse of alcohol. And with good reason, since alcohol adds nothing to nutrition but calories. But there *is* one way a dieter can enjoy liquor without paying the price — and that's to cook with it. Alcohol evaporates when it cooks and leaves little in the way of calories — but leaves lots in the way of flavor.

Sweet wines, of course, will leave behind sugar calories, so the calorie-cautious cook should choose only the driest table wines for cooking. Beer used in cooking will also give up its alcohol calories but the carbohydrate calories will remain. Low-calorie beers that are also low-carbohydrate are a good alternative in recipes calling for beer. "Hard" liquor — distilled spirits like scotch, bourbon, plain brandy, and rum — has no carbohydrate calories to remain after cooking. Neither does vodka, but since vodka has no flavor there is little point in using it in cooking.

Of course, liquor that is used in uncooked recipes still retains all its alcohol and alcohol calories — rum or brandy in an unbaked refrigerator pie filling, for example. Rum or brandy extract would be a better choice for dieters.

Recipes

Japanese Skewered Lamb

2 lbs. lean boneless lamb	2 tbsp. sherry
¼ cup soy sauce	2 garlic cloves
1 tbsp. honey	¼ tsp. ground ginger
2 tbsp. vinegar	1½ cups bouillon

Before cooking: Cut the lamb into strips that are ⅛ inch thick, ½ inch wide and 3 inches long across the grain. Combine the remaining ingredients (crushing the garlic with a garlic press), and pour the mixture over the meat. Turn the meat to coat it well and let it stand uncovered for 1 hour at room temperature — or covered overnight in the refrigerator. Turn the meat occasionally so it gets seasoned evenly.

Weave the meat onto skewers. Broil them about 4 inches from the heat source for about 2 minutes on each side. *Makes 8 servings*

	Calories	Carbo-hydrate (gm)	Protein (gm)	Total Fat (gm)	Saturated Fat (gm)	Choles-terol (mg)
Total	1986.3	28.7	248.1	83.6	41.8	926.8
Per Serving	248.3	3.6	31.0	10.5	5.2	115.9

gm=grams; mg=milligrams. Nutritional figures are approximate. Figures are based on findings of U.S. Department of Agriculture.

Stir-Fried Chicken and Snow Peas

2 large whole chicken
  breasts
2 tbsp. soy sauce
2 tbsp. sherry
1 tsp. ground ginger
1 clove garlic

1 tbsp. corn or
  safflower oil
1 cup sliced onions
1 cup sliced
  mushrooms
7 oz. package frozen
  snow peas

Before cooking: Bone and skin the chicken breasts. Cut the meat into bite-size strips. Blend the soy sauce, sherry, ginger, and garlic (crush the garlic with a garlic press) together in a bowl. Add the chicken to the bowl and let the mixture sit uncovered at room temperature for 30 minutes. Let the snow peas thaw.

Heat the oil in a non-stick skillet, rotating the pan to spread it evenly. Add the chicken, onions, mushrooms, and snow peas. Sauté the chicken and vegetables for about 5 minutes, stirring constantly, until the chicken is tender and the vegetables are crisp.

Makes 4 servings

	Calories	Carbo-hydrate (gm)	Protein (gm)	Total Fat (gm)	Saturated Fat (gm)	Choles-terol (mg)
Total	746.7	47.4	84.8	23.0	5.0	204.0
Per Serving	186.7	11.9	21.2	5.8	1.3	51.0

Chinese Chicken Packets

4 whole chicken
  breasts
2 thin slices of boiled
  ham
1 tbsp. soy sauce
2 tbsp. sherry

1 tbsp. chopped
  green onion
1 tsp. cornstarch
1/4 tsp. ground ginger
  dash garlic
  powder

Before cooking: Bone and skin the chicken breasts. Slice each breast diagonally into 3 long pieces. Trim the fat from the ham and cut each slice into 3 portions. Combine the soy sauce, sherry, onion, cornstarch, ginger, and garlic powder in a bowl. Pour this mixture over the chicken and ham and let it stand at room temperature, uncovered, for 30 minutes or longer.

Cut 6 rectangles of aluminum foil, about 6 inches x 12 inches. Place a portion of ham on each piece of foil. On top of the ham place 2 pieces of chicken side by side. Spoon any remaining marinade over the meat. Fold the foil over to make square packets, using a double fold at the edges. Place the packets on a baking sheet and bake them at 400° for 20 minutes. Serve in the packets. *Makes 6 servings*

	Calories	Carbo-hydrate (gm)	Protein (gm)	Total Fat (gm)	Saturated Fat (gm)	Choles-terol (mg)
Total	913.6	9.1	155.1	24.0	11.0	483.0
Per Serving	152.3	1.5	25.9	4.0	1.8	80.5

Apple-Wine Broiled Chicken

2 lbs. broiler-fryer chicken
1 tsp. salt

$^1/_4$ cup apple juice
$^1/_4$ cup dry white wine

Before cooking: Split the chicken in half lengthwise.

Place the chicken skin side down on a broiler rack and season it with half the salt. Combine the apple juice and wine, and pour half the mixture into the cavities of the chicken. Broil the chicken about 10 inches from the heat source for about 30 minutes. Then turn the chicken over, season it with the rest of the salt, and brush it with the remaining wine mixture. Broil it for 30 minutes longer until it is tender. *Makes 4 servings*

	Calories	Carbo-hydrate (gm)	Protein (gm)	Total Fat (gm)	Saturated Fat (gm)	Choles-terol (mg)
Total	942.9	9.8	130.3	34.3	13.7	555.7
Per Serving	235.7	2.5	32.6	8.6	3.4	138.9

gm=grams; mg=milligrams. Nutritional figures are approximate. Figures are based on findings of U.S. Department of Agriculture.

Coq Au Vin

3 lbs. broiler-fryer
   chicken pieces
1 cup chicken broth
1/2 cup Burgundy or
   other dry red wine
1 lb. (about 16) small
   white onions
4 oz. can sliced
   mushrooms

1 bay leaf
1 large garlic clove
1/4 tsp. poultry
   seasoning
1/4 tsp. salt
2 tbsp. flour

Before cooking: Skim the fat from the broth by chilling it until the fat rises to the top and can be whisked off. Peel the onions. Drain the mushrooms. Mince the garlic.

Brown the chicken skin side down in a large, heavy non-stick skillet. Do not add any oil to the pan because the chicken will release enough of its own fat for frying. Pour off the fat that accumulates in the pan. Then add 2/3 cup of the broth, the wine, onions, mushrooms, and seasonings to the skillet. Turn the chicken pieces. Cover the pan, and cook the contents over low heat for about 45 minutes until the chicken is tender. Blend the other 1/3 cup broth with the flour in a cup until it is smooth. Then slowly stir this mixture into the sauce. Continue to cook the chicken mixture, stirring, until the sauce has thickened.   *Makes 8 servings*

	Calories	Carbo-hydrate (gm)	Protein (gm)	Total Fat (gm)	Saturated Fat (gm)	Choles-terol (mg)
Total	1672.6	65.6	211.0	51.9	20.5	845.0
Per Serving	209.1	8.2	26.4	6.5	2.6	105.6

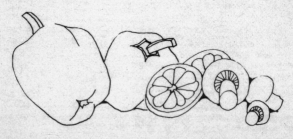

CONSUMER GUIDE

Chicken in Wine Sauce

2 whole chicken
   breasts
1/2 lb. Canadian bacon
1/2 lb. fresh mushrooms
1/2 cup chopped green
   pepper
1 tbsp. diet margarine
1/4 cup flour

1 cup chicken broth
13 oz. evaporated
   skim milk
1/3 cup dry white wine
1/2 tsp. salt
1/4 tsp. white pepper
1/4 tsp. nutmeg

Before cooking: Simmer the chicken breasts. For directions, see the introduction to "Chicken." When the chicken has cooled, dice the chicken meat. Cut the Canadian bacon into cubes, and slice the mushrooms. Skim the chicken broth of fat by using a bulb-type baster, or by chilling the broth until the fat rises to the surface and can be lifted away.

Combine the diced chicken and Canadian bacon. Melt the margarine and sauté the mushrooms and peppers for 5 minutes in a non-stick skillet. Add the mushrooms and peppers to the chicken mixture. Blend the flour with the chicken broth and milk in a saucepan. Bring this mixture to a boil, stirring it to keep it smooth. Add the meat and vegetables to the saucepan and also add the wine, salt, pepper, and nutmeg. Simmer the entire mixture for 3 minutes. *Makes 6 servings*

Special note: Use the water in which you simmer the chicken as your broth. Or you may used canned bouillon undiluted, or 2 chicken bouillon cubes mixed with 1 cup water.

	Calories	Carbo-hydrate (gm)	Protein (gm)	Total Fat (gm)	Saturated Fat (gm)	Choles-terol (mg)
Total	1972.0	101.2	179.5	89.5	33.6	534.7
Per Serving	328.7	16.9	29.9	14.9	5.6	89.1

gm = grams; mg = milligrams. Nutritional figures are approximate. Figures are based on findings of U.S. Department of Agriculture.

Chicken Romanoff

3 whole chicken breasts	¼ cup sherry or other dry white wine
1 tbsp. diet margarine	2 tsp. arrowroot or cornstarch
1½ tsp. salt	2 tbsp. cold water
1 onion	1 cup yogurt
½ lb. mushrooms	1½ tsp. paprika

Before cooking: Bone the chicken breasts, and remove the skin. Cut the meat into strips. Chop the onion into fine pieces and slice the mushrooms.

Melt the margarine in a non-stick skillet over medium heat. Add the chicken and season it with the salt. Cook the chicken, stirring constantly, for 3 minutes. Then add the onion and mushrooms and continue to cook the mixture for 2 minutes longer, continuing to stir. Add the sherry, cover the pan, and cook for an additional 4 minutes. Blend together the arrowroot and water in a cup. Add this to the skillet and continue cooking, stirring rapidly, until the sauce has thickened. Stir in the yogurt and paprika, continuing to cook just until the mixture is heated through. Do not let it boil. *Makes 6 servings*

	Calories	Carbo-hydrate (gm)	Protein (gm)	Total Fat (gm)	Saturated Fat (gm)	Choles-terol (mg)
Total	955.6	57.2	123.5	24.5	9.0	326.0
Per Serving	159.3	9.5	20.6	4.1	1.5	54.3

Chicken Cacciatore Casserole

2 lbs. broiler-fryer chicken pieces	10½ oz. can condensed tomato soup
8 small white onions	½ cup water
1 medium green pepper	2 tbsp. dry white wine
4 oz. can sliced mushrooms	½ tsp. oregano
1 small garlic clove	

Before cooking: Cut the green pepper into strips. Mince the garlic clove. Drain the mushrooms.

Arrange the chicken pieces in a single layer in a casserole. Bake the chicken uncovered at 450° for 30 minutes. Pour off the fat that accumulates in the casserole. Then add the onions, green pepper, mushrooms, and garlic. Blend together the tomato soup, water, wine, and oregano in a bowl. Pour this mixture over the chicken and vegetables. Bake the casserole uncovered at 350° for about 30 minutes.

Makes 6 servings

	Calories	Carbo-hydrate (gm)	Protein (gm)	Total Fat (gm)	Saturated Fat (gm)	Choles-terol (mg)
Total	1323.8	90.8	147.5	42.2	13.7	555.7
Per Serving	220.6	15.1	24.6	7.0	2.3	92.6

Sherried Veal With Mushrooms

2 lbs. lean veal shoulder
1 tbsp. diet margarine
1/2 cup sliced onion
3/4 cup sherry
1 1/2 tsp. garlic salt

1/4 tsp. coarse-ground pepper
1 lb. fresh mushrooms
2 tbsp. chopped fresh parsley

Before cooking: Cut the meat into 1-inch cubes, trimming away all fat. Slice the mushrooms.

Melt the margarine in a large, non-stick skillet. Add the meat and brown it over moderate heat. Then add the onion, sherry, salt, and pepper. Cover the pan, and simmer the contents for 45 minutes or until the veal is almost tender. Add the mushrooms, cover the pan, and simmer the mixture for 15 minutes longer. Just before serving, stir in the parsley.   *Makes 6 servings*

	Calories	Carbo-hydrate (gm)	Protein (gm)	Total Fat (gm)	Saturated Fat (gm)	Choles-terol (mg)
Total	1741.8	66.8	217.4	53.7	22.3	640.2
Per Serving	290.3	11.1	36.2	9.0	3.7	106.7

gm=grams; mg=milligrams. Nutritional figures are approximate. Figures are based on findings of U.S. Department of Agriculture.

Korean Beef (Bul Kogi)

1½ lbs. flank steak
⅓ cup soy sauce
3 tbsp. cream sherry
2 tbsp. onion flakes

1 tsp. garlic powder
1 tbsp. corn or
  safflower oil
¼ cup sliced green
  onions
3 tsp. sesame seeds

Before cooking: Have the steak partially frozen for easier handling. Slice it in thirds, lengthwise. Then slice each third across the grain into ¼-inch slices. Toast the sesame seeds by stirring them quickly over high heat in a non-stick skillet. Or place them on a cookie sheet in a 450° oven until they are golden. They must be watched carefully or they will burn. Combine the meat, soy sauce, sherry, onion, and garlic in a bowl. Refrigerate and cover for several hours.

Heat the oil over high heat in a large non-stick skillet. Add the steak strips and stir-fry them quickly until they are seared. Be careful not to overcook. Remove the meat to a platter and sprinkle with the green onions and toasted sesame seeds.

Makes 6 servings

	Calories	Carbo-hydrate (gm)	Protein (gm)	Total Fat (gm)	Saturated Fat (gm)	Choles-terol (mg)
Total	1596.6	16.4	218.0	58.5	21.6	620.0
Per Serving	266.1	2.7	36.3	9.8	3.6	103.3

Wine-Basted Roast Tenderloin with Mushrooms

2 lbs. beef tenderloin
  salt (or garlic salt or
    onion salt)
  coarse ground pepper

1 cup dry red wine
4 oz. can sliced
  mushrooms
2 tsp. arrowroot or
  cornstarch

Before cooking: Trim the meat of all visible fat. Drain the mushrooms, saving the liquid.

Season the meat liberally with salt and pepper. Insert a meat thermometer so that the tip is in the center of the roast. (By all means, do not forget to use a thermometer; tenderloin is too expensive to ruin by overcooking). Place the roast on a rack in a non-stick roasting pan and roast it in a pre-heated 450° oven for 30 to 35 minutes — until the thermometer reads 125°. Baste every 10 minutes with the wine. Remove the roast to a platter.

Using a bulb-type baster, skim all the fat from the pan juices. In a cup, combine the arrowroot (or cornstarch) with the juice from the mushrooms. Then stir this into the roasting pan, scraping well. Cook the sauce over moderate heat until it thickens and simmers. Then add the mushrooms. Slice the roast thinly, and serve it with the sauce.   *Makes 8 servings*

	Calories	Carbo-hydrate (gm)	Protein (gm)	Total Fat (gm)	Saturated Fat (gm)	Choles-terol (mg)
Total	2082.8	18.1	291.8	64.0	32.0	816.0
Per Serving	260.4	2.3	36.5	8.0	4.0	102.0

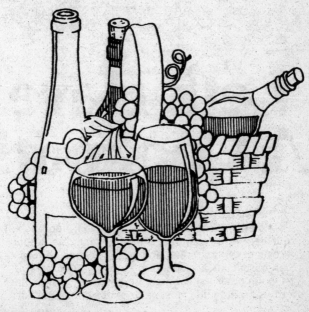

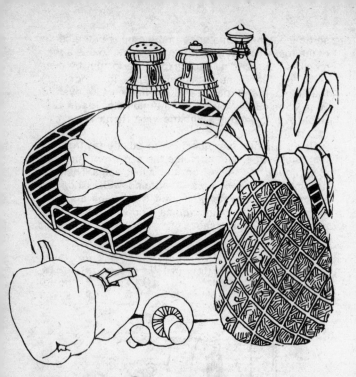

Let's Have
A Cookout!

C ooking over the coals can be a calorie-saver or a
dietary disaster, depending on your approach. If
your backyard repertoire is mainly limited to hotdogs
— or steaks, spareribs, and sugar-packed sauces —
then barbecues are bound to be bikini-stretchers.

On the other hand, barbecuing is really just another
form of broiling, the most calorie-safe cooking of all. If

you choose your ingredients with a sharp eye for calorie counts, there is no reason why your rotisserie or hibachi cannot prove to be an effective weapon in your war against overweight.

The first rule is to expand your horizons. Most backyard chefs limit their choices to steaks and fatty hamburger, with less emphasis on poultry, seafood, and the leaner cuts of meat. And most sauces or bastes — bottled or homemade — are generally packed with fats and sugars, which add unneeded calories.

Many of the recipes throughout this book call for broiling. In all cases, broiling can be done outside over hot coals for an additional flavor treat.

Recipes

Chicken-in-a-Packet

2 chicken breasts	2 tsp. salt
4 small raw carrots	¼ tsp. pepper
4 raw medium-sized white potatoes	½ tsp. oregano

Before cooking: Split the breasts in half. Cut the carrots in sticks. Peel the potatoes.

Tear off 4 pieces of heavy-duty aluminum foil, approximately 18 inches square. Place 1 piece of chicken, 1 potato, and ¼ of the carrot sticks on each piece of foil. Sprinkle salt, pepper, and oregano over all. Wrap the foil tightly around the food and cook it in a covered grill for approximately 1 hour until the chicken is tender. *Makes 4 servings*

	Calories	Carbo-hydrate (gm)	Protein (gm)	Total Fat (gm)	Saturated Fat (gm)	Choles-terol (mg)
Total	776.0	104.0	80.0	8.0	4.0	204.0
Per Serving	194.0	26.0	20.0	2.0	1.0	51.0

---

gm=grams; mg=milligrams. Nutritional figures are approximate. Figures are based on findings of U.S. Department of Agriculture.

Soy-Broiled Chicken

2 lbs. broiler-fryer
    chicken, split in half
    lengthwise
$1/4$ cup soy sauce
4 tbsp. fresh lemon
    juice

$1/2$ tsp. salt
$1/4$ tsp. pepper
$1/2$ tsp. paprika

Make a sauce by combining the soy sauce, lemon juice, salt, pepper, and paprika. Place the chicken on a grill skin side up and brush some sauce on the chicken. Broil the chicken approximately 10 inches from the coals for about 45 minutes until tender, basting as needed.   *Makes 4 servings*

	Calories	Carbo-hydrate (gm)	Protein (gm)	Total Fat (gm)	Saturated Fat (gm)	Choles-terol (mg)
Total	975.0	9.0	164.3	24.0	8.0	536.0
Per Serving	243.8	2.3	41.1	6.0	2.0	134.0

Chinese-Broiled Breast Steaks of Turkey

6 turkey breast steaks,
    cut to $1 1/2$ inches
    thick
1 tsp. grated fresh
    ginger or ground
    ginger
1 tsp. dry mustard

1 tbsp. honey
$1/2$ cup soy sauce
1 tbsp. corn or
    safflower oil
3 minced garlic
    cloves

Before cooking: Combine all of the ingredients, except the turkey, in a glass bowl. Pour this mixture over the turkey steaks, cover them, and refrigerate them for several hours or overnight.

Drain the steaks and cook them quickly on both sides on a barbecue grill, allowing about 8 minutes per side. Brush them occasionally with the marinade, if you like.   *Makes 6 servings*

Special hint: If turkey breast steaks are not available, have a butcher cut a turkey breast crosswise into $1 1/2$-

inch thick steaks. Frozen breasts can be cut also, and thawed when ready to use.

	Calories	Carbo-hydrate (gm)	Protein (gm)	Total Fat (gm)	Saturated Fat (gm)	Choles-terol (mg)
Total	1477.4	25.0	234.4	41.4	7.9	528.2
Per Serving	246.2	4.2	39.1	6.9	1.3	88.0

Mediterranean-Style Shish Kebab

1½ lbs. boneless leg of lamb
12 bay leaves
12 slices lemon peel
2 large tomatoes
2 medium onions

2 medium green peppers
¼ cup diet Italian salad dressing
salt
pepper

Before cooking: Cut the lamb into 1½-inch cubes, trimming off all fat. Cut each tomato and onion into 6 wedges, and each green pepper into 6 pieces.

On one set of skewers, alternate the lamb, bay leaves, and lemon peel. On a second set of skewers, arrange the tomatoes. And on a third set of skewers, alternate the onion and green pepper. Brush all of the meat and vegetables with the salad dressing. Grill the lamb kebabs and the onion and green pepper kebabs 3 to 5 inches from the hot coals for 5 to 7 minutes on each side, or until the lamb has reached the desired doneness and the onion and pepper are brown and tender. Grill the tomatoes for about 3 minutes on each side. Baste the lamb and vegetables frequently with the salad dressing. Season with salt and pepper to taste before serving. *Makes 6 servings*

	Calories	Carbo-hydrate (gm)	Protein (gm)	Total Fat (gm)	Saturated Fat (gm)	Choles-terol (mg)
Total	1497.5	52.9	202.9	52.0	28.8	681.6
Per Serving	249.6	8.8	33.8	8.7	4.8	113.6

gm=grams; mg=milligrams. Nutritional figures are approximate. Figures are based on findings of U.S. Department of Agriculture.

Hawaiian Beef Kebabs

2 lbs. lean round steak,
  cut 2 inches thick
1½ tsp. dry mustard
¾ tsp. ground ginger
⅛ tsp. ground pepper
⅛ tsp. garlic powder

6 tbsp. soy sauce
3 tbsp. fresh lemon
  juice
16 cherry tomatoes
16 wedges green
  pepper
16 whole fresh
  mushrooms

Before cooking: Trim the meat of all visible fat and slice
it into ¼-inch strips. Place the strips in a shallow pan
or dish. Combine the mustard, ginger, pepper, garlic
powder, soy sauce, and lemon juice. Mix these ingredients well and pour the mixture over the steak strips.
Cover the dish and allow the meat to marinate in the
refrigerator for at least 4 hours.

Thread the marinated steak strips on metal skewers,
alternating them with the tomatoes, green pepper, and
mushrooms. Brush the meat and vegetables with the
marinade and place the skewers over hot coals for 3
minutes. Then, turn the skewers, brush with the
marinade, and cook them for 3 to 4 minutes longer.

Makes 8 servings

	Calories	Carbo-hydrate (gm)	Protein (gm)	Total Fat (gm)	Saturated Fat (gm)	Choles-terol (mg)
Total	2214.8	99.5	310.3	54.1	26.7	826.5
Per Serving	276.9	12.4	38.8	6.8	3.3	103.3

Italian Beef Kebabs

2 lbs. lean top round
  steak
1 cup diet Italian salad
  dressing

2 medium zucchini
12 cherry tomatoes

Before cooking: Cut the meat into 1½-inch cubes, trimming off all fat. Cut the zucchini into 1-inch slices. Put
the beef cubes in a bowl and pour the dressing over
them. Stir to coat the meat thoroughly. Cover the meat

tightly and refrigerate it for 10 hours or overnight, stirring once or twice.

Drain the marinade from the meat, but reserve it. Thread 4 metal skewers alternately with the beef cubes, zucchini, and tomatoes. Brush them with the marinade. Place the kebabs over hot coals and broil them for 12 to 18 minutes, depending upon degree of doneness desired, turning and brushing them with the marinade occasionally. *Makes 8 servings*

	Calories	Carbohydrate (gm)	Protein (gm)	Total Fat (gm)	Saturated Fat (gm)	Cholesterol (mg)
Total	2133.3	61.6	294.1	69.3	26.7	826.5
Per Serving	266.7	7.7	36.8	8.7	3.3	103.3

Polynesian Skewered Veal and Pineapple

1½ lbs. lean veal steak
16 oz. can juice-packed
    pineapple chunks
3 tbsp. cider vinegar

1 tsp. salt
½ tsp. pepper
½ tsp. marjoram

Before cooking: Cut the veal into cubes, trimming off all fat. Put the veal cubes in a ceramic bowl. Add the vinegar and seasonings. Add just enough drained pineapple juice (from the can of chunks) to cover all the meat. Cover the bowl and marinate the veal in the refrigerator all day or overnight.

Drain the meat and thread it on skewers, alternating it with the pineapple chunks. Broil the meat and pineapple for 15 to 20 minutes over hot coals, turning the skewers frequently. *Makes 6 servings*

	Calories	Carbohydrate (gm)	Protein (gm)	Total Fat (gm)	Saturated Fat (gm)	Cholesterol (mg)
Total	1329.7	70.9	137.7	56.0	24.0	480.0
Per Serving	221.6	11.8	23.0	9.3	4.0	80.0

gm=grams; mg=milligrams. Nutritional figures are approximate. Figures are based on findings of U.S. Department of Agriculture.

Luscious Leftovers

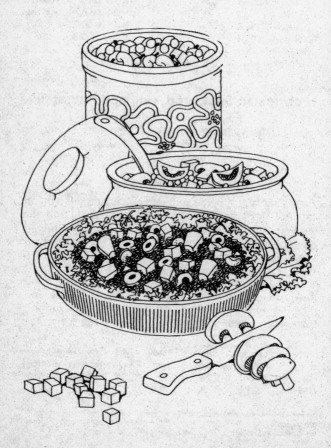

The word *leftover* has an unpleasant hand-me-down sound to it. We prefer to think of them as "planned-overs," food purposely prepared in double quantities to simplify meal-planning another day. True "leftovers" should be avoided. The weight-wise cook never, but never, makes more food than needed lest she lead her family into the temptation to overeat. It is better to cook too little than too much, when weight is a problem.

Even if your family is small, do not hesitate to cook a large roast, multiple chickens, or a big turkey. The remaining meat can serve as the perfect departure for second-day meals. The advantage of recycled roasts is that most of the fat has already been cooked out, and the remaining fat can be trimmed away before the cooked meat is combined with other ingredients.

One way to avoid any suggestion of "leftovers" is to store the cooked meat in your freezer for a few weeks before it takes another curtain call at the family dinner table.

Recipes

Pineapple Chicken Salad

2 cups cubed cooked
  chicken
2 cups cubed fresh
  pineapple
1/2 cup diet mayonnaise

1 cup diced celery
1/2 cup toasted soy
  nuts

Chill all of the ingredients, combine them, and toss them lightly.   *Makes 4 servings*

	Calories	Carbo-hydrate (gm)	Protein (gm)	Total Fat (gm)	Saturated Fat (gm)	Choles-terol (mg)
Total	1156.9	60.0	133.9	42.5	6.0	447.9
Per Serving	289.2	15.0	33.5	10.6	1.5	112.0

gm=grams; mg=milligrams. Nutritional figures are approximate. Figures are based on findings of U.S. Department of Agriculture.

Winter Chicken Salad

1 cup diced cooked
   broiler-fryer
   chicken, loosely
   packed
1/4 cup diet Italian salad
   dressing

1 cup canned wax
   beans, drained
1/2 cup thinly sliced
   onion
crisp salad greens

Combine all of the ingredients except the salad greens and refrigerate the mixture for 2 hours or more. Serve the salad on the crisp salad greens.

Makes 3 servings

	Calories	Carbo- hydrate (gm)	Protein (gm)	Total Fat (gm)	Saturated Fat (gm)	Choles- terol (mg)
Total	442.1	18.0	62.4	12.6	2.9	192.3
Per Serving	147.4	6.0	20.8	4.2	1.0	64.1

Nutty Chicken Mold

1 cup diced broiler-fryer
   chicken, loosely
   packed
4- serving envelope of
   lime-flavored, low-
   calorie gelatin
1 3/4 cups water

1/8 tsp. ground ginger
8 oz. can pineapple
   tidbits, packed
   in juice
3 tbsp. dry-roasted
   cashews
lettuce leaves

Before cooking: Drain the pineapple. Chop the cashews.

Prepare the gelatin with the water as directed on the package, stirring in the ginger. Chill the gelatin until it has slightly thickened; then fold in the chicken, pineapple, and nuts. Pour the mixture into a 1-quart mold, and chill it until it is firm. Un-mold the gelatin onto the lettuce.

Makes 4 servings

	Calories	Carbo- hydrate (gm)	Protein (gm)	Total Fat (gm)	Saturated Fat (gm)	Choles- terol (mg)
Total	607.6	76.5	40.1	16.5	3.5	95.8
Per Serving	151.9	19.1	10.0	4.1	0.9	24.0

Creamy Chicken Salad Ring

2½ cups chopped cooked
    broiler-fryer
    chicken, loosely
    packed
2 tbsp. unflavored
    gelatin (2
    envelopes)
½ cup cold water
2½ cups tomato juice
2 chicken bouillon
    cubes
⅓ cup lemon juice
½ tsp. onion powder

¼ tsp. salt
2 cups plain yogurt
⅓ cup crumbled bleu
    cheese
1 cup finely chopped
    celery
5 tbsp. slivered
    almonds
⅓ cup chopped
    green pepper
    salad greens
1 tomato
1 cucumber

Before cooking: Toast the almonds by spreading them out on a cookie sheet and baking them at 400°. Watch them carefully so they don't burn. Cut the tomato into thin wedges and cut the cucumber into spears.

Soften the gelatin in the water. In a saucepan heat 1 cup of the tomato juice, the bouillon cubes, and the softened gelatin. Stir until the gelatin is dissolved. Then add the remaining tomato juice, the lemon juice, onion powder, and salt. Chill this mixture until it is partially set. Meanwhile, combine the yogurt and bleu cheese. When the gelatin mixture is partially set, fold in the yogurt mixture. Also fold in the chicken, celery, almonds, and green pepper. Turn the whole mixture into a 7-cup mold, and chill it until it is firm. Serve the mold on the salad greens, and garnish it with the tomato wedges and cucumber spears.

Makes 10 servings

	Calories	Carbo-hydrate (gm)	Protein (gm)	Total Fat (gm)	Saturated Fat (gm)	Choles-terol (mg)
Total	1978.3	130.0	227.7	97.7	34.0	601.3
Per Serving	197.8	13.0	22.8	9.8	3.4	60.1

gm=grams; mg=milligrams. Nutritional figures are approximate. Figures are based on findings of U.S. Department of Agriculture.

Curried Chicken and Rice Salad

1 cup boiling water
1 cup packaged pre-
cooked rice
1 tsp. curry
1 tsp. salt
2 cups cooked boned
chicken or turkey,
diced

2 medium tomatoes
2 tbsp. slivered
almonds
1/4 cup sliced green
onion
5 tbsp. any flavor
low-calorie
salad dressing
lettuce

Before preparing: Cut the tomato into wedges. Toast
the almonds by spreading them on a baking sheet and
placing them in a 400° oven until they are brown.

Combine the boiling water, rice, curry, and salt.
Allow the mixture to cool and then toss in all the remaining ingredients, except the lettuce. Chill the mixture and serve it on lettuce. *Makes 4 servings*

	Calories	Carbo-hydrate (gm)	Protein (gm)	Total Fat (gm)	Saturated Fat (gm)	Choles-terol (mg)
Total	908.5	79.1	78.5	30.0	4.1	263.1
Per Serving	227.1	19.8	19.6	7.5	1.0	65.8

Chickenburgers

2 cups ground cooked
broiler-fryer
chicken, loosely
packed
1/2 tsp. salt
2 eggs, beaten

2 tsp. instant minced
onion
1/4 cup chili sauce
6 hamburger buns

Combine all of the ingredients and shape the mixture into 6 patties. Broil the patties about 5 minutes on
each side just until they are heated through. Serve the
Chickenburgers on buns. *Makes 6 servings*

	Calories	Carbo-hydrate (gm)	Protein (gm)	Total Fat (gm)	Saturated Fat (gm)	Choles-terol (mg)
Total	1334.0	143.6	96.8	34.0	13.3	739.1
Per Serving	222.3	23.9	16.1	5.7	2.2	123.2

Chicken Salad Waikiki

2 cups cooked broiler-
fryer chicken, cut in
chunks, loosely
packed
1/4 cup diet mayonnaise
1/4 cup pineapple tidbits,
juice-packed

1/2 cup chopped
celery
2 tbsp. slivered
almonds
1 tsp. soy sauce
4 crisp lettuce
leaves

Drain the pineapple. Add all of the rest of the ingredients except the lettuce and mix well. Serve the salad on the lettuce leaves. *Makes 4 servings*

	Calories	Carbo-hydrate (gm)	Protein (gm)	Total Fat (gm)	Saturated Fat (gm)	Choles-terol (mg)
Total	898.1	20.7	118.6	35.2	6.5	415.9
Per Serving	224.5	5.2	29.7	8.8	1.6	104.0

Supper Chicken Salad

4 cups diced cooked
broiler-fryer
chicken, loosely
packed
2 cups diced celery
1/2 red or green pepper
2 tbsp. lemon juice

1 cup diet
mayonnaise
1 tsp. salt
1/8 tsp. pepper

Chop the red or green pepper and combine it with the rest of the ingredients. Chill the mixture before serving. *Makes 8 servings*

	Calories	Carbo-hydrate (gm)	Protein (gm)	Total Fat (gm)	Saturated Fat (gm)	Choles-terol (mg)
Total	1684.4	32.6	229.4	66.4	11.5	896.5
Per Serving	210.1	4.1	28.7	8.3	1.4	112.1

gm=grams; mg=milligrams. Nutritional figures are approximate. Figures are based on findings of U.S. Department of Agriculture.

Chicken Chop Suey

2 cups diced cooked
broiler-fryer
chicken, loosely
packed
1 tbsp. diet margarine
1/2 cup sliced onion
1 cup sliced celery
1 green pepper

1/2 cup chicken broth
4 oz. can
mushrooms
16 oz. can bean
sprouts
2 tsp. cornstarch
2 tbsp. soy sauce
salt

Before cooking: Skim the fat from the chicken broth by chilling it until the fat rises to the top and can be whisked away. Drain the mushrooms and bean sprouts. Cut the green pepper into strips.

Melt the margarine in a non-stick skillet and sauté the onions, celery, and green pepper. Add the chicken broth, mushrooms, bean sprouts, and salt and bring the mixture to a boil. Blend the cornstarch with the soy sauce in a cup. Add this mixture to the skillet and continue cooking, stirring constantly, until the sauce has thickened slightly. Then add the chicken. Continue cooking just until the chicken is heated through.

Makes 6 servings

	Calories	Carbo-hydrate (gm)	Protein (gm)	Total Fat (gm)	Saturated Fat (gm)	Choles-terol (mg)
Total	951.1	60.5	129.6	22.5	6.3	364.0
Per Serving	158.5	10.1	21.6	3.8	1.1	60.7

Quick Turkey Chow Mein

2 cups cubed cooked
turkey, loosely
packed
2 chicken bouillon
cubes
1 1/2 cups boiling water
1 1/2 tbsp. cornstarch

2 tbsp. cold water
3 tbsp. soy sauce
1 lb. can chow mein
vegetables

Before cooking: Drain the chow mein vegetables and rinse them in water.

Dissolve the bouillon cubes in the boiling water in a saucepan. Combine the cornstarch and cold water in a cup and stir until the mixture is smooth. Then add the cornstarch mixture to the saucepan. Bring the entire mixture to a boil, stirring constantly, and then allow it to simmer for 5 minutes. Add the soy sauce, chow mein vegetables, and turkey, and continue to cook just until the mixture is heated through. *Makes 3 servings*

	Calories	Carbo-hydrate (gm)	Protein (gm)	Total Fat (gm)	Saturated Fat (gm)	Choles-terol (mg)
Total	714.8	64.3	120.3	31.2	9.7	254.5
Per Serving	238.3	21.4	40.1	10.4	3.2	84.8

Turkey Hash

3 cups diced cooked turkey, loosely packed	1/3 cup evaporated skim milk
3/4 cup cooked potatoes, diced	1 1/2 tsp. Worcestershire sauce
3 tbsp. chopped onion	1/2 tsp. salt
2 tbsp. diet margarine	1/8 tsp. pepper

Melt the margarine in a heavy, non-stick skillet and saute' the potatoes and onions until they are brown. Then stir in the remaining ingredients. Cook the mixture over low heat for about 10 minutes, stirring frequently, until the mixture is hot and well combined.
Makes 4 servings

Special note: If you do not have leftover potatoes, you may use canned potatoes or frozen slices that have been defrosted.

	Calories	Carbo-hydrate (gm)	Protein (gm)	Total Fat (gm)	Saturated Fat (gm)	Choles-terol (mg)
Total	1149.8	23.3	154.0	46.0	14.7	432.4
Per Serving	287.5	5.8	38.5	11.5	3.7	108.1

gm=grams; mg=milligrams. Nutritional figures are approximate. Figures are based on findings of U.S. Department of Agriculture.

Turkey Hurry Curry

3 cups diced cooked
turkey, loosely
packed
1 tbsp. diet margarine
1/2 cup finely chopped
onion
1 to 2 tbsp. curry
powder

2/3 cup water
10 1/2 oz. can condensed
cream of
chicken soup
lemon juice

Melt the margarine in a non-stick skillet and sauté the onions until they are tender. Stir in the curry powder and continue to heat the onions for a few seconds. Add the water and soup. Heat the mixture through, stirring continuously. Then add the turkey. Heat the mixture just until the turkey is heated through. Just before serving, add lemon juice according to your own taste. *Makes 6 servings*

	Calories	Carbo-hydrate (gm)	Protein (gm)	Total Fat (gm)	Saturated Fat (gm)	Choles-terol (mg)
Total	1191.8	27.2	155.2	49.2	12.7	433.0
Per Serving	198.6	4.5	25.9	8.2	2.1	72.2

Diced Turkey Cantonese

1 cup diced cooked
turkey, loosely
packed
1 cup diagonally-sliced
celery
1 cup thinly sliced
carrots
1 medium onion,
chopped
2 tbsp. slivered
almonds
2 tbsp. diet margarine
3/4 cup canned pineapple
chunks, packed in
juice

1/4 tsp. salt
1 tbsp. cornstarch
1/4 tsp. ground ginger
1/4 tsp. nutmeg
1 tbsp. soy sauce
1 tsp. lemon juice
5 oz. can water
chestnuts, thinly
sliced

Melt the margarine in a large non-stick skillet and sauté the celery, carrots, onion, and almonds until the nuts are lightly browned. Drain the pineapple, saving the juice. Add enough water to the juice to make 1¼ cups, and pour the mixture into the skillet. Add the salt, cornstarch, ginger, nutmeg, soy sauce, and lemon juice to the saucepan; and cook the mixture slowly, stirring constantly, until it has thickened. Then add the pineapple chunks, turkey, and water chestnuts. Continue cooking just until everything is heated through. Serve Diced Turkey Cantonese with Skinny Rice (the recipe is in "Potatoes, Pasta, and Rice").

Makes 4 servings

	Calories	Carbo-hydrate (gm)	Protein (gm)	Total Fat (gm)	Saturated Fat (gm)	Choles-terol (mg)
Total	842.4	94.5	56.5	30.6	5.7	127.3
Per Serving	210.6	23.6	14.1	7.7	1.4	31.8

Turkey Curry Salad with Fruit Garnish

2½ cups diced cooked
    turkey, loosely
    packed
⅓ cup plain yogurt
⅓ cup diet mayonnaise
1 tbsp. lemon juice
1 tsp. salt
1 tsp. curry powder
1½ cups diced celery

2 tbsp. slivered
    almonds
6 large lettuce
    leaves
½ cup seedless
    grapes, halved
1 cup canned
    pineapple
    chunks, packed
    in juice

Combine all of the ingredients except the almonds, lettuce, and fruit. Mix them lightly and chill them until serving time. Serve the salad on the lettuce leaves and garnish it with the almonds, grapes and pineapple chunks.

Makes 6 servings

	Calories	Carbo-hydrate (gm)	Protein (gm)	Total Fat (gm)	Saturated Fat (gm)	Choles-terol (mg)
Total	1634.6	69.9	204.1	59.3	13.8	595.7
Per Serving	272.4	11.6	34.0	9.9	2.3	99.3

gm=grams; mg=milligrams. Nutritional figures are approximate. Figures are based on findings of U.S. Department of Agriculture.

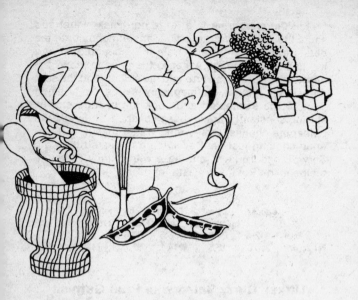

Turkey Divan

2 lbs. cooked turkey white meat or turkey roast	2 cups chicken stock
	3 tbsp. sherry
	salt
1 large bunch broccoli	pepper
4 tbsp. flour	1/4 cup grated
1/2 cup skim milk	Parmesan cheese

Before cooking: Cut the turkey into thin slices. Wash and drain the broccoli. Cook it in boiling salted water for about 10 minutes until it is tender. Drain it and keep it hot.

Make a sauce as follows: Put the flour in a saucepan. Over low heat, gradually add the chicken stock, stirring constantly until the mixture is thick and smooth. Then stir in the milk and sherry, and season it with salt and pepper according to your own taste.

Place the cooked broccoli on a hot oven-safe platter and pour half the sauce over it. To the remaining sauce, add the Parmesan cheese. Arrange the slices of turkey over the broccoli. Then cover the turkey slices with the remaining sauce. Set the dish under the broiler until the sauce bubbles and has lightly browned.

Makes 8 servings

Special note: If you do not have chicken stock, you may use canned stock. But don't forget to skim the fat by using a bulb-type baster. Also, if fresh broccoli isn't available, use 3 packages of frozen whole stalks.

	Calories	Carbo-hydrate (gm)	Protein (gm)	Total Fat (gm)	Saturated Fat (gm)	Choles-terol (mg)
Total	2403.2	81.7	374.7	63.5	21.1	799.1
Per Serving	300.4	10.2	46.8	7.9	2.6	99.9

Lamb 'N Macaroni Salad

3 cups diced cooked lean lamb, loosely packed
1 tbsp. salt
3 qts. boiling water
2 cups elbow macaroni
1 cup diced celery
1/2 cup diet mayonnaise

1/4 cup drained sweet pickle relish
2 tbsp. chopped onion
1 tsp. salt
1/8 tsp. pepper
8 large lettuce leaves

Add the salt to the rapidly boiling water. Gradually add the macaroni so that the water continues to boil. Cook the macaroni, uncovered, stirring it occasionally, until it is tender. Then drain it in a colander and rinse it with cold water. Combine the remaining ingredients and toss them with the macaroni. Chill the entire mixture and serve it on lettuce leaves. *Makes 8 servings*

	Calories	Carbo-hydrate (gm)	Protein (gm)	Total Fat (gm)	Saturated Fat (gm)	Choles-terol (mg)
Total	2125.7	175.3	214.8	60.5	28.8	713.6
Per Serving	265.7	21.9	26.9	7.6	3.6	89.2

---

gm=grams; mg=milligrams. Nutritional figures are approximate. Figures are based on findings of U.S. Department of Agriculture.

Greek Lamb and Vegetable Salad

2 cups cooked lamb,
  cut in julienne
  strips, loosely
  packed
2 tbsp. olive oil
2 tbsp. dry red wine
2 tbsp. lemon juice

garlic salt
pepper
1 tsp. crushed mint
  leaves
2 medium
  cucumbers
3 black olives
4 cups shredded
  lettuce

Before cooking: Dice the cucumbers. Slice the olives. Combine the oil, wine, lemon juice, garlic salt, pepper, and mint. Pour the mixture over the lamb strips, and let it sit at room temperature for several hours.

Add the cucumbers, and olives to the meat, and toss the mixture well. Arrange the meat and vegetables on the shredded lettuce.   *Makes 4 servings*

Diet hint: The heart-wise cook will want to use corn or safflower oil instead of olive oil — a savings of 2 grams of saturated fat.

	Calories	Carbo-hydrate (gm)	Protein (gm)	Total Fat (gm)	Saturated Fat (gm)	Choles-terol (mg)
Total	1002.6	26.4	82.9	58.6	17.8	294.4
Per Serving	250.7	6.6	20.7	14.7	4.5	73.6

Lamb and Rice Salad

3 cups cold cooked rice
2 cups cubed cooked
  lamb
1 medium tomato, diced
1/2 cup chopped red
  onion
1/2 cup chopped parsley

1/2 cup diet Italian
  salad dressing
3 tbsp. lemon juice
1/2 tsp. salt
1/4 tsp. pepper
  salad greens

242   CONSUMER GUIDE

Combine all of the ingredients, except the salad greens, in a bowl and mix them well. Chill the salad before serving it on the salad greens.

Makes 6 servings

	Calories	Carbo-hydrate (gm)	Protein (gm)	Total Fat (gm)	Saturated Fat (gm)	Choles-terol (mg)
Total	1412.8	166.6	107.1	31.0	13.8	326.6
Per Serving	235.5	27.8	17.9	5.2	2.3	54.4

Lamb Salad

1 lb. cooked lean leg of lamb
2 tbsp. chopped parsley
1 tbsp. instant minced onion
1 1/2 tsp. salt
1/4 tsp. pepper
1/3 cup vinegar

2 tbsp. corn or safflower oil
1/2 tsp. oregano
3 cups torn lettuce
2 medium tomatoes
1 cup chopped celery
1 cup cubed cooked potatoes

Before cooking: Dice the lamb and dice the tomatoes.
Combine the parsley, onion, salt, pepper, vinegar, oil, and oregano in a bowl. Add the lamb, and mix well. Chill this mixture for 1 hour, turning the lamb occasionally. Meanwhile, combine the rest of the ingredients, toss them lightly, and chill them also. Before serving, add the lamb mixture to the salad greens mixture and toss everything lightly but thoroughly.

Makes 6 servings

	Calories	Carbo-hydrate (gm)	Protein (gm)	Total Fat (gm)	Saturated Fat (gm)	Choles-terol (mg)
Total	1288.0	52.7	135.2	60.0	21.2	454.4
Per Serving	214.7	8.8	22.5	10.0	3.5	75.7

gm=grams; mg=milligrams. Nutritional figures are approximate. Figures are based on findings of U.S. Department of Agriculture.

North Carolina "Barbecued" Pork

3 lbs. leftover roast
   pork
  Sauce:
3 tbsp. catsup
3 tbsp. vinegar
1 tbsp. fresh lemon
  juice
2 tbsp. Worcestershire
  sauce

¼ cup water
1 tsp. salt
3 tbsp. brown sugar
  substitute
1 tsp. chili powder
1 tsp. paprika

Slice the roast, trimming off all fat; and cut the slices into 1- or 2-inch pieces. Place the pieces in a baking dish. Combine the sauce ingredients in a saucepan and bring the mixture to boil. Pour the sauce over the pork and heat it in the oven for 15 minutes at 325°. Do not allow the pork to dry out.   *Makes 12 servings*

	Calories	Carbo-hydrate (gm)	Protein (gm)	Total Fat (gm)	Saturated Fat (gm)	Choles-terol (mg)
Total	5011.6	16.2	336.1	384.0	144.0	1216.0
Per Serving	417.6	1.4	28.0	32.0	12.0	101.3

Ham and Cottage Cheese Filled Rolls

1 egg
1 cup 99% fat-free
  cottage cheese,
  drained
1 cup ground boiled
  ham
6 tbsp. shredded
  cheddar cheese

½ cup chopped
  onion
¼ cup catsup
2 tbsp. chopped
  green pepper
6 brown 'n serve
  club rolls
6 green pepper
  strips

Before preparing: Hard-boil the egg, and then separate the egg white and yolk. Press the yolk through a sieve and set it aside. Chop the egg white.

Combine the cottage cheese, ham, cheddar cheese,

onion, catsup, green pepper, and chopped egg white in a bowl. Cut a thin slice from the top of each roll, scoop out the bready center of the roll, leaving a thin shell. Fill the shells with the cottage cheese mixture, mounding it on top. Place them on a baking sheet and bake them for about 15 minutes at 375° until the roll is golden brown. Sprinkle the tops with egg yolk, and garnish each serving with a green pepper strip.

Makes 6 servings

	Calories	Carbo-hydrate (gm)	Protein (gm)	Total Fat (gm)	Saturated Fat (gm)	Choles-terol (mg)
Total	1773.5	140.6	110.9	81.0	33.2	523.9
Per Serving	295.6	23.4	18.5	13.5	5.5	87.2

Main Course Hot Ham and Potato Salad

1 cup lean boiled ham, diced
1 tbsp. diet margarine
2 potatoes
1/2 cup chopped onion

10 3/4 oz. can condensed cream of celery soup
4 tbsp. imitation sour cream
1/4 tsp. caraway seeds (optional)

Before preparing: Peel the potatoes and boil them. Cut the boiled potatoes into cubes and set them aside.

Melt the margarine in a non-stick skillet and sauté the ham and onions for 5 minutes. Add the soup, sour cream, and caraway seeds, and blend well. Then gently mix in the potatoes. Continue cooking until the mixture is heated thoroughly, but do not boil.

Makes 4 servings

	Calories	Carbo-hydrate (gm)	Protein (gm)	Total Fat (gm)	Saturated Fat (gm)	Choles-terol (mg)
Total	883.0	69.0	58.6	42.9	15.1	151.2
Per Serving	220.8	17.3	14.7	10.7	3.8	37.8

gm=grams; mg=milligrams. Nutritional figures are approximate. Figures are based on findings of U.S. Department of Agriculture.

Main Course Beef Stroganoff Salad

1 lb. cold cooked lean
   beef round, sliced
2 tbsp. dry sherry
3 tbsp. wine vinegar
1/2 tsp. prepared mustard

1 tbsp. catsup
1/4 cup yogurt
1/4 cup fresh sliced
   mushrooms
2 potatoes

Marinate the beef for 2 hours in a mixture of the sherry, vinegar, mustard, and catsup. In the meantime, peel the potatoes, boil them, dice them, and then put them aside. After the meat has marinated, mix the yogurt in with beef and marinade. Toss mixture with potatoes and mushrooms. Chill for serving.   *Makes 4 servings*

	Calories	Carbo-hydrate (gm)	Protein (gm)	Total Fat (gm)	Saturated Fat (gm)	Choles-terol (mg)
Total	1012.0	55.2	150.1	19.1	6.4	426.0
Per Serving	253.0	13.8	37.5	4.8	1.6	106.5

Roast Beef Salad

1 lb. leftover lean roast
   beef, thinly sliced
1 red onion
2 tbsp. corn or safflower
   oil
1/4 cup wine vinegar
1/4 cup chopped parsley

1 tbsp. capers
1 tsp. oregano
2 tsp. prepared
   mustard
1/2 tsp. garlic salt
1/4 tsp. pepper
1 large or 2 small
   heads of lettuce

Slice the onion, and combine it with all the ingredients, except the lettuce. Cover the mixture and let it marinate in the refrigerator for 3 hours or longer. At serving time, shred the lettuce and toss it with the rest of the salad.   *Makes 6 servings*

	Calories	Carbo-hydrate (gm)	Protein (gm)	Total Fat (gm)	Saturated Fat (gm)	Choles-terol (mg)
Total	1716.3	88.3	131.5	90.2	28.7	408.9
Per Serving	286.1	14.7	21.9	15.0	4.8	68.2

gm=grams; mg=milligrams. Nutritional figures are approximate. Figures are based on findings of U.S. Department of Agriculture.

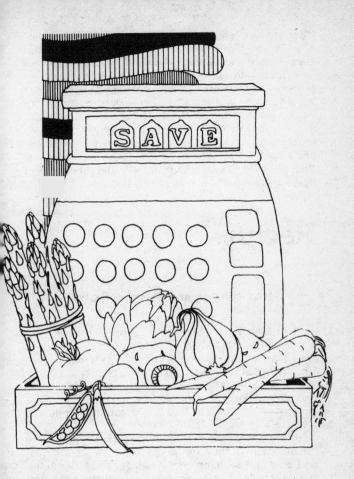

Budget~
Stretchers

Unfortunately, many packaged casserole mixes, "budget" recipes, and cafeteria concoctions are starch-laden, nutritionally-neutered pound-provokers — loaded with fat, but stingy on appetite-appeasing protein. Moreover, some packaged hamburger stretchers are not even a bargain — often costing more per pound than the meat they're supposed to replace.

But it is possible to eat inexpensively — and low-calorically. If you have to pinch pennies while counting calories, here are some low- or no-meat recipes that will help you tighten your belt, both literally and figuratively.

Recipes

Hamburger and Noodle Skillet

1 lb. lean ground beef
1 cup chopped onion
1 tbsp. diet margarine
1½ tsp. poultry seasoning
1 tsp. garlic salt
¼ tsp. pepper

6 oz. uncooked
   noodles
3 cups tomato juice
⅓ cup coarsely
   chopped green
   pepper
1 cup plain yogurt

Melt the margarine in a non-stick skillet, and sauté the onions until they are golden. Add the ground beef and continue sauteing until it has browned. Stir in the seasonings and noodles. Add the tomato juice and green pepper. Cover the pan and simmer the contents for about 30 minutes until the noodles are tender, stirring occasionally. Stir in the yogurt and continue cooking just until the yogurt is heated through.

Makes 6 servings

	Calories	Carbo-hydrate (gm)	Protein (gm)	Total Fat (gm)	Saturated Fat (gm)	Choles-terol (mg)
Total	1531.1	89.2	145.6	65.2	30.7	493.9
Per Serving	255.2	14.9	24.3	10.9	5.1	82.3

Hamburger Stroganoff with Noodles

1 lb. round steak,
    trimmed of fat, and
    ground
2 onions
1 cup water
4 cups tomato juice

2 tsp. garlic salt
1/4 tsp. pepper
2 tsp. Worcester-
    shire sauce
6 oz. curly egg
    noodles
1 cup plain yogurt

Before cooking: Chop the onions.

Saute the beef and onions in a large non-stick skillet. Do not add any oil because the meat will release enough of its own fat for frying. When the meat is brown, add 1 cup water to the skillet and bring it to a boil. Then drain all the liquid from the pan. This will remove the remaining fat from the meat. Stir in the tomato juice, salt, pepper, and Worcestershire sauce, and heat this mixture until it is boiling. Then add the noodles just a few at a time — so that the mixture continues to boil. When all the noodles have been added, cover the skillet, reduce the heat, and simmer the contents for 10 minutes or longer, stirring occasionally, until they are tender. Then stir in the yogurt, and continue cooking just until the yogurt is heated through but is not boiling. *Makes 6 servings*

	Calories	Carbo-hydrate (gm)	Protein (gm)	Total Fat (gm)	Saturated Fat (gm)	Choles-terol (mg)
Total	1501.8	142.6	175.4	27.5	9.7	535.8
Per Serving	250.3	23.8	29.2	4.6	1.6	89.3

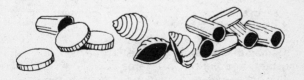

gm=grams; mg=milligrams. Nutritional figures are approximate. Figures are based on findings of U.S. Department of Agriculture.

Chili Mexicana

1 lb. ground beef
1 cup water
3 tbsp. instant chopped
   onion
1 tsp. garlic powder
2 tbsp. chili powder

1 tsp. salt
14½ oz. can whole
   tomatoes,
   undrained
1 lb. 14 oz. can red
   kidney beans,
   undrained

Brown the meat in a non-stick skillet. Do not add any oil because the meat will release enough of its own fat for frying. When the meat is brown, add 1 cup water to the pan and let it come to a boil. Then drain the liquid from the pan. This will remove the rest of the fat from the meat. Add all of the remaining ingredients, except the beans, cover the pan, and let the mixture simmer for 1 hour. Then add the beans, and continue simmering, uncovered, for about 15 minutes — until most of the liquid has evaporated.   *Makes 6 servings*

	Calories	Carbo-hydrate (gm)	Protein (gm)	Total Fat (gm)	Saturated Fat (gm)	Choles-terol (mg)
Total	1946.7	177.5	182.9	58.9	26.7	426.4
Per Serving	324.5	29.6	30.5	9.8	4.5	71.1

Cottage Meat Loaf

1¼ lbs. lean round steak,
   ground
1 egg, slightly beaten
1½ tsp. Worcestershire
   sauce
1 tsp. salt
¾ tsp. dry mustard

⅛ tsp. pepper
1 cup 99% fat-free
   cottage cheese
½ cup minced onion
¼ cup minced green
   pepper

Combine the egg, Worcestershire sauce, salt, mustard, and pepper in a large bowl. Then add the meat, cottage cheese, onion, and green pepper. Mix everything together lightly, but thoroughly. Shape the mixture into a loaf and place it in a shallow baking pan. Bake it at 350° for 50 to 60 minutes. Let the meat

loaf stand for a few minutes before removing it from the
pan to serve. *Makes 6 servings*

	Calories	Carbo-hydrate (gm)	Protein (gm)	Total Fat (gm)	Saturated Fat (gm)	Choles-terol (mg)
Total	1210.1	12.0	215.1	30.2	10.6	797.5
Per Serving	201.7	2.0	35.9	5.0	1.8	132.9

Beef-Noodle Casserole

1 lb. lean round steak,
   trimmed of fat and
   ground
8 oz. package medium
   noodles
1/3 cup sliced green
   onions
1/3 cup chopped green
   pepper

6 oz. can tomato
   paste
1/2 cup yogurt
1/4 tsp. salt
1 cup 99% fat-free
   cottage cheese
8 oz. can tomato
   sauce

Cook the noodles according to the directions on the
package. Meanwhile, heat a large non-stick skillet.
Add the meat and brown it slowly. Do not add any oil to
the pan because the meat will release enough of its
own fat for frying. After the meat is browned, pour off
the fat that has accumulated in the pan. Then add the
onions and green pepper, and continue cooking until
they are tender. Set the meat aside. Stir the tomato
paste, yogurt, and salt together in a large bowl; add
the cooked and drained noodles and the cottage
cheese. In a baking dish, place half the meat mixture.
Add the noodle mixture and top with the remaining
meat mixture. Pour the tomato sauce over all. Bake the
casserole at 350° for 30 to 35 minutes until it is heated
through. *Makes 8 servings*

	Calories	Carbo-hydrate (gm)	Protein (gm)	Total Fat (gm)	Saturated Fat (gm)	Choles-terol (mg)
Total	1501.2	119.4	195.8	25.0	9.5	520.4
Per Serving	187.7	14.9	24.5	3.1	1.2	65.1

gm=grams; mg=milligrams. Nutritional figures are approximate. Figures
are based on findings of U.S. Department of Agriculture.

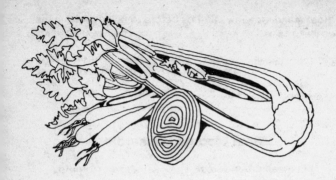

Hi-Protein Swedish Meat Balls

1 lb. lean ground round steak	$^1/_8$ tsp. pepper
1 cup soy granules	$^1/_4$ tsp. nutmeg
1 cup skim milk	1 cup beef broth, canned or bouillon
1 egg, well beaten	
2 medium onions	1 tbsp. flour
2 tsp. salt	2 tbsp. cold water

Before cooking: If you are using canned broth, chill it until the fat rises to the top, hardens, and can be lifted off. Chop the onions.

Combine the meat with the soy granules, milk, egg, onions and seasonings. Mix them together well, and form the meat into 1-inch balls. Spray a non-stick skillet with spray-on vegetable coating for no-fat frying. Heat the pan and brown the meat balls over moderate heat. Add the broth to the skillet, stirring and scraping the pan well. In a cup, combine the flour with 2 tablespoons cold water. Mix them together well and then stir the flour mixture into the skillet. Bring the contents of the skillet to a boil, cooking and stirring, until the sauce has thickened. Then cover the pan, lower the heat and simmer the meat balls for about 20 minutes, adding more water if necessary. If you like, you may add a few drops of brown gravy coloring.

Makes 6 servings

Diet hint: To save an extra 50 calories (about 8 per serving), use 2 egg whites instead of 1 whole egg.

	Calories	Carbohydrate (gm)	Protein (gm)	Total Fat (gm)	Saturated Fat (gm)	Cholesterol (mg)
Total	1472.6	71.9	234.7	60.3	9.1	702.0
Per Serving	245.4	12.0	39.1	10.1	1.5	117.0

Skillet Chili and Macaroni

³/₄ lb. lean ground beef
1 onion
1 green pepper
2 cups water
8 oz. protein-enriched elbow macaroni

16 oz. can of kidney beans and liquid
2 (8 oz.) cans tomato sauce
1 tsp. chili powder
1 tsp. salt
¹/₂ cup shredded cheddar cheese (2 oz.)

Before cooking: Chop the onion and green pepper.

Brown the ground beef, onion, and green pepper in a large non-stick skillet. Do not add any oil to the pan because the meat will release enough of its own fat for frying. After the meat and vegetables are brown add 1 cup water to the pan and let it come to a boil. Then drain off the liquid from the pan. This will remove the remaining fat from the meat. Next, add an additional cup of water to the pan and all of the remaining ingredients — except the cheese. Simmer this mixture for about 15 minutes, stirring constantly, until most of the liquid has evaporated. Then sprinkle the cheese over the top of the meat and continue heating until it has melted. *Makes 8 servings*

	Calories	Carbohydrate (gm)	Protein (gm)	Total Fat (gm)	Saturated Fat (gm)	Cholesterol (mg)
Total	1961.3	202.7	154.4	63.1	30.0	376.0
Per Serving	245.2	25.3	19.3	7.9	3.8	47.0

---

gm=grams; mg=milligrams. Nutritional figures are approximate. Figures are based on findings of U.S. Department of Agriculture.

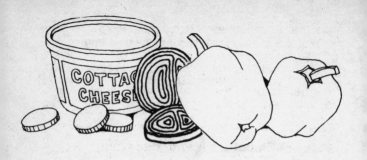

Lasagna

1 lb. lean round steak, trimmed of fat and ground
8 oz. protein-enriched lasagna noodles
1 cup 99% fat-free cottage cheese
1 egg
3 tbsp. extra-sharp grated Romano cheese
1 tsp. garlic salt
¼ tsp. pepper
1 tsp. oregano
2 tbsp. parsley
1½ cups canned tomato sauce
1 tbsp. Italian seasoned bread crumbs

Brown the meat in a skillet, breaking it up as it cooks. Do not add oil to the pan because the meat will release enough of its own fat for frying. Drain off any accumulated fat after the meat has browned. At the same time, cook the noodles in boiling salted water for about 18 minutes until they are tender. Drain them and rinse them well. In a bowl, combine the cottage cheese, egg, Romano cheese, garlic salt, pepper, oregano and parsley. In a 2-quart shallow baking dish, arrange the noodles, meat, cheese mixture and tomato sauce in layers. Sprinkle the bread crumbs evenly over the top. Bake the lasagna in a 350° oven for 30 to 45 minutes.   *Makes 8 servings*

	Calories	Carbo-hydrate (gm)	Protein (gm)	Total Fat (gm)	Saturated Fat (gm)	Choles-terol (mg)
Total	2118.1	130.9	204.0	83.4	41.5	870.6
Per Serving	264.8	16.4	25.5	10.4	5.2	108.8

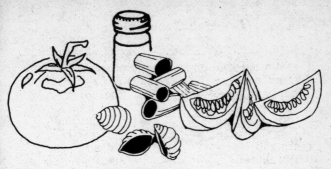

Tacos

1 lb. lean round steak,
    trimmed of fat and
    ground
1 onion
1 cup canned corn with
    sweet peppers
8 oz. can Spanish-style
    tomato sauce
    sugar substitute to
    equal 1 tbsp.

1/2 tsp. oregano
1/8 tsp. chili powder
1/2 tsp. ground cumin
1/2 tsp. garlic salt
6 tacos shells
    (packaged or
    frozen)

Before cooking: Chop the onion. Drain the corn and peppers.

Brown the ground beef and onion in a non-stick skillet. Do not add any oil to the pan because the meat will release enough of its own fat for frying. After the meat has browned, drain off the fat that has accumulated in the pan. Then stir in the corn, tomato sauce, oregano, chili powder, cumin and garlic salt. Simmer the entire mixture, uncovered, for 15 to 20 minutes until all of the sauce is absorbed. Then stir in the sugar substitute. Serve the taco filling in the tacos shells.

Makes 6 servings

	Calories	Carbo-hydrate (gm)	Protein (gm)	Total Fat (gm)	Saturated Fat (gm)	Choles-terol (mg)
Total	1312.0	114.9	156.4	39.2	14.3	413.5
Per Serving	218.7	19.2	26.1	6.5	2.4	68.9

gm=grams; mg=milligrams. Nutritional figures are approximate. Figures are based on findings of U.S. Department of Agriculture.

Goulash Casserole

1½ lbs. round steak,
    trimmed of fat, and
    ground
1 cup high-protein
    cereal,
    unsweetened
1 egg, slightly beaten
1 tsp. salt
⅛ tsp. nutmeg

⅛ tsp. thyme
⅛ tsp. pepper
2 (10¾ oz.) cans
    condensed
    tomato soup
½ cup "V-8" juice
2 cups cooked
    protein-enriched
    macaroni
5 tbsp. shredded
    cheddar cheese

Before cooking: Cook the macaroni, according to the directions on the package, to yield 2 cups.

Combine the beef, cereal, egg and seasonings in a large bowl. Shape the meat mixture into 24 meat balls and set them on a non-stick baking sheet. Place them in a 450° oven — or under the broiler — just until the meat is brown. Transfer the meat balls to a casserole, and add the soup, "V-8" juice and macaroni. Bake the casserole at 400° for 35 minutes, stirring occasionally. Then sprinkle the cheese over the top and continue to bake for about 5 minutes — until the cheese has melted. *Makes 8 servings*

	Calories	Carbo-hydrate (gm)	Protein (gm)	Total Fat (gm)	Saturated Fat (gm)	Choles-terol (mg)
Total	2335.6	171.6	260.9	70.4	21.9	944.8
Per Serving	292.0	21.5	32.6	8.8	2.7	118.1

Lamb Loaf

1 lb. lean ground lamb
1 cup crushed protein
    cereal, such as
    Special K
1 cup skim milk
¼ cup chopped green
    peppers
¼ cup chopped onions

¼ cup catsup
2 Tbsp. finely
    chopped
    pimiento
1½ tsp. salt
½ tsp. paprika
¼ tsp. black pepper

Combine the meat and cereal, and mix them well. Add the rest of the ingredients to the meat, mixing thoroughly. Then press the meat into a loaf pan, and bake it at 350° for 45 minutes to 1 hour.

Makes 6 servings

	Calories	Carbo-hydrate (gm)	Protein (gm)	Total Fat (gm)	Saturated Fat (gm)	Choles-terol (mg)
Total	1089.5	49.5	142.6	32.4	19.2	459.4
Per Serving	181.6	8.3	23.8	5.4	3.2	76.6

Fresh Mushroom Cheese Quiche

"Single Crust Pie Pastry" (see recipe in "Unforbidden Sweets")
1 cup shredded Swiss cheese
2 tbsp. flour
2 eggs, beaten
³/₄ cup skim milk
¹/₂ tsp. dried summer savory, crumbled
¹/₂ tsp. salt
¹/₄ tsp. pepper
2 cups fresh sliced mushrooms

Before cooking: Prepare a "Single Crust Pie Pastry." The recipe is in "Unforbidden Sweets." After the dough has been chilled according to the directions, roll it out and place it in a 9-inch pie pan. Flute the edges.

Toss the shredded cheese with the flour in a bowl. Then add the beaten eggs, milk and seasonings, and fold in the sliced mushrooms. Turn this mixture into the pastry-lined pan and bake the quiche at 350° for about 1 hour until it has browned.

Makes 6 servings

	Calories	Carbo-hydrate (gm)	Protein (gm)	Total Fat (gm)	Saturated Fat (gm)	Choles-terol (mg)
Total	1712.2	79.9	98.0	105.6	38.0	747.8
Per Serving	285.4	13.3	16.3	17.6	6.3	124.6

gm=grams; mg=milligrams. Nutritional figures are approximate. Figures are based on findings of U.S. Department of Agriculture.

Egg Foo Yong (Chinese Omelets)

3½ oz. finely-diced, chicken, tuna, shrimp or lobster

4 eggs soy sauce or Chinese gravy

2 tbsp. minced onions

¼ cup sliced water chestnuts

1 cup bean sprouts (or substitute onions, chestnuts and bean sprouts with 2½ cups canned mixed Chinese vegetables)

Toss the onion, water chestnuts and bean sprouts (or the mixed Chinese vegetables) together in a bowl with the chicken or fish. Beat the eggs in another bowl. Spray a non-stick skillet with spray-on vegetable coating for no-fat frying and heat the pan. Pour ¼ cup of the beaten eggs and ¼ cup of the vegetable-meat mixture into the skillet. Cook them over moderate heat until the egg has set; then flip one-half of the omelet over the other half. Continue to cook the omelet for another 1 or 2 minutes until the egg has set completely. Remove the omelet to a platter and place it in a 200° oven to keep warm. Repeat the same process 5 more times to make 6 omelets. Serve the Egg Foo Yong with soy sauce or Chinese gravy. *Makes 6 servings*

	Calories	Carbo-hydrate (gm)	Protein (gm)	Total Fat (gm)	Saturated Fat (gm)	Choles-terol (mg)
Total	527.6	16.5	51.9	27.5	9.2	1085.7
Per Serving	87.9	2.8	8.7	4.6	1.5	181.0

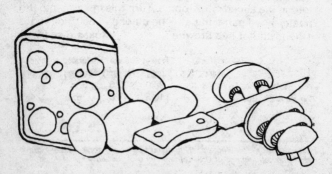

Hi-Protein Pizza

1½ cup soy pancake mix
2 tbsp. corn or safflower oil
2 eggs
¼ cup skim milk
¼ tsp. salt
16 oz. can tomatoes in puree
oregano or mixed Italian seasonings
1 cup shredded part-skim mozzarella (pizza cheese)

4 tbsp. extra-sharp grated Romano
½ tsp. garlic salt
¼ tsp. black pepper
¼ tsp. crushed red pepper
1 cup sliced mushrooms or onion or green pepper or thinly sliced zucchini (optional)

To make the crust, mix together the pancake mix, oil, eggs, milk and salt. Knead them enough so that the dough isn't sticky. Spray a 14-inch non-stick pizza pan with spray-on vegetable coating and press the dough onto the pan until it is completely covered. Bake the crust in a preheated 400° oven for about 8 minutes and then remove it from the oven.

Break up the tomatoes with a fork and spread them (with the puree) evenly over the crust. Then sprinkle on the seasonings, cheeses and optional toppings, and return the pizza to the hot oven just until the cheese is melted and bubbly. To serve, cut the pizza into wedges.   *Makes 6 servings*

Special note: Hi-Protein Pizza can be cut into much smaller wedges to be served as a delicious appetizer or party snack.

	Calories	Carbo-hydrate (gm)	Protein (gm)	Total Fat (gm)	Saturated Fat (gm)	Choles-terol (mg)
Total	1938.5	186.6	148.1	166.6	22.0	642.0
Per Serving	323.1	31.1	24.7	27.8	3.7	107.0

---

gm=grams; mg=milligrams. Nutritional figures are approximate. Figures are based on findings of U.S. Department of Agriculture.

Skinny Salads And Dressings

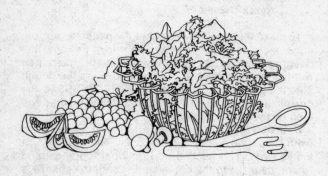

Salads — everybody knows — are slimming. Or are they? Although the business end of a salad is slim, the toppings and trimmings are often a weight-inflating wipeout. A whole bowlful of shredded lettuce weighs in at less than 100 calories, but two tablespoons of bottled French dressing add 120 calories or more. Real French dressing — the kind you make with oil and vinegar — fluctuates in calories depending on the ratio of oil to vinegar you use. The oil portion weighs in at 125 calories per tablespoon. And if you like mayonnaise-based dressings, remember that mayonnaise is almost as fattening as butter: close to 1600 calories a cupful.

Luckily for waistline-watchers, salad dressing makers have come to the rescue with a variety of slimmed-down toppings with only a fraction of the usual fat and calories. Low-cal versions of nearly every favorite are available: French, Italian, Russian, Bleu Cheese, Caesar, Coleslaw and Mayonnaise. Name it and you'll find it somewhere.

The savings are not to be sneered at. Consider, for example, the caloric comparison of a tuna salad made with a 7-ounce can of water-packed tuna and 5 tablespoons diet mayonnaise: total, 320 calories. The same tuna salad made with oil-packed tuna and regular mayonnaise would add up to a whopping 1077 calories.

Because salads are chock full of vitamins, appetite-appeasing bulk and regularity-producing roughage, they should be a daily part of every dieter's slim-down plan. Here's a variety of salad ideas — proof that salads can be delicious and exciting.

For do-it-yourself dressing makers, we also have included a number of de-calorized variations of fattening favorites — all designed to take salad dressings off the "forbidden" list.

Recipes

Waldorf Salad

3 red apples	5 tbsp. vanilla yogurt
1/8 tsp. salt	2 cups diced celery
5 tbsp. diet mayonnaise	4 tbsp. chopped walnuts

Core and dice the apples and combine them with all of the ingredients except the nuts. Chill the salad before serving. When you are ready to serve the salad, garnish it with the nuts. *Makes 6 servings*

	Calories	Carbo-hydrate (gm)	Protein (gm)	Total Fat (gm)	Saturated Fat (gm)	Choles-terol (mg)
Total	576.3	79.8	9.0	30.0	1.6	46.2
Per Serving	96.1	13.3	1.5	5.0	0.3	7.7

gm=grams; mg=milligrams. Nutritional figures are approximate. Figures are based on findings of U.S. Department of Agriculture.

Pineapple Waldorf Salad

4 small or 2 large tart
apples
2 cups pineapple
chunks, packed in
juice

2 cups chopped
celery
4 tbsp. chopped
walnuts
1/2 cup diet
mayonnaise

Drain the pineapple. Peel the apples and chop them.
Combine the pineapple chunks and apple pieces with
the rest of the ingredients. Chill the salad before serving.   *Makes 10 servings*

	Calories	Carbo-hydrate (gm)	Protein (gm)	Total Fat (gm)	Saturated Fat (gm)	Choles-terol (mg)
Total	823.7	136.8	6.5	34.8	1.0	64.0
Per Serving	82.4	13.7	0.7	3.5	0.1	6.4

Cran-Apple Cream Cheese Salad

4- serving envelope
cherry-flavored
diet gelatin
1 cup boiling water
1/2 cup orange juice
8 oz. low-calorie cream
cheese

8 oz. can jellied
cranberry sauce
1/2 tsp. grated orange
peel
1/4 tsp. salt
3 cups chopped red
apples,
unpeeled
1 cup 99% fat-free
cottage cheese
lettuce leaves

Pour the boiling water over the gelatin in a bowl, and
stir until it dissolves. Stir in the orange juice. In another
bowl beat the cream cheese until it is soft and creamy.
Very gradually beat in the cranberry sauce until the
mixture is smooth. Beat in the orange peel and salt.
Then gradually beat in the gelatin mixture. Chill the
mixture until it has a jelly-like consistency. Then fold in
2 cups of the apples. Turn the mixture into a ring mold,

and chill it until it is firm. When ready to serve, turn the mold out onto a lettuce-lined plate. Combine the cottage cheese with the remaining 1 cup of apple and spoon this mixture into the center of the mold.

Makes 8 servings

Special hint: To prevent discoloration of remaining chopped apple, sprinkle with lemon juice and store in refrigerator until serving time.

	Calories	Carbo-hydrate (gm)	Protein (gm)	Total Fat (gm)	Saturated Fat (gm)	Choles-terol (mg)
Total	1428.1	182.7	53.0	51.3	33.2	187.4
Per Serving	178.5	22.8	6.6	6.4	4.2	23.4

Two-Bean Salad

16 oz. can sliced green
beans
16 oz. can French-style
sliced yellow beans
1/4 cup onion flakes
1 cup diced celery

1/2 envelope French
salad dressing
mix
1 cup buttermilk
2 tbsp. finely
chopped
pimiento
1/2 tsp. oregano
dash of salt

Before preparing: Drain the green beans and yellow beans.

Mix the beans, onion flakes and celery in a bowl. In another bowl, combine the salad dressing mix with the buttermilk. Add the rest of the ingredients. Pour this mixture over the beans and toss lightly. Chill the bean salad for several hours before serving.

Makes 8 servings

	Calories	Carbo-hydrate (gm)	Protein (gm)	Total Fat (gm)	Saturated Fat (gm)	Choles-terol (mg)
Total	313.3	63.8	21.1	0.3	0.0	5.0
Per Serving	39.2	8.0	2.6	0.0	0.0	0.6

gm=grams; mg=milligrams. Nutritional figures are approximate. Figures are based on findings of U.S. Department of Agriculture.

Marrakesh Salad

1 small onion
2 large green peppers
3 medium tomatoes
1 tbsp. olive oil
3 tbsp. wine vinegar

2 tsp. ground cumin
3 tbsp. dry wine
1 tsp. salt
1 tsp. pepper
1 tbsp. chopped parsley

Before preparing: Cut the onion into thin slices. Cut the green pepper into 1-inch squares. Peel the tomatoes and cut them into cubes. Tomatoes can be easily peeled if they are first plunged into boiling water.

Combine the oil, vinegar, cumin, wine, salt, pepper and parsley in a bowl. Then add the onion, green pepper and tomato cubes. Toss the mixture well, and refrigerate it until it is thoroughly chilled. When serving, sprinkle more chopped parsley over the top as garnish.   *Makes 6 servings*

	Calories	Carbohydrate (gm)	Protein (gm)	Total Fat (gm)	Saturated Fat (gm)	Cholesterol (mg)
Total	335.6	44.7	9.0	14.0	2.0	0.0
Per Serving	55.9	7.5	1.5	2.3	0.3	0.0

Chinese Celery Tomato Salad

2 cups finely chopped Chinese celery cabbage
1/2 tsp. garlic salt
2 medium tomatoes

1/2 tsp. dry mustard
1 tbsp. water
1 tbsp. soy sauce
1 tbsp. corn oil

Chop the tomatoes finely and mix them with the rest of the ingredients. Chill the salad before serving.
                                   Makes 6 servings

	Calories	Carbohydrate (gm)	Protein (gm)	Total Fat (gm)	Saturated Fat (gm)	Cholesterol (mg)
Total	235.0	23.0	7.0	14.0	1.0	0.0
Per Serving	39.2	3.8	1.2	2.3	0.2	0.0

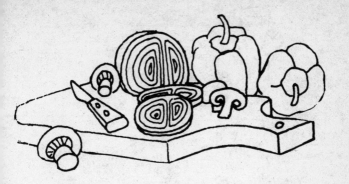

Mushroom Salad

1 lb. fresh mushrooms
1 cup diced celery
1 cup diced green
 pepper
2 tbsp. finely chopped
 onion
1 tbsp. olive oil

1 tbsp. wine vinegar
2 tsp. salt
¹/₈ tsp. ground black
 pepper
2 tbsp. lemon juice

Before preparing: Rinse the mushrooms and pat them dry. Cut them into slices.

Place the sliced mushrooms, celery, green pepper and onion in a salad bowl. Mix the remaining ingredients in another bowl. Then pour this mixture over the vegetables and toss gently.   *Makes 6 servings*

Diet hint: The heart-conscious person can save 1 gram of saturated fat by using corn or safflower oil instead of olive oil.

	Calories	Carbo-hydrate (gm)	Protein (gm)	Total Fat (gm)	Saturated Fat (gm)	Choles-terol (mg)
Total	509.0	69.9	36.4	19.0	2.0	0.0
Per Serving	84.8	11.7	6.1	3.2	0.3	0.0

gm=grams; mg=milligrams. Nutritional figures are approximate. Figures are based on findings of U.S. Department of Agriculture.

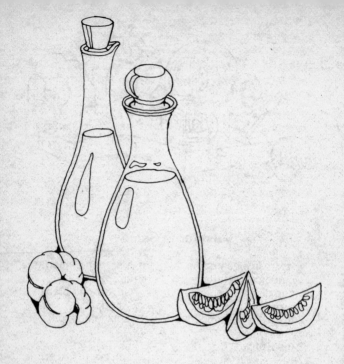

Tomato-Cucumber Vinaigrette

3 tbsp. vinegar
1 tbsp. corn or safflower
   oil
$1/2$ tsp. sugar
$1/2$ tsp. salt
$1/4$ tsp. ground black
   pepper

$1/4$ tsp. basil
1 tsp. instant minced
   onion
1 medium cucumber
3 large tomatoes

Before preparing: Peel and slice the cucumber. Slice
the tomatoes and place them in the refrigerator.
  Combine the vinegar, oil, sugar, salt, pepper, basil

and onion in a jar or shaker. Shake the mixture well and pour it over the cucumber slices. Cover this mixture and chill it for 1 hour. Before serving, pour the cucumber mixture over the sliced tomatoes and mix gently. *Makes 8 servings*

	Calories	Carbo-hydrate (gm)	Protein (gm)	Total Fat (gm)	Saturated Fat (gm)	Choles-terol (mg)
Total	409.2	66.8	13.1	14.0	1.0	0.0
Per Serving	51.2	8.4	1.6	1.8	0.1	0.0

Cottage Shrimp Mold

1 lb. frozen shelled
   deveined shrimp
2 tbsp. (2 envelopes)
   unflavored gelatin
3/4 cup water

2 cups 99% fat-free
   cottage cheese
1 cup yogurt
1 cup chili sauce
1/4 cup finely chopped
   celery
salad greens

Before preparing: Cook the shrimp according to the directions on the package, and then cut them into pieces. Save a few shrimp and split them lengthwise instead of cutting them in pieces.

Place the water in a small saucepan. Sprinkle the gelatin over it and let it stand for a few minutes until it softens. Then heat the water slowly, stirring constantly, until the gelatin has dissolved. Allow it to cool slightly. In a large bowl, combine the cottage cheese, yogurt, chili sauce, celery, cut-up shrimp and gelatin; and blend them thoroughly. Arrange the split shrimp in a mold and then fill the mold with the cottage cheese mixture. Chill the mold until it is firm. Unmold it onto salad greens. *Makes 8 servings*

	Calories	Carbo-hydrate (gm)	Protein (gm)	Total Fat (gm)	Saturated Fat (gm)	Choles-terol (mg)
Total	1205.2	95.9	160.0	13.3	4.4	741.1
Per Serving	150.7	12.0	20.0	1.7	0.6	92.6

gm=grams; mg=milligrams. Nutritional figures are approximate. Figures are based on findings of U.S. Department of Agriculture.

Cottage Cheese Garden Salad

1¹/₂ cups 99% fat-free
    cottage cheese
5 tbsp. diet mayonnaise
1¹/₂ tsp. salt
1 cup shredded carrot
2 cups thinly-sliced
    celery

1 cup diced
    cucumber,
    unpeeled
¹/₂ cup chopped
    green or red
    pepper
¹/₄ cup sliced
    radishes
¹/₄ cup chopped
    onion
8 large lettuce
    leaves

Combine the ingredients and chill them before serving. Serve the salad on the lettuce leaves.

Makes 8 servings

	Calories	Carbo-hydrate (gm)	Protein (gm)	Total Fat (gm)	Saturated Fat (gm)	Choles-terol (mg)
Total	482.3	46.1	48.7	13.0	1.8	69.1
Per Serving	60.3	5.8	6.1	1.6	0.2	8.6

Stuffed Tomatoes

6 medium tomatoes
2 cups 99% fat-free
    cottage cheese
¹/₄ cup chopped
    pimiento-stuffed
    olives
¹/₄ cup shredded carrot

¹/₄ cup chopped
    pecans
2 tbsp. chopped
    onion
6 large lettuce
    leaves

Before preparing: Turn the tomatoes stem end down and cut each one into 6 sections, cutting only ²/₃ of the way down. Gently spread the sections apart. Chill the tomatoes before filling them.

Combine the cottage cheese, olives, carrot, pecans and onion in a bowl. Toss the mixture lightly. Just before serving, place the tomatoes on the lettuce and fill them with the cottage cheese mixture.

Makes 6 servings

	Calories	Carbo-hydrate (gm)	Protein (gm)	Total Fat (gm)	Saturated Fat (gm)	Choles-terol (mg)
Total	845.2	73.8	75.3	29.3	3.7	38.8
Per Serving	140.9	12.3	12.6	4.9	0.6	6.5

Cottage Cheese Asparagus Mold

1 tbsp. unflavored gelatin (1 envelope)	2 tbsp. lemon juice
1/4 cup water	1/2 tsp. prepared mustard
14 1/2 oz. can cut asparagus	1/2 tsp. salt
1 1/2 cups 99% fat-free cottage cheese	1/4 cup chopped blanched almonds
	salad greens

Before cooking: Force the cottage cheese through a sieve to remove the lumps or beat it in a blender. Drain the asparagus, reserving the liquid. Add enough water to the liquid to make 1 cup.

Sprinkle the gelatin over the 1/4 cup water to soften it. In a 1-quart saucepan, bring the liquid and water from the asparagus to a boil. Stir in the softened gelatin until it is dissolved and let the mixture cool slightly. Combine the cottage cheese, lemon juice, mustard, salt, almonds and asparagus in a bowl. Add this mixture to the saucepan. Turn the contents of the saucepan into a mold and chill it until it is firm. Unmold it onto salad greens.

Makes 8 servings

	Calories	Carbo-hydrate (gm)	Protein (gm)	Total Fat (gm)	Saturated Fat (gm)	Choles-terol (mg)
Total	608.6	34.8	65.9	24.0	3.3	29.1
Per Serving	76.1	4.4	8.2	3.0	0.4	3.6

---

gm=grams; mg=milligrams. Nutritional figures are approximate. Figures are based on findings of U.S. Department of Agriculture.

Celery Slaw

4 cups thinly-sliced celery	1 tbsp. cider vinegar
1/3 cup coarsely shredded carrots	2 tsp. salt
3 tbsp. raisins	1/2 tsp. ground white pepper
3 tbsp. coarsely chopped walnuts	2/3 cup plain yogurt

Combine the celery, carrots, raisins, and walnuts in a large bowl. Set this mixture aside. Blend the vinegar, salt and pepper together in a bowl. Stir in the yogurt. Pour the dressing over the celery mixture and toss lightly. If you like, you can serve the Celery Slaw on lettuce leaves. *Makes 8 servings*

	Calories	Carbo-hydrate (gm)	Protein (gm)	Total Fat (gm)	Saturated Fat (gm)	Choles-terol (mg)
Total	546.8	106.5	10.9	16.9	2.1	13.2
Per Serving	68.4	13.3	1.4	2.1	0.3	1.7

Orchard Coleslaw

1/4 cup evaporated skim milk	1/4 tsp. celery seeds
1/4 cup diet mayonnaise	1 tsp. salt
2 tbsp. cider vinegar	1 large red apple
1 tsp. dry mustard	6 lightly packed cups shredded green cabbage (about a 2 1/4 lb. head)
sugar substitute to equal 2 tbsp.	

Before preparing: Dice the apple, but don't peel it.
Whisk all of the ingredients, except the apple and cabbage, together in a medium mixing bowl. Then mix in the apple and cabbage. Cover the coleslaw and chill it until ready to serve. *Makes 6 servings*

	Calories	Carbo-hydrate (gm)	Protein (gm)	Total Fat (gm)	Saturated Fat (gm)	Choles-terol (mg)
Total	358.2	60.0	10.5	13.0	2.7	51.5
Per Serving	59.7	10.0	1.8	2.2	0.5	8.6

Crunchy Salad

4- serving envelope
lemon-flavored diet
gelatin
1 cup boiling water
1 cup cold water

1 tbsp. instant
onions
3/4 cup finely
shredded green
cabbage
1/4 cup diced
cucumber
1/4 cup toasted soy
nuts

Dissolve the gelatin in the boiling water. Then add the cold water. Chill the gelatin until it is thick but not set. Then fold in the remaining ingredients. Pour the mixture into a 1-quart mold and chill it until it is firm.

Makes 6 servings

	Calories	Carbo-hydrate (gm)	Protein (gm)	Total Fat (gm)	Saturated Fat (gm)	Choles-terol (mg)
Total	281.4	46.6	16.0	4.7	0.2	0.0
Per Serving	46.9	7.8	2.7	0.8	0.0	0.0

Coleslaw

4 cups shredded
cabbage
1/2 small onion

4 tbsp. diet
mayonnaise
4 tbsp. plain or
lemon yogurt

Mince the onion and combine it with the other ingredients. Chill the coleslaw before serving it.

Makes 4 servings

	Calories	Carbo-hydrate (gm)	Protein (gm)	Total Fat (gm)	Saturated Fat (gm)	Choles-terol (mg)
Total	211.3	32.3	7.0	9.0	0.5	37.0
Per Serving	52.8	8.1	1.8	2.3	0.1	9.3

---

gm=grams; mg=milligrams. Nutritional figures are approximate. Figures are based on findings of U.S. Department of Agriculture.

Confetti Coleslaw

5 cups finely shredded
    green cabbage
1 cup shredded raw
    carrot
1 red apple
1/4 cup chopped green
    pepper
1/2 cup evaporated skim
    milk

sugar substitute to
    equal 3 tbsp.
1/4 tsp. salt
1/8 tsp. pepper
1/4 cup cider vinegar

Before preparing: Peel the apple, core it and dice it.
   Combine the apple with the cabbage, carrot and
green pepper. Blend evaporated skim milk, the sugar
substitute, salt and pepper together in a small bowl.
Gradually stir in the vinegar. Pour the dressing over
the vegetables, and toss lightly to blend. Cover the
coleslaw and chill it until you are ready to serve.
Makes 6 servings

	Calories	Carbo-hydrate (gm)	Protein (gm)	Total Fat (gm)	Saturated Fat (gm)	Choles-terol (mg)
Total	390.3	70.0	16.3	10.0	5.5	39.0
Per Serving	65.1	11.7	2.7	1.7	0.9	6.5

Thousand Island Dressing

1 small dill pickle
1 tbsp. catsup

1 tbsp. parsley
1/2 cup diet
    mayonnaise

Chop the pickle and mix it with the rest of the ingredients. Chill the dressing before serving.
Makes 12 tablespoons
(6 servings)

	Calories	Carbo-hydrate (gm)	Protein (gm)	Total Fat (gm)	Saturated Fat (gm)	Choles-terol (mg)
Total	186.0	13.0	1.0	16.0	0.0	64.0
Per Serving	31.0	2.2	0.2	2.7	0.0	10.7

Thousand Island Dressing II

1 cup diet mayonnaise
¼ cup chili sauce
3 tbsp. chopped green
    pepper

1 tbsp. finely
    chopped
    pimiento
2 tbsp. chopped
    onion

Combine all of the ingredients and mix them thoroughly. Chill the dressing before serving. If the dressing becomes too thick, stir in 1 or 2 tablespoons skim milk (there are about 6 calories in 1 tablespoon skim milk). *Makes 24 tablespoons*
(12 servings)

	Calories	Carbo-hydrate (gm)	Protein (gm)	Total Fat (gm)	Saturated Fat (gm)	Choles-terol (mg)
Total	397.0	35.2	0.7	32.2	0.0	128.0
Per Serving	33.1	2.9	0.1	2.7	0.0	10.7

Two-Cheese Salad Dressing

1½ cups 99% fat-free
    cottage cheese
½ cup diet French
    dressing

¼ cup crumbled bleu
    cheese
1 tbsp. prepared
    horseradish

Beat the cottage cheese at the highest speed of the electric mixer until it is fairly smooth. Slowly beat in the French dressing, bleu cheese, and horseradish. Cover the dressing and chill it before serving. Two-Cheese Dressing is delicious on tossed salads. *Makes 32 tablespoons*
(16 servings)

	Calories	Carbo-hydrate (gm)	Protein (gm)	Total Fat (gm)	Saturated Fat (gm)	Choles-terol (mg)
Total	549.7	12.5	60.2	25.8	14.5	89.8
Per Serving	34.4	0.8	3.8	1.6	0.9	5.6

gm=grams; mg=milligrams. Nutritional figures are approximate. Figures are based on findings of U.S. Department of Agriculture.

Bleu Cheese Salad Dressing

³/₄ cup diet mayonnaise
³/₄ cup plain yogurt
3 oz. bleu cheese
2 tbsp. vinegar

1 tsp. Worcestershire sauce
sugar substitute to equal 2 tsp.
¹/₂ tsp. salt or garlic salt
¹/₈ tsp. pepper

Crumble the bleu cheese and mix it with the rest of the ingredients. Chill the dressing before serving.

*Makes 28 tablespoons
(14 servings)*

	Calories	Carbohydrate (gm)	Protein (gm)	Total Fat (gm)	Saturated Fat (gm)	Cholesterol (mg)
Total	650.8	26.8	24.0	54.0	16.5	183.0
Per Serving	46.5	1.9	1.7	3.9	1.2	13.1

Cottage Dill Dressing

1 cup 99% fat-free cottage cheese
1 tbsp. lemon juice
1 tsp. dill weed
¹/₂ tsp. celery salt

¹/₂ tsp. sugar
¹/₈ tsp. grated lemon peel
2 tbsp. skim milk

Beat the cottage cheese in a small mixing bowl at the highest speed of the electric mixer until it is fairly smooth. Then slowly beat in the lemon juice, dill weed, celery salt, sugar and lemon peel. Blend in the milk. Cover the dressing and chill it until serving. Use this as a dressing for tossed salds.

*Makes 20 tablespoons
(10 servings)*

	Calories	Carbohydrate (gm)	Protein (gm)	Total Fat (gm)	Saturated Fat (gm)	Cholesterol (mg)
Total	210.7	12.8	31.3	2.0	1.2	20.1
Per Serving	21.1	1.3	3.1	0.2	0.1	2.0

Oriental Wine Salad Dressing

¼ cup sake or sherry	2 tbsp. lemon juice
1 tbsp. corn or safflower oil	2 tbsp. finely chopped parsley
1 tbsp. Japanese soy sauce	1 tbsp. sesame seeds
2 tsp. grated lemon peel	1 tsp. honey

Before preparing: Toast the sesame seeds by sprinkling them on a cookie sheet and baking them at 400° until they are brown. Watch them carefully so they don't burn.

Combine all of the ingredients in a bowl and mix them until they are well-blended. Cover the dressing and refrigerate it until you are ready to use it. Mix it again before serving. *Makes 10 tablespoons (5 servings)*

	Calories	Carbo-hydrate (gm)	Protein (gm)	Total Fat (gm)	Saturated Fat (gm)	Choles-terol (mg)
Total	278.1	15.1	3.9	18.4	1.6	0.0
Per Serving	55.6	3.0	0.8	3.7	0.3	0.0

Fruit Dressing

1 cup plain yogurt	½ cup aerosol whipped cream

Gently fold the whipped cream into the yogurt. Serve with fresh pineapple, blueberries or strawberries. *Makes 20 tablespoons (10 servings)*

	Calories	Carbo-hydrate (gm)	Protein (gm)	Total Fat (gm)	Saturated Fat (gm)	Choles-terol (mg)
Total	205.0	13.0	8.0	12.0	2.0	20.0
Per Serving	20.5	1.3	0.8	1.2	0.2	2.0

---

gm=grams; mg=milligrams. Nutritional figures are approximate. Figures are based on findings of U.S. Department of Agriculture.

Lemon Dressing

1 tsp. unflavored
  gelatin
1 tbsp. cold water
1/4 cup boiling water
  sugar substitute to
  equal 2 tbsp.
1/2 tsp. garlic salt

1/2 cup freshly-
  squeezed lemon
  juice
dash of red pepper
1 tsp. prepared
  mustard
1/2 tsp. Worcester-
  shire sauce

Sprinkle the gelatin over the cold water in a cup to
soften it. When the gelatin has softened, place it in a
bowl and add the boiling water, stirring until the
gelatin is completely dissolved. Then beat in the remaining ingredients. The dressing should be stored in
the refrigerator but served at room temperature.

Makes 16 tablespoons
(8 servings)

	Calories	Carbo-hydrate (gm)	Protein (gm)	Total Fat (gm)	Saturated Fat (gm)	Choles-terol (mg)
Total	38.3	10.0	2.5	0.0	0.0	0.0
Per Serving	4.8	1.3	0.3	0.0	0.0	0.0

Citrus Dressing

1/4 cup orange juice
1/4 cup freshly-squeezed
  lemon juice
2 tbsp. corn or safflower
  oil
1/2 tsp. paprika

1 tsp. salt
1/2 tsp. garlic powder
1/8 tsp. black pepper

Place the ingredients in a blender and blend them
until thoroughly mixed. Chill the dressing before serving.

Makes 10 tablespoons
(5 servings)

	Calories	Carbo-hydrate (gm)	Protein (gm)	Total Fat (gm)	Saturated Fat (gm)	Choles-terol (mg)
Total	292.5	11.5	0.8	28.3	2.0	0.0
Per Serving	58.5	2.3	0.2	5.7	0.4	0.0

Citrus Dressing II

2 tbsp. flour
1/2 tsp. salt
1/2 tsp. dry mustard
1 1/4 cups orange juice

1/4 cup lemon juice
1 1/2 tsp. liquid
sweetener
2 egg yolks, beaten

Combine the flour, salt and mustard in the top of a double boiler. Gradually stir in the orange juice, lemon juice, liquid sweetener and beaten egg yolks. Cook the entire mixture over boiling water, stirring constantly, until it has thickened. Chill the dressing before serving.

Makes 20 tablespoons
(10 servings)

	Calories	Carbo-hydrate (gm)	Protein (gm)	Total Fat (gm)	Saturated Fat (gm)	Choles-terol (mg)
Total	336.2	50.8	10.6	11.4	4.0	504.0
Per Serving	33.6	5.1	1.1	1.1	0.4	50.4

Creamy Fruit-Mint Dressing

1 1/2 cups 99% fat-free
cottage cheese
1/4 cup unsweetened
pineapple juice
2 tbsp. lemon juice

1 envelope French
salad dressing
mix
2 tsp. finely chopped
mint

Beat the cottage cheese at the highest speed of the electric mixer until it is fairly smooth. Then slowly beat in the pineapple juice, lemon juice, salad dressing mix and mint. Cover the dressing and chill it before serving. Use this as a dressing for fruit salads.

Makes 32 tablespoons
(16 servings)

	Calories	Carbo-hydrate (gm)	Protein (gm)	Total Fat (gm)	Saturated Fat (gm)	Choles-terol (mg)
Total	311.6	20.1	45.4	3.0	1.8	29.1
Per Serving	19.5	1.3	2.8	0.5	0.1	1.8

gm=grams; mg=milligrams. Nutritional figures are approximate. Figures are based on findings of U.S. Department of Agriculture.

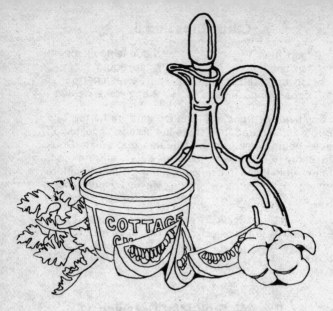

Spiced Orange Dressing

1 cup 99% fat-free	½ tsp. sugar
cottage cheese	¼ tsp. salt
½ tsp. grated orange	⅛ tsp. cinnamon
peel	
¼ cup orange juice	

Beat the cottage cheese in a small mixing bowl at the highest speed of the electric mixer until it is fairly smooth. Then slowly beat in the orange peel, juice, sugar, salt and cinnamon. Cover the dressing and chill it. Allow the dressing to stand at room temperature for a few minutes before serving it. Spiced Orange Dressing is a delicious dressing for fruit salads.   *Makes 20 tablespoons*
(10 servings)

	Calories	Carbo-hydrate (gm)	Protein (gm)	Total Fat (gm)	Saturated Fat (gm)	Choles-terol (mg)
Total	216.2	14.8	30.5	2.3	1.2	19.4
Per Serving	21.6	1.5	3.1	0.2	0.1	1.9

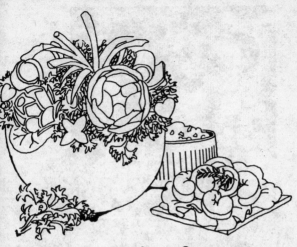

Cranberry Sauce

4 cups fresh
    cranberries
2 cups water
1 tbsp. unflavored
    gelatin

6 tbsp. sugar
    sugar substitute to
      equal ½ cup

Combine all of the ingredients, except the sugar substitute, in a saucepan. Cook and stir the mixture over moderate heat until the gelatin has dissolved and the mixture begins to simmer. Then cover the pot, and simmer the contents over very low heat until the cranberries are tender and have popped open. Remove the pot from the heat and stir in the sweetener. Chill the mixture until it sets.　　　　　*Makes 8 servings*

	Calories	Carbo-hydrate (gm)	Protein (gm)	Total Fat (gm)	Saturated Fat (gm)	Cholesterol (mg)
Total	527.8	125.9	6.0	4.6	0.0	0.0
Per Serving	66.0	15.7	0.8	0.6	0.0	0.0

gm=grams; mg=milligrams. Nutritional figures are approximate. Figures are based on findings of U.S. Department of Agriculture.

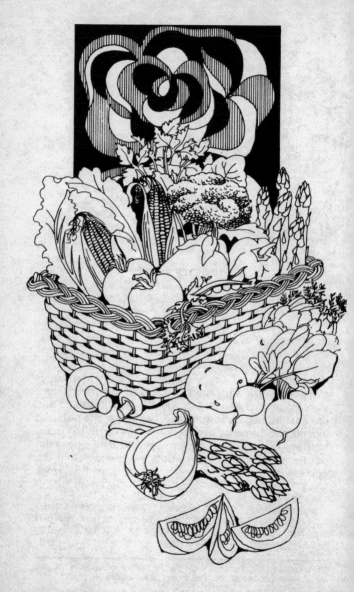

280

Vegetables From A To Z

Vegetables, unfortunately, are a victim of their own virtue. Anything that is good for you is bound to be a bore — or so it must seem if you grew up in a home where clean plates were equated with Godliness.

Many an adult aversion to vegetables got its start when Mama began negotiating deals over parsnips and pudding: "Finish your spinach or you don't get any pie." Right then and there Junior decided that dessert must be more valuable than vegetables . . . . and that when he grew up to be an insurance salesman, nobody was going to dictate how much broccoli he had to eat before starting on the seven-layer cake. As a result, many an otherwise intelligent and mature adult still operates on a two-year-old level where vegetables are concerned, insisting that he dislikes varieties he may never have even tried or tasted.

Maybe Mother's vegetables tasted awful because she didn't know how to cook them (most people — and most restaurants — don't). If you have never tried a certain vegetable — or have tried it only once, or only one way — you haven't given it a fair chance. You may be depriving yourself of a food friend that can stand you in good stead for the rest of your slim days.

Become a Vegetable Adventurer

- Try a new variety every week. When you shop at the supermarket, inspect the produce section for vegetables you have never tried before and give it a go.
- Combine them. Put together a blend of old favorites with a vegetable you've never tasted or one you decided you disliked back when you were 10 years old.
- Try it raw if it is usually served cooked. Or cook a vegetable that is normally served in salad — braised celery is delicious and so are raw mushrooms.
- Try vegetables in season, preferably from a local farm. The deteriorated taste and texture of stored or processed produce may be what turns you off.
- Stir-fry vegetables the Oriental way. One tablespoon of diet margarine (50 calories) is all you need to stir up a skilletful of crisp onions and green beans liberally laced with soy sauce.
- Simmer vegetables in soup or stock — from which you have skimmed the fat.
- Try cooking vegetables in wine — the alcohol calories evaporate.
- Add perennial favorites — like chopped onions or sliced green pepper — for a fresh taste, especially when cooking canned or frozen vegetables.
- Cook vegetables in canned unsweetened fruit juice — apple, orange, or pineapple are some you might try.
- Turn the cooking water into a low-cal sauce. Stir a little flour into skim milk and stir it into the saucepan after the vegetables are cooked. A cream sauce without the cream — or cream calories.
- Spice and season your vegetables by adding a small amount of bottled diet dressing to the cooking water. The water evaporates as the vegetables simmer and leaves behind a tangy sauce — no butter needed.

Vegetables Do's and Don'ts

• Do use a sharp knife when preparing vegetables — for fewer bruises and less loss of nutrients.

• Don't pare, peel, slice, or cut up fresh vegetables until just before cooking — to preserve nutrients.

• Do use as little water as possible — to retain both flavor and nutrients. If possible, cook them in so little water that no draining is needed — and no loss of vitamins. But watch the pot carefully so they don't stick. Frozen vegetables can be cooked with no added water at all. Two outer leaves from a head of lettuce placed in the bottom of the pot will provide enough moisture for frozen vegetables.

• Don't overcook vegetables. Every known vegetable is better undercooked — cooked only till crunchy.

• Do use a pot with a tight-fitting lid to steam green vegetables.

• Do keep the heat low when steaming vegetables. Otherwise, the steam will escape.

• Do steam white, yellow, and red vegetables. Place them on a rack over boiling water, and cover the pot with a tight lid. (This method takes longer than boiling the vegetables, but is well worth it in the savings of nutrients.)

• Do add $1/2$ to 1 teaspoon salt to the pot for each six servings of vegetables. Try seasoned salt — butter, onion, garlic, or celery. A little butter-flavored salt added to the cooking water gives vegetables a buttery flavor — without the butter and without the butter calories.

• Don't use soda for preserving color while cooking vegetables. It makes them mushy and flavorless. You can preserve color by undercooking.

• Do cook strongly flavored vegetables (cabbage, broccoli, cauliflower, Brussels sprouts, turnips) in an uncovered pan. Add additional water if needed to prevent burning.

• Do add butter-flavored salt and freshly ground pepper to vegetables just before serving. Herbs and spices as seasonings go a long way, and the calorie contribution is fractional.

FRESH VEGETABLE GUIDE

Vegetable	Maximum Cooking Time in Minutes
Asparagus	10 to 20 (whole spears)
	5 to 15 (cuts and tips)
Beans, lima	25 to 30
Beans, snap (green or wax)	12 to 16 (1-inch pieces)
Beets	30 to 45 (young, whole)
	45 to 90 (older, whole)
	15 to 25 (sliced or diced)
Broccoli	10 to 15 (heavy stalk split)
Brussels sprouts	15 to 20
Cabbage	3 to 10 (shredded)
	10 to 15 (wedges)
Carrots	15 to 20 (young, whole)
	20 to 30 (older, whole)
	10 to 20 (sliced or diced)
Cauliflower	8 to 15 (separated)
	15 to 25 (whole)
Celery	15 to 18 (cut-up)
Corn	5 to 15 (on cob)
Kale	10 to 15
Okra	10 to 14
Onions, mature	15 to 30
Parsnips	20 to 40 (whole)
	8 to 15 (quartered)
Peas	12 to 16
Potatoes	25 to 40 (whole, medium)
	20 to 25 (quartered)
	10 to 15 (diced)
Spinach	3 to 10
Squash, summer	8 to 15 (sliced)
Squash, winter	15 to 20 (cut-up)
Tomatoes	7 to 15 (cut-up)
Turnip greens	10 to 30
Turnips	20 to 30 (whole)
	10 to 20 (cut-up)

FRESH VEGETABLE GUIDE

**Pounds To Buy
for 8 Servings**

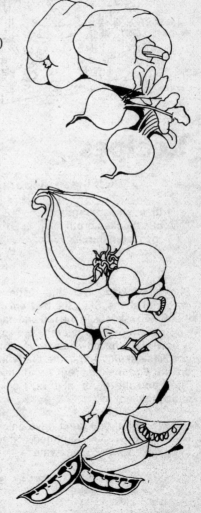

2½ for spears
1¾ (cuts and tips)
2¾ in pods
1

2½ with tops or
1½ without tops

2
1½
1¼
1½
1½ without tops

1½ without tops
2
2
1½
3 in husks
1¼ untrimmed
1¼
1¾
1½
1½
3 in pods
1½
1½
1¼
1½ prepackaged
1½
2½
1¼
2¾ prepackaged
1¾ without tops
1¾

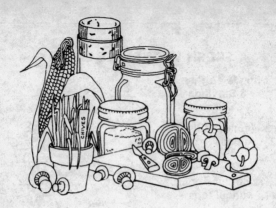

Recipes

Chinese Asparagus

1 lb. fresh asparagus	2 tbsp. soy sauce
½ cup chicken broth	1 tbsp. diet
1 tbsp. cornstarch	margarine
	½ cup chopped
	onion

Before cooking: Cut the asparagus into ¼-inch diagonal slices. Skim the fat from the broth by chilling it until the fat rises to the top and can be whisked away.

Mix the broth, cornstarch, and soy sauce together in a bowl. Set the bowl aside. Heat the margarine in a non-stick skillet and sauté the onion until it is golden brown. Add the asparagus and stir-fry it for 3 minutes. Then add the broth mixture. Cook and stir until the sauce is clear.   *Makes 4 servings*

Special hint: If you don't have chicken broth, you can use canned broth undiluted, or a chicken bouillon cube mixed with ½ cup water.

	Calories	Carbo-hydrate (gm)	Protein (gm)	Total Fat (gm)	Saturated Fat (gm)	Choles-terol (mg)
Total	218.8	30.7	14.4	6.0	1.0	18.3
Per Serving	54.7	7.7	3.6	1.5	0.3	4.6

Artichokes with Peas

9 oz. package frozen
artichoke hearts
3 cups thinly-sliced
celery
1/2 cup boiling water
1/2 tsp. salt

10 oz. package frozen
peas
2 tsp. lemon juice
1/4 tsp. butter salt

Cook the artichokes and celery in a covered saucepan for 3 minutes in boiling water to which the salt has been added. Then add the peas, and return the liquid to boiling. Cover the pot and cook the vegetables for 5 minutes more. Drain them well. Add the lemon juice and butter salt before serving.

Makes 8 servings

	Calories	Carbo-hydrate (gm)	Protein (gm)	Total Fat (gm)	Saturated Fat (gm)	Choles-terol (mg)
Total	305.0	77.8	21.7	0.0	0.0	0.0
Per Serving	38.1	9.7	2.7	0.0	0.0	0.0

Pickled Beets

1 lb. can sliced beets
1/4 cup cider vinegar

1 tsp. whole mixed
pickling spice
sugar substitute to
equal 2 tbsp.

Drain the liquid from the beets into a small saucepan. Add the vinegar and pickling spice to the liquid, and boil it gently for 5 minutes. Remove the pot from the heat and add the beets and sugar substitute. Cover the pot and let it stand for several hours. At serving time, reheat the beets, then drain off the liquid.

Makes 4 servings

	Calories	Carbo-hydrate (gm)	Protein (gm)	Total Fat (gm)	Saturated Fat (gm)	Choles-terol (mg)
Total	158.7	38.6	3.6	0.0	0.0	0.0
Per Serving	39.7	9.7	0.9	0.0	0.0	0.0

gm=grams; mg=milligrams. Nutritional figures are approximate. Figures are based on findings of U.S. Department of Agriculture.

Marinated Beets

2 cups canned julienne-
cut beets, drained
1/2 cup cider vinegar
1 tbsp. grated onion

1 mashed garlic
clove
few drops of liquid
sweetener
1 tbsp. pickling
spice

Before preparing: Tie the pickling spice in a small piece of gauze, so it can be removed before serving.

Mix all of the ingredients in a bowl, cover the bowl and refrigerate it for several days. Remove the pickling spices before serving.　　　　　*Makes 4 servings*

	Calories	Carbo-hydrate (gm)	Protein (gm)	Total Fat (gm)	Saturated Fat (gm)	Choles-terol (mg)
Total	222.9	56.1	5.1	0.0	0.0	0.0
Per Serving	55.7	14.0	1.3	0.0	0.0	0.0

Beets in Sour Cream

3 cups halved cooked
beets
4 tbsp. low-fat non-
dairy sour cream
substitute
1 tbsp. vinegar

3/4 tsp. sugar
1/2 tsp. salt
dash of cayenne

To cook the beets, boil them in salted water until they are tender. Drain them and cut them in half. Combine all of the ingredients, except the beets, in a bowl. Mix the sauce well and add it to the beets. Heat the beets with the sauce slowly, stirring to coat.

Makes 6 servings

	Calories	Carbo-hydrate (gm)	Protein (gm)	Total Fat (gm)	Saturated Fat (gm)	Choles-terol (mg)
Total	382.3	66.2	8.1	9.7	8.8	0.0
Per Serving	63.7	11.0	1.4	1.6	1.3	0.0

Beets with Orange Sauce

³/₄ tsp. salt
2 tbsp. cornstarch
³/₄ cup orange juice
2 tbsp. lemon juice

sugar substitute to
equal ¹/₄ cup
3 cups canned
sliced beets,
drained

Mix salt, cornstarch, and orange juice in a saucepan. Cook the mixture, stirring constantly, until it has thickened. Then remove it from the heat. Stir in the lemon juice and sugar substitute. Pour the sauce over the beets, and stir carefully. Heat the mixture through and serve. *Makes 6 servings*

	Calories	Carbo-hydrate (gm)	Protein (gm)	Total Fat (gm)	Saturated Fat (gm)	Choles-terol (mg)
Total	352.9	81.7	6.6	0.8	0.0	0.0
Per Serving	58.8	13.6	1.1	0.1	0.0	0.0

Deviled Beets

3 cups diced canned
beets
1 tbsp. diet margarine
¹/₄ tsp. dry mustard
¹/₄ tsp. ground cloves
2 tbsp. vinegar

1 tbsp. brown sugar
¹/₂ tsp. salt
¹/₂ tsp. paprika
1 tsp. Worcester-
shire sauce

Melt the diet margarine over low heat in a non-stick skillet. Add the rest of the ingredients, except the beets, and stir to combine. Then add the beets and continue cooking until they are hot — about 5 minutes. *Makes 6 servings*

	Calories	Carbo-hydrate (gm)	Protein (gm)	Total Fat (gm)	Saturated Fat (gm)	Choles-terol (mg)
Total	405.4	84.4	6.0	6.0	1.0	0.0
Per Serving	67.6	14.1	1.0	1.0	0.2	0.0

gm=grams; mg=milligrams. Nutritional figures are approximate. Figures are based on findings of U.S. Department of Agriculture.

Broccoli Italienne

1 bunch broccoli
1 tbsp. olive oil
1 garlic clove
3 tbsp. minced onion

3 tbsp. water
¾ tsp. salt
pinch of cayenne
½ tsp. oregano

Before cooking: Wash the broccoli and with a vegetable peeler remove the thin layer of skin on the stems. Split each stem lengthwise into quarters and then cut the strips into 1-inch pieces. Cut the flowerets into coarse pieces. Peel and chop the garlic clove.

Heat the oil in a large non-stick skillet. Sauté the garlic and onion slowly until they are tender. Then add the broccoli, water, salt, cayenne, and oregano. Cover the pan tightly and cook the broccoli slowly for about 15 minutes until it is tender.   *Makes 6 servings*

Diet hint: The heart-conscious cook should substitute corn or safflower oil for the olive oil to save 1 gram of saturated fat. Also, if fresh broccoli isn't available, you may use 3 packages of frozen broccoli spears for this recipe.

	Calories	Carbo-hydrate (gm)	Protein (gm)	Total Fat (gm)	Saturated Fat (gm)	Choles-terol (mg)
Total	343.2	39.3	28.5	18.7	2.0	0.0
Per Serving	57.2	6.6	4.8	3.1	0.3	0.0

Broccoli with Lemon Butter

2 packages frozen
    broccoli
1 tbsp. margarine
1 tsp. arrowroot or
    cornstarch

2 tbsp. fresh lemon
    juice
¾ cup cold water
5 or 6 drops of
    yellow food
    coloring

Cook the broccoli according to the directions on the package. In the meantime, melt the margarine in a small saucepan and stir in the arrowroot or cornstarch. Add the lemon juice and water and cook the mixture over moderate heat until it simmers. Stir in the food coloring a drop at a time until the sauce is buttery yellow. Serve the sauce over the broccoli.

Makes 6 servings

	Calories	Carbo-hydrate (gm)	Protein (gm)	Total Fat (gm)	Saturated Fat (gm)	Choles-terol (mg)
Total	252.2	29.2	18.9	11.0	2.0	0.0
Per Serving	42.0	4.9	3.2	1.8	0.3	0.0

Oriental Broccoli with Mushrooms

2 packages frozen
broccoli spears
1 small onion
1/2 cup cold water
1 tsp. arrowroot or
cornstarch

1 tsp. beef bouillon
or 1 bouillon
cube
1 tbsp. soy sauce
8 oz. can mushroom
stems and
pieces

Before cooking: Allow the broccoli to partially thaw and slice it into 1-inch diagonal pieces. Slice the onion.

Combine the arrowroot (or cornstarch) in a saucepan with the bouillon, water, and soy sauce. Bring the mixture to a boil and then add the rest of the ingredients. Cook and stir the vegetables over moderate heat, uncovered, for about 2 minutes until the sauce thickens and simmers and the vegetables are just crunchy. Serve immediately. *Makes 6 servings*

	Calories	Carbo-hydrate (gm)	Protein (gm)	Total Fat (gm)	Saturated Fat (gm)	Choles-terol (mg)
Total	265.6	47.1	29.8	4.2	0.0	3.0
Per Serving	44.3	7.9	5.0	0.7	0.0	0.5

---

gm=grams; mg=milligrams. Nutritional figures are approximate. Figures are based on findings of U.S. Department of Agriculture.

Zesty Broccoli

1 bunch broccoli
¼ cup boiling water
  salted
⅓ cup diet mayonnaise
⅓ cup plain yogurt

1 tsp. onion flakes
dash of cayenne
¾ tsp. salt

Before cooking: Cut the broccoli into 1-inch pieces.
  Add the broccoli to the boiling salted water, cover the pan and cook it until the broccoli is barely tender. In a bowl, combine the mayonnaise, yogurt, onion flakes, cayenne, and salt. Serve the sauce over the hot broccoli. *Makes 4 servings*

Special hint: If fresh broccoli is not available, you may use 2 packages of frozen broccoli spears.

	Calories	Carbo-hydrate (gm)	Protein (gm)	Total Fat (gm)	Saturated Fat (gm)	Choles-terol (mg)
Total	362.5	47.9	30.8	16.7	0.7	49.2
Per Serving	90.6	12.0	7.7	4.2	0.2	12.3

Curried Sprouts

10 oz. package frozen
  Brussels sprouts
3 tbsp. diet mayonnaise
1 tbsp. grated
  Parmesan cheese

pinch of celery
  seed
pinch of curry

Cook the Brussels sprouts according to the directions on the package. In the meantime, blend the mayonnaise, cheese, celery seed, and curry in a bowl. Drain the sprouts, and serve the sauce as a topping. *Makes 3 servings*

	Calories	Carbo-hydrate (gm)	Protein (gm)	Total Fat (gm)	Saturated Fat (gm)	Choles-terol (mg)
Total	248.0	23.6	21.2	13.4	3.0	40.2
Per Serving	82.7	7.9	7.1	4.5	1.0	13.4

Saucy Brussels Sprouts

3 packages frozen
  Brussels sprouts
1/2 cup chopped onion
1 tbsp. flour
1 tsp. salt

2 tsp. prepared
  mustard
1 cup plain yogurt
1 tsp. parsley flakes
  or 1 tbsp.
  chopped fresh
  parsley

Simmer the Brussels sprouts in 1 or 2 tbsp. water just until they are tender. Combine the rest of the ingredients in a separate saucepan, stirring until they are blended. Cook and stir the sauce over moderate heat until it thickens and bubbles. Serve the sauce over the Brussels sprouts. *Makes 8 servings*

	Calories	Carbo-hydrate (gm)	Protein (gm)	Total Fat (gm)	Saturated Fat (gm)	Choles-terol (mg)
Total	549.7	97.3	48.0	9.6	2.0	20.0
Per Serving	68.7	12.2	6.0	1.2	0.3	2.5

Red Cabbage and Applesauce

1 lb. head red cabbage
1/2 cup sliced onion
2 cups unsweetened
  applesauce

1 tsp. salt
pinch of coarsely
  ground pepper
1 tbsp. caraway
  seeds

Shred the cabbage and combine it with the rest of the ingredients in a saucepan. Cover the pot and simmer the mixture over very low heat for 30 to 40 minutes, stirring occasionally. *Makes 6 servings*

	Calories	Carbo-hydrate (gm)	Protein (gm)	Total Fat (gm)	Saturated Fat (gm)	Choles-terol (mg)
Total	348.0	89.0	9.4	0.0	0.0	0.0
Per Serving	58.0	14.8	1.6	0.0	0.0	0.0

gm=grams; mg=milligrams. Nutritional figures are approximate. Figures are based on findings of U.S. Department of Agriculture.

Red Cabbage with Apples

10 cups shredded red
    cabbage
2 cooking apples
2 tbsp. salt
1/2 cup cider vinegar

1/2 cup cold water
sugar substitute to
    equal 1/2 cup
1 tbsp. flour

Before cooking: Peel the apples and slice them thinly.
Combine the cabbage, apples, salt, vinegar, and
water in a large skillet. Cover the pan, and cook the
contents over moderate heat for 20 to 25 minutes, stirring occasionally, until the cabbage is tender but still
crisp. Sprinkle the flour and sugar substitute over the
cabbage, and continue cooking and stirring until the
mixture thickens. *Makes 8 servings*

	Calories	Carbo-hydrate (gm)	Protein (gm)	Total Fat (gm)	Saturated Fat (gm)	Choles-terol (mg)
Total	375.3	99.7	10.8	0.1	0.0	0.0
Per Serving	46.9	12.5	1.4	0.0	0.0	0.0

Sweet and Sour Red Cabbage

1 large head red
    cabbage (about 3
    lbs.)
1 tbsp. flour
1 tsp. salt
3 tbsp. lemon juice

2 tbsp. brown sugar
1/2 cup crushed
    pineapple
sugar substitute to
    equal 1/4 cup

Wash the cabbage and shred it fine. Place the cabbage in a heavy pot and sprinkle it with the flour, salt,
brown sugar, and lemon juice. Add the pineapple, and
stir well. Cover the pot and simmer the contents over
low heat for 30 minutes, stirring occasionally. Remove
the pot from the heat and stir in the sugar substitute.
Makes 8 servings

	Calories	Carbo-hydrate (gm)	Protein (gm)	Total Fat (gm)	Saturated Fat (gm)	Choles-terol (mg)
Total	596.6	150.4	20.7	0.1	0.0	0.0
Per Serving	74.6	18.8	2.6	0.0	0.0	0.0

Creole Cabbage

1 head green cabbage
¼ cup chopped onion
¼ cup chopped green
   pepper
8 oz. can tomatoes,
   undrained

½ tsp. salt
1 cup water
dash of pepper

Cut the head of cabbage into quarters and combine it with the rest of the ingredients in a saucepan. Cover the pan and simmer the contents for 10 minutes.

Makes 4 servings

	Calories	Carbohydrate (gm)	Protein (gm)	Total Fat (gm)	Saturated Fat (gm)	Cholesterol (mg)
Total	179.0	36.3	48.9	1.0	0.0	0.0
Per Serving	44.8	9.1	12.2	0.3	0.0	0.0

Carrots in Pineapple Sauce

3 cups sliced carrots,
   fresh or frozen
6 oz. can unsweetened
   pineapple juice
½ tsp. arrowroot or
   cornstarch

½ cup water
¼ tsp. cinnamon
salt
pepper

Combine all the ingredients in a saucepan. Cover the pan tightly and simmer the mixture until the carrots are nearly tender. Then uncover the pan and continue to simmer, stirring occasionally, until nearly all of the liquid has evaporated.

Makes 4 servings

	Calories	Carbohydrate (gm)	Protein (gm)	Total Fat (gm)	Saturated Fat (gm)	Cholesterol (mg)
Total	224.9	56.4	6.8	0.0	0.0	0.0
Per Serving	56.2	14.1	1.7	0.0	0.0	0.0

---

gm=grams; mg=milligrams. Nutritional figures are approximate. Figures are based on findings of U.S. Department of Agriculture.

Maple-Glazed Carrots

1 lb. can carrots,
drained

2 tbsp. sugar-free
maple syrup
1 tsp. butter-flavored
salt

Combine all of the ingredients in a saucepan. Cover the pan and simmer the mixture over low heat for about 10 minutes, stirring occasionally.   *Makes 4 servings*

	Calories	Carbo-hydrate (gm)	Protein (gm)	Total Fat (gm)	Saturated Fat (gm)	Choles-terol (mg)
Total	161.1	38.0	4.6	0.0	0.0	0.0
Per Serving	40.3	9.5	1.2	0.0	0.0	0.0

Glazed Carrots and Brussels Sprouts

1 lb. carrots
2 packages (10 oz.)
frozen Brussels
sprouts
2 tbsp. chopped onion
10¹/₂ oz. can condensed
consommé

¹/₃ cup apple juice
2 tsp. lemon juice
2 tbsp. cornstarch
1 tbsp. brown sugar
substitute
generous dash of
ground clove

Cut the carrots into 1¹/₂-inch pieces and boil them until they are tender. Cook the Brussels sprouts according to the directions on the package. Combine the carrots and Brussels sprouts; add the remaining ingredients, except the sugar substitute, and cook the entire mixture, stirring until the sauce has thickened. Remove the pan from the heat and add the sugar substitute.
Makes 8 servings

	Calories	Carbo-hydrate (gm)	Protein (gm)	Total Fat (gm)	Saturated Fat (gm)	Choles-terol (mg)
Total	514.7	103.2	45.6	3.6	0.0	62.9
Per Serving	64.3	12.9	5.7	0.5	0.0	7.9

Cauliflower with Quick Cheese Sauce

2 packages frozen
  cauliflower
10¾ oz. can condensed
  cheddar cheese
  soup

¼ cup skim milk
  generous dash of
  nutmeg

Cook the cauliflower according to the directions on the package. In the meantime, blend the soup, milk, and nutmeg in a saucepan. Cook and stir the sauce until it is bubbling. Drain the cauliflower and serve it hot with the sauce over it. *Makes 6 servings*

	Calories	Carbo-hydrate (gm)	Protein (gm)	Total Fat (gm)	Saturated Fat (gm)	Choles-terol (mg)
Total	525.8	52.1	29.2	25.8	12.9	65.8
Per Serving	87.6	8.7	5.0	4.3	2.2	11.0

Cauliflower with "Sour Cream"

2 packages (10 oz.)
  frozen cauliflower
salt
pepper
paprika

½ cup non-dairy low-
  fat sour cream
  substitute
4 tbsp. bread crumbs

Cook the cauliflower according to the directions on the package until it is just tender. Season it with salt, pepper, and paprika. Place the cauliflower in a non-stick baking dish, cover it with the imitation sour cream and bread crumbs and bake it at 350° just until it is brown. *Makes 6 servings*

	Calories	Carbo-hydrate (gm)	Protein (gm)	Total Fat (gm)	Saturated Fat (gm)	Choles-terol (mg)
Total	434.3	50.2	21.8	20.3	17.8	1.3
Per Serving	72.4	8.4	3.6	3.4	3.0	0.2

gm=grams; mg=milligrams. Nutritional figures are approximate. Figures are based on findings of U.S. Department of Agriculture.

Cauliflower and Carrots Almondine

1 small head
    cauliflower
2 cups diagonally-
    sliced carrots
4 tbsp. slivered,
    blanched almonds

2 tsp. lemon juice
    coarsely ground
    pepper

Before cooking: Break the cauliflower into flowerets.
Cook the cauliflower and carrots in a small amount
of boiling, salted water for about 15 minutes until they
are just tender. Then drain them. Place the almonds in
a non-stick skillet over moderate heat for about 1
minute until they are lightly browned. Remove them
from the heat and stir in the lemon juice. Pour the
lemon and almonds over the vegetables and sprinkle
them generously with the pepper.   *Makes 8 servings*

	Calories	Carbo-hydrate (gm)	Protein (gm)	Total Fat (gm)	Saturated Fat (gm)	Choles-terol (mg)
Total	411.4	51.1	24.5	19.3	1.5	0.0
Per Serving	51.4	6.4	3.1	2.4	0.2	0.0

Creamed Cauliflower with Cheese

1 large cauliflower
    (2¹/₄-2¹/₂ lbs.)
1 cup salted water
4¹/₂ tsp. butter-flavored
    salt
3 tbsp. flour

white pepper
¹/₂ tsp. dry mustard
1¹/₂ cups skim milk
1 cup lightly packed
    grated American
    cheese

Break the cauliflower into flowerets and wash them
well in cold water. Add the cauliflower to a saucepan
with the salted water and bring it to a boil. Boil the
cauliflower for 5 to 10 minutes until it is tender-crisp.
Then drain it. Combine the flour, mustard, salt, and
pepper in a saucepan over a low heat. Add the milk.
Cook this mixture, stirring constantly, until it has
thickened. Then mix in the cauliflower and reheat. Just
before serving, sprinkle the cheese over the top.

Makes 8 servings

	Calories	Carbo-hydrate (gm)	Protein (gm)	Total Fat (gm)	Saturated Fat (gm)	Choles-terol (mg)
Total	1471.8	78.2	105.2	80.2	48.0	263.5
Per Serving	184.0	9.8	13.2	10.0	6.0	32.9

Celery Italiano

½ cup minced onion
1 minced clove of garlic
4 cups celery cut into 2-inch chunks

15 oz. can tomato sauce
1¼ tsp. salt
1¼ tsp. basil

Combine all of the ingredients in a medium saucepan and bring the mixture to the boiling point. Then lower the heat, cover the pot, and simmer the celery for about 10 minutes until it is tender-crisp.

Makes 6 servings

	Calories	Carbo-hydrate (gm)	Protein (gm)	Total Fat (gm)	Saturated Fat (gm)	Choles-terol (mg)
Total	215.9	60.0	6.9	0.7	0.0	0.0
Per Serving	36.0	10.0	1.2	0.1	0.0	0.0

Creamed Celery

2 cups thinly-sliced celery
1 cup boiling water
2 tbsp. flour
¼ tsp. paprika

1 cup skim milk
salt
white pepper

Boil the celery in the water just until it is tender-crisp. Then drain it. Combine the flour, paprika, salt, pepper, and milk, and add this to the celery. Heat the entire mixture slowly until it is creamy.

Makes 4 servings

	Calories	Carbo-hydrate (gm)	Protein (gm)	Total Fat (gm)	Saturated Fat (gm)	Choles-terol (mg)
Total	174.6	35.4	10.6	0.1	0.0	5.0
Per Serving	43.7	8.9	2.7	0.0	0.0	1.3

gm=grams; mg=milligrams. Nutritional figures are approximate. Figures are based on findings of U.S. Department of Agriculture.

Braised Celery

4 bunches of celery
1 onion
2 carrots

2 cans (10½ oz.)
chicken broth
water

Before cooking: Trim and slice the celery, slice the onion, and scrub and slice the carrots. Skim the fat from the broth by chilling it until the fat rises to the top and can be whisked away.

Place the onion and carrot slices in a large skillet and arrange the celery on top. Add the broth and just enough water to cover the vegetables. Cover the skillet and bring the mixture to a boil. Then lower the heat and simmer for about 45 minutes until the vegetables are tender.

Makes 8 servings

	Calories	Carbo-hydrate (gm)	Protein (gm)	Total Fat (gm)	Saturated Fat (gm)	Choles-terol (mg)
Total	375.3	102.5	19.7	0.0	0.0	73.4
Per Serving	46.9	12.8	2.5	0.0	0.0	9.2

Hi-Protein Corn Casserole

2 cups skim milk
1 onion
2 red or green peppers
1½ cups canned or frozen
corn

2 eggs
2 tsp. butter-flavored
salt
pinch of pepper

Before cooking: If frozen corn is used, first cook and drain it according to the directions on the package.

Scald the milk. Stir in the rest of the ingredients and turn the whole mixture into a casserole. Bake the casserole in a preheated 325° oven for about 1¼ hours until a knife inserted in the center comes out clean.

Makes 8 servings

	Calories	Carbo-hydrate (gm)	Protein (gm)	Total Fat (gm)	Saturated Fat (gm)	Choles-terol (mg)
Total	713.0	112.0	46.0	13.5	4.0	514.0
Per Serving	89.1	14.0	5.8	1.7	0.5	64.3

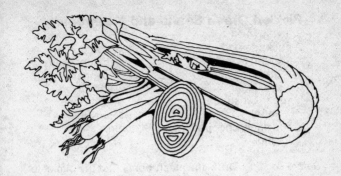

Eggplant Parmesan

1 eggplant
3 tbsp. Italian-
   seasoned bread
   crumbs
1¹/₂ tbsp. grated
   Parmesan cheese
¹/₂ tsp. garlic salt

pinch of cayenne
8 oz. can tomato
   sauce
3 thin slices
   Mozzarella
   cheese (3 oz.)

Before cooking: Peel the eggplant and cut it into ¹/₄-inch cubes.

Mix the bread crumbs, Parmesan cheese, garlic salt, and cayenne together in a bowl. Arrange the eggplant in the bottom of a baking dish. Spread the bread crumb mixture over this and then pour on the tomato sauce. Top with the slices of Mozzarella cheese. Bake the mixture at 325° for 25 minutes.   *Makes 6 servings*

	Calories	Carbo-hydrate (gm)	Protein (gm)	Total Fat (gm)	Saturated Fat (gm)	Choles-terol (mg)
Total	556.6	43.6	65.2	25.4	8.2	82.0
Per Serving	92.8	7.3	10.9	4.2	1.4	13.7

gm=grams; mg=milligrams. Nutritional figures are approximate. Figures are based on findings of U.S. Department of Agriculture.

Pickled Green Beans and Mushrooms

2 packages (10 oz.
  each) frozen cut
  green beans
$^1/_2$ cup vinegar
  sugar substitute to
  equal $^3/_4$ cup
$^1/_2$ cup finely chopped
  onion

$^1/_2$ tsp. salt
$^1/_2$ tsp. celery seed
$^1/_2$ tsp. pepper
4 oz. can sliced
  mushrooms
2 oz. pimiento
1 onion

Before cooking: Drain the mushrooms. Cut the pimiento and onion into slices.

Cook the beans according to the directions on the package. Drain the beans, saving 1 cup of the liquid. Add all the remaining ingredients to the liquid, except the pimiento and onion slices. Pour the liquid over the beans and toss lightly to mix. Chill the bean mixture for several hours to marinate it. Serve the beans hot or cold, garnished with the pimiento and onion slices.

Makes 8 servings

	Calories	Carbo-hydrate (gm)	Protein (gm)	Total Fat (gm)	Saturated Fat (gm)	Choles-terol (mg)
Total	283.1	72.3	16.3	1.8	0.0	0.0
Per Serving	35.4	9.0	2.0	0.2	0.0	0.0

Green Beans with Bacon

1 lb. fresh green beans,
  French-cut or 9 oz.
  package frozen
  beans
$^1/_4$ cup boiling water
1 tbsp. diet margarine

$^1/_2$ cup finely-diced
  Canadian bacon
1 clove garlic
$^1/_2$ tsp. salt
$^1/_4$ tsp. pepper
1 tomato

Before cooking: Mince the garlic clove. Cut the tomato into wedges.

Cook the fresh or frozen green beans in the water until they are tender. Then drain them. Melt the margarine in a non-stick skillet and sauté the bacon and garlic until they are brown. Add the beans, salt, and pepper to the skillet, and top with the tomato wedges. Cover the pan and heat the contents through.

Makes 4 servings

Diet hint: The calorie-conscious cook can save 50 calories (about 12 per serving) by omitting the diet margarine. Spray a non-stick skillet with spray-on vegetable coating, so you can brown the bacon and garlic without calories.

	Calories	Carbo-hydrate (gm)	Protein (gm)	Total Fat (gm)	Saturated Fat (gm)	Choles-terol (mg)
Total	351.1	25.0	25.1	18.5	4.3	58.9
Per Serving	87.8	6.3	6.3	4.6	1.1	14.7

Hot Green Bean Salad

¹/₄ cup diet Italian salad
    dressing
2 packages (9 oz.)
    frozen cut green
    beans

¹/₂ cup diced celery
1 large onion
2 tsp. dill

Before cooking: Allow the green beans to partially thaw. Slice the onion, and separate the slices into rings.

Combine the salad dressing, green beans, and celery in a non-stick skillet. Cover the pan, and cook just until the beans are fully thawed, separating them with a fork as they cook. Then add the onion and dill, and continue cooking for about 3 minutes, stirring occasionally, just until the vegetables are tender but still crisp.

Makes 6 servings

	Calories	Carbo-hydrate (gm)	Protein (gm)	Total Fat (gm)	Saturated Fat (gm)	Choles-terol (mg)
Total	220.7	46.4	11.1	4.0	0.0	0.0
Per Serving	36.8	7.7	1.9	0.7	0.0	0.0

---

gm=grams; mg=milligrams. Nutritional figures are approximate. Figures are based on findings of U.S. Department of Agriculture.

Green Beans Español

3 cups canned French-
style green beans
2 tbsp. minced onion
2 tbsp. minced green
pepper
2½ cups canned tomato
pieces
1 tsp. chili powder

pinch of cayenne
1 tsp. salt
⅛ tsp. pepper
6 tbsp. grated
Parmesan
cheese

Before cooking: Drain the beans and tomatoes.

Place the beans in a 1½-quart casserole. Combine
the onion, green pepper, tomatoes, and seasonings in
a bowl. Pour this mixture over the beans. Sprinkle the
cheese over all. Cover the casserole and bake it at
350° for about 20 minutes.   *Makes 6 servings*

	Calories	Carbo-hydrate (gm)	Protein (gm)	Total Fat (gm)	Saturated Fat (gm)	Choles-terol (mg)
Total	689.6	51.3	54.5	34.9	18.0	97.2
Per Serving	114.9	8.6	9.1	5.8	3.0	16.2

Parmesan Beans

1 lb. fresh green beans
1 cup boiling water
½ tsp. salt

2 tbsp. diet Italian
salad dressing
3 tbsp. grated
Parmesan
cheese

Before cooking: Wash the beans in cold water and cut
them into 1-inch diagonal pieces.

Add the salt and beans to the boiling water, cover
the pan, and cook until the beans are just tender — 8 or
9 minutes. Drain the beans and stir in the salad dressing and cheese.   *Makes 6 servings*

	Calories	Carbo-hydrate (gm)	Protein (gm)	Total Fat (gm)	Saturated Fat (gm)	Choles-terol (mg)
Total	357.7	26.9	28.8	18.2	9.0	48.6
Per Serving	59.6	4.5	4.8	3.0	1.5	8.1

Green Beans Milano

1/2 cup chicken broth
2 lbs. fresh green beans
1 tomato

1/2 tsp. oregano
1 medium garlic
clove

Before cooking: Skim the fat from the broth by chilling it until the fat rises to the top and can be whisked away. (If you do not have chicken broth, use canned chicken broth.) Peel the tomato by first plunging it in boiling water; then chop it. Mince the garlic.

Combine all of the ingredients in a saucepan. Cook the mixture over low heat for about 20 minutes until the vegetables are tender. *Makes 8 servings*

	Calories	Carbo-hydrate (gm)	Protein (gm)	Total Fat (gm)	Saturated Fat (gm)	Choles-terol (mg)
Total	265.7	60.2	17.8	0.0	0.0	7.0
Per Serving	33.2	7.5	2.2	0.0	0.0	0.9

Sweet-Sour Beans

4 cups canned wax
beans
1 cup water
1/2 cup vinegar

sugar substitute to
equal 1/2 cup
2 cloves
1 stick of cinnamon

Before cooking: Drain the beans.

Combine the water, vinegar, and spices in a saucepan, bring the mixture to a boil. Then lower the heat, and simmer it for 4 to 5 minutes. Remove the pan from the heat, and stir in the sugar substitute. Pour the vinegar mixture over the drained beans, and allow it to cool. Serve the beans chilled. *Makes 6 servings*

	Calories	Carbo-hydrate (gm)	Protein (gm)	Total Fat (gm)	Saturated Fat (gm)	Choles-terol (mg)
Total	128.0	32.0	8.0	0.0	0.0	0.0
Per Serving	21.3	5.3	1.3	0.0	0.0	0.0

gm=grams; mg=milligrams. Nutritional figures are approximate. Figures are based on findings of U.S. Department of Agriculture.

Javanese Mushroom Soup

1/4 lb. fresh mushrooms
2 cans (10 1/2 oz. each) condensed chicken broth
2 soup cans water
1/2 cup finely chopped onion
1/8 tsp. ground cinnamon
1/8 tsp. ground nutmeg
1/8 tsp. salt
1/8 tsp. ground black pepper
1 tsp. cornstarch
1 tbsp. cold water

Before cooking: Skim the fat from the broth by chilling it until the fat rises to the top and can be whisked away. Rinse the mushrooms, pat them dry, and chop them finely.

Combine the mushrooms, broth, 2 cans of water, onion, cinnamon, nutmeg, salt, and pepper in a medium-sized saucepan. Bring this mixture to a boil; then reduce the heat, cover the pan, and simmer it for 15 minutes. Mix the cornstarch with the 1 tablespoon water, and slowly stir this into the hot soup. Continue cooking until the soup has slightly thickened and has cleared. If you like, serve the soup with toasted onion flakes sprinkled over the top. *Makes 6 servings*

	Calories	Carbo-hydrate (gm)	Protein (gm)	Total Fat (gm)	Saturated Fat (gm)	Choles-terol (mg)
Total	227.5	31.1	25.5	1.3	0.0	73.4
Per Serving	37.9	5.2	4.3	0.2	0.0	12.2

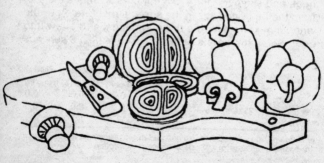

Mushrooms Sautéed in White Wine

1/2 lb. fresh mushrooms
1 tbsp. diet margarine

2 tbsp. dry white
wine

Slice the mushrooms and combine them with the rest of the ingredients in a non-stick skillet. Cook and stir them over high heat until the liquid evaporates and the mushrooms are lightly browned. *Makes 6 servings*

Special note: If fresh mushrooms are not available, you may use a 3- or 4-oz. can of mushroom stems and pieces, undrained.

	Calories	Carbo-hydrate (gm)	Protein (gm)	Total Fat (gm)	Saturated Fat (gm)	Choles-terol (mg)
Total	244.7	28.7	17.5	8.5	1.0	0.0
Per Serving	40.8	4.8	2.9	1.4	0.2	0.0

Chinese Style Mushrooms

1 lb. fresh mushrooms
1 tbsp. diet margarine
2 tbsp. soy sauce

2 tbsp. water
1 tbsp. cornstarch

Before cooking: Wash the mushrooms, and cut them into thin slices.

Melt the margarine in a non-stick skillet. Add the mushrooms and cook them for 3 minutes, stirring as needed. Combine the rest of the ingredients in a cup, and then stir this mixture in with the mushrooms. Continue to cook and stir for about 2 minutes until the sauce is clear. *Makes 4 servings*

	Calories	Carbo-hydrate (gm)	Protein (gm)	Total Fat (gm)	Saturated Fat (gm)	Choles-terol (mg)
Total	220.4	28.4	14.9	7.8	1.0	0.0
Per Serving	55.1	7.1	3.7	2.0	0.3	0.0

---

gm=grams; mg=milligrams. Nutritional figures are approximate. Figures are based on findings of U.S. Department of Agriculture.

Minted Peas

2 cups shelled peas
½ cup chopped green
  onion
1 tbsp. diet margarine
2 tbsp. water

1 tbsp. finely
  chopped fresh
  mint leaves
1 tsp. lemon juice
¼ tsp. salt

Melt the margarine in a non-stick skillet and sauté the onions until they are tender. Then add the rest of the ingredients. Cover the pan, and simmer the contents for 7 or 8 minutes. Add a little water, if necessary, to keep the peas from burning. *Makes 4 servings*

	Calories	Carbo-hydrate (gm)	Protein (gm)	Total Fat (gm)	Saturated Fat (gm)	Choles-terol (mg)
Total	301.2	43.4	19.0	8.0	1.0	0.0
Per Serving	75.3	10.9	4.8	2.0	0.3	0.0

Peas and Cauliflower

1 package frozen
  cauliflower
1 package frozen peas
¼ tsp. butter salt

¼ tsp. pepper
2 tbsp. chopped
  pimiento

Cook the vegetables according to the directions on the package. Stir in the pimiento and season with the salt and pepper. *Makes 4 servings*

	Calories	Carbo-hydrate (gm)	Protein (gm)	Total Fat (gm)	Saturated Fat (gm)	Choles-terol (mg)
Total	255.6	46.4	21.3	0.3	0.0	0.0
Per Serving	63.9	11.6	5.3	0.1	0.0	0.0

Italian Fried Peppers

5 Italian frying peppers
1 medium onion
2 cloves garlic
2 tbsp. water

2 tsp. olive oil
½ tsp. Italian
  seasoning
salt
pepper

Before cooking: Cut the tops off the peppers. Cut the peppers into slices, discarding the inner pulp and seeds. Peel and slice the onion. Mince the garlic cloves.

Combine all of the ingredients in a non-stick skillet. Cover the pan and cook the contents over moderate heat for 2 minutes. Then remove the cover and continue cooking until the moisture has evaporated and the vegetables begin to brown slightly.

Makes 4 servings

	Calories	Carbo-hydrate (gm)	Protein (gm)	Total Fat (gm)	Saturated Fat (gm)	Choles-terol (mg)
Total	197.5	25.0	7.0	9.2	1.3	0.0
Per Serving	49.4	6.3	1.8	2.3	0.3	0.0

Stir-Fried Peppers

4 Italian frying peppers   1 tbsp. water
1 large onion   1 tsp. olive oil
2 tbsp. soy sauce

Before cooking: Slice the tops from the peppers. Cut the peppers into strips, removing the inner pulp and seeds. Peel and slice the onion, breaking the slices into rings.

Place all of the ingredients in a non-stick skillet. Cover the pan and simmer the contents for 2 minutes. Then remove the cover and continue cooking until the moisture evaporates and the vegetables just begin to brown slightly in the oil that will remain in the pan.

Makes 4 servings

	Calories	Carbo-hydrate (gm)	Protein (gm)	Total Fat (gm)	Saturated Fat (gm)	Choles-terol (mg)
Total	181.3	29.0	9.0	4.6	0.7	0.0
Per Serving	45.3	7.3	2.3	1.2	0.2	0.0

---

gm=grams; mg=milligrams. Nutritional figures are approximate. Figures are based on findings of U.S. Department of Agriculture.

Skillet Pepper and Tomatoes

1 tbsp. diet margarine
1 1/2 cups sliced sweet
    onions
2 green peppers
3 medium tomatoes

1 tsp. salt
1/4 tsp. pepper
1/4 tsp. oregano

Before cooking: Cut the green peppers into thin strips. Peel the tomatoes by first plunging them into boiling water, and cut each one into 8 wedges.

Melt the diet margarine in a non-stick skillet over low heat. Add the onions and sauté them until tender. Add the green pepper and tomatoes and the seasonings. Cover the skillet and simmer the contents for about 10 minutes — just until the peppers are tender-crisp. *Makes 6 servings*

	Calories	Carbo-hydrate (gm)	Protein (gm)	Total Fat (gm)	Saturated Fat (gm)	Choles-terol (mg)
Total	260.0	48.0	11.0	6.0	1.0	0.0
Per Serving	43.3	8.0	1.8	1.0	0.2	0.0

Green Peppers and Tomatoes

1 tsp. olive oil
1/2 cup thinly-sliced
    onion
2 cloves garlic, minced
1 lb. can tomatoes
2 tsp. sugar

1 tsp. salt
1/4 tsp. pepper
1/2 tsp. basil
4 cups green pepper
    cut in strips

Heat the oil in a large non-stick skillet and sauté the onion and garlic until they are tender. Add the tomatoes (with the liquid) and the seasonings. Simmer the mixture uncovered and then add the green pepper. Continue simmering until the green pepper is tender but still crisp. *Makes 6 servings*

	Calories	Carbo-hydrate (gm)	Protein (gm)	Total Fat (gm)	Saturated Fat (gm)	Choles-terol (mg)
Total	245.1	43.6	8.7	6.5	0.7	0.0
Per Serving	40.9	7.3	1.5	1.1	0.1	0.0

Baked Rutabagas

2 lbs. rutabagas
1½ tsp. butter-flavored
   salt

⅓ cup water

Spray a casserole with spray-on vegetable coating. Pare and dice the rutabagas and place the pieces in the casserole with the other ingredients. Cover the casserole and bake the rutabagas at 350° for about 1 hour until they are tender. *Makes 6 servings*

	Calories	Carbo-hydrate (gm)	Protein (gm)	Total Fat (gm)	Saturated Fat (gm)	Choles-terol (mg)
Total	319.9	73.1	9.1	0.0	0.0	0.0
Per Serving	53.3	12.2	1.5	0.0	0.0	0.0

Rutabaga-Onion Casserole

2 lbs. rutabagas
3 cups thinly-sliced
   onion
salt

pepper
1 chicken bouillon
   cube
½ cup boiling water

Pare the rutabaga and cut it into thin slices. Arrange alternate layers of rutabaga and onion slices in a 2½-quart casserole. Sprinkle each layer lightly with salt and pepper. Dissolve the bouillon cube in the boiling water and pour the bouillon over the vegetables. Cover the casserole, and bake at 350° for about 1¼ hours until the rutabagas are tender. *Makes 6 servings*

	Calories	Carbo-hydrate (gm)	Protein (gm)	Total Fat (gm)	Saturated Fat (gm)	Choles-terol (mg)
Total	446.9	121.6	24.8	7.0	2.0	0.0
Per Serving	74.5	20.3	4.1	1.2	0.3	0.0

---

gm=grams; mg=milligrams. Nutritional figures are approximate. Figures are based on findings of U.S. Department of Agriculture.

Oriental Spinach

2 tsp. lemon juice
1½ tbsp. soy sauce
sugar substitute to
equal 1 tsp.
1 tbsp. corn oil
1½ cups diagonally-
sliced celery

6 oz. can sliced
mushrooms,
drained
½ cup thinly-sliced
onion
6 cups washed fresh
spinach leaves

Combine the lemon juice, soy sauce, and sugar substitute in a cup and set it aside. Heat the oil in a non-stick skillet. Add the celery, mushrooms, and onion, and stir-fry them for 1 minute. Then add the spinach and lemon-juice mixture. Stir-fry the vegetables for about 2 minutes longer until the celery and onion are tender-crisp and the spinach is just limp. Do not overcook! *Makes 4 servings*

Diet hint: The careful calorie-counter can save an extra 75 calories by using diet margarine instead of corn oil.

	Calories	Carbo-hydrate (gm)	Protein (gm)	Total Fat (gm)	Saturated Fat (gm)	Choles-terol (mg)
Total	482.9	61.0	39.8	20.0	1.0	0.0
Per Serving	120.7	15.3	10.0	5.0	0.3	0.0

Mashed Acorn Squash

2 medium acorn squash
1 tbsp. skim milk
½ tsp. cinnamon

½ tsp. allspice
½ tsp. butter-flavored
salt

Cut the acorn squash in half and place the halves, cut side down, in a baking pan. Bake them for about 30 minutes at 400° until they are tender. Scoop the squash from shells, and place in bowl. Mash the squash, stirring in the remaining ingredients. *Makes 8 servings*

	Calories	Carbo-hydrate (gm)	Protein (gm)	Total Fat (gm)	Saturated Fat (gm)	Choles-terol (mg)
Total	503.3	123.3	15.8	3.8	0.0	0.3
Per Serving	62.9	15.4	2.0	0.5	0.0	0.0

Sesame Spinach

1½ lbs. fresh spinach
½ tsp. butter-flavored
   salt

2 tbsp. sesame
   seeds

Before cooking: Toast sesame seeds by sprinkling them on a cookie sheet and baking them at 400° until they are brown. Watch them carefully so they do not burn. Cut tough stems off spinach and wash carefully.

Place the spinach in a saucepan with just the water that clings to the leaves. Add the salt. Cook the spinach over moderate heat, uncovered, just until it is tender. Sprinkle the sesame seeds over the cooked spinach. *Makes 4 servings*

	Calories	Carbo-hydrate (gm)	Protein (gm)	Total Fat (gm)	Saturated Fat (gm)	Choles-terol (mg)
Total	256.1	27.2	22.8	12.7	1.3	0.0
Per Serving	64.0	6.8	5.7	3.2	0.3	0.0

Orange Simmered Squash

¾ lb. yellow summer
   squash
6 oz. can unsweetened
   orange juice

½ tsp. arrowroot or
   cornstarch
2 green onions
   salt
   pepper

Slice the squash and green onions, combining them with the rest of the ingredients in a shallow saucepan. Leaving the pan uncovered, simmer the contents, stirring occasionally, until most of the liquid has evaporated. *Makes 4 servings*

	Calories	Carbo-hydrate (gm)	Protein (gm)	Total Fat (gm)	Saturated Fat (gm)	Choles-terol (mg)
Total	148.2	34.8	5.0	0.0	0.0	0.0
Per Serving	37.1	8.7	1.3	0.0	0.0	0.0

gm=grams; mg=milligrams. Nutritional figures are approximate. Figures are based on findings of U.S. Department of Agriculture.

Baked Squash Casserole

2 lbs. yellow summer
  squash
1/4 cup water
3 tbsp. chopped onion
3 eggs, beaten
1/2 tsp. hot pepper sauce

2 tsp. parsley flakes
salt
pepper
5 tbsp. cracker
  crumbs

Slice the squash into 1/2-inch pieces and boil it for about 3 minutes in the water until it is tender. Drain the squash and add the onion, eggs, and seasonings. Mix until well-blended. Pour the mixture into a 1-quart casserole that has been sprayed with spray-on vegetable coating. Sprinkle the cracker crumbs over the top. Bake the casserole uncovered at 350° for 35 to 40 minutes until the squash is brown. *Makes 6 servings*

	Calories	Carbo-hydrate (gm)	Protein (gm)	Total Fat (gm)	Saturated Fat (gm)	Choles-terol (mg)
Total	438.2	41.8	28.2	19.3	6.0	756.0
Per Serving	73.0	7.0	4.7	3.2	1.0	126.0

Baked Acorn Squash

3 small acorn squash
1 tsp. salt

5 tbsp. diet
  margarine
5 tbsp. diet maple
  syrup

Wash the squash and cut them in half, discarding the seeds. Sprinkle the surface of the squash with salt and place them cut side down in a baking dish. Bake them at 400° for 25 minutes. Combine the margarine and syrup. Turn the squash cut side up and spoon the syrup mixture into each cavity. Bake them for about 30 minutes longer until they are tender. *Makes 6 servings*

	Calories	Carbo-hydrate (gm)	Protein (gm)	Total Fat (gm)	Saturated Fat (gm)	Choles-terol (mg)
Total	895.0	159.0	18.0	34.5	5.0	0.0
Per Serving	149.2	26.5	3.0	5.8	0.8	0.0

Baked Tomatoes

2 large ripe tomatoes   minced parsley
liquid sweetener   salt
minced green onion   pepper

Slice the tomatoes in half and place each half on a large square of double-thick foil. Sprinkle the surface of the tomato with sweetener, green onion, parsley, salt, and pepper. Bring the foil up and around the tomato half. Seal the sides of the foil, but leave a space at the top for steam to escape. Bake the tomatoes at 350° for 20 minutes.   *Makes 4 servings*

	Calories	Carbo-hydrate (gm)	Protein (gm)	Total Fat (gm)	Saturated Fat (gm)	Choles-terol (mg)
Total	82.2	18.3	4.1	0.0	0.0	0.0
Per Serving	20.6	4.6	1.0	0.0	0.0	0.0

Stewed Tomatoes

2 lbs. tomatoes   1½ tsp. garlic salt
4 green onions   ¼ tsp. seasoned
                    pepper

Before cooking: Peel the tomatoes by first plunging them in boiling water. Chop the green onions.

Cut the tomatoes into wedges and place them in a saucepan. Add the remaining ingredients and cook them over moderate heat for 10 minutes, stirring occasionally.   *Makes 6 servings*

	Calories	Carbo-hydrate (gm)	Protein (gm)	Total Fat (gm)	Saturated Fat (gm)	Choles-terol (mg)
Total	192.4	43.6	9.7	0.0	0.0	0.0
Per Serving	32.1	7.3	1.6	0.0	0.0	0.0

---

gm=grams; mg=milligrams. Nutritional figures are approximate. Figures are based on findings of U.S. Department of Agriculture.

Tomato-Spinach Bake

4 tbsp. flour
1 tbsp. chopped onion
1 lb. can tomatoes
1 cup cooked spinach,
    well-drained

1 cup 99% fat-free
    cottage cheese
2 eggs, beaten
1 tsp. salt

Combine the flour, onion, and tomatoes (with the liquid) in a saucepan. Cook the mixture over moderate heat until it has thickened slightly. Then add the remaining ingredients and mix well. Pour the entire mixture into a 1½-quart casserole that has been sprayed with spray-on vegetable coating. Bake the casserole for 20 minutes at 325°. *Makes 6 servings*

	Calories	Carbo-hydrate (gm)	Protein (gm)	Total Fat (gm)	Saturated Fat (gm)	Cholesterol (mg)
Total	594.2	55.0	54.1	17.2	5.2	523.4
Per Serving	99.0	9.2	9.0	2.9	0.9	87.2

Broiled Tomatoes

6 medium tomatoes
¼ cup diet mayonnaise

2 oz. Swiss cheese
½ tsp. paprika

Before cooking: Grate the Swiss cheese medium fine.
Cut each tomato in half. Mix the mayonnaise, cheese, and paprika together, and spread this mixture over the cut surface of the tomatoes. Broil the tomatoes for about 5 minutes until the tops are brown. *Makes 6 servings*

	Calories	Carbo-hydrate (gm)	Protein (gm)	Total Fat (gm)	Saturated Fat (gm)	Cholesterol (mg)
Total	527.9	58.0	27.4	23.4	7.7	88.7
Per Serving	88.0	9.7	4.6	3.9	1.3	14.8

Skillet Vegetables

1 tbsp. diet margarine
2 cups diagonally
  sliced carrots
2 cups snap beans,
  broken into 1-inch
  pieces

2 cups sliced
  summer squash
1 cup thinly-sliced
  onion
1/2 tsp. salt
  ground black
  pepper

Melt the margarine in a non-stick skillet. Add the vegetables and salt. Cover the pan, and cook the vegetables for 10 to 15 minutes until they are crisp-tender, stirring occasionally. Season with the pepper according to your taste and serve the vegetables hot.

Makes 6 servings

	Calories	Carbo-hydrate (gm)	Protein (gm)	Total Fat (gm)	Saturated Fat (gm)	Choles-terol (mg)
Total	290.0	58.0	14.0	6.0	1.0	0.0
Per Serving	48.3	9.7	2.3	1.0	0.2	0.0

Beefy Vegetables

1 package frozen
  vegetables
1/2 cup water

1 beef bouillon
  cube

Place the water in a saucepan and bring it to a boil. Add the bouillon cube and vegetables, separating the beans with a fork. Heat the liquid to boiling. Lower the heat, and simmer the vegetables until they are tender.

Makes 3 servings

	Calories	Carbo-hydrate (gm)	Protein (gm)	Total Fat (gm)	Saturated Fat (gm)	Choles-terol (mg)
Total	188.0	37.2	9.6	0.0	0.0	3.0
Per Serving	62.7	12.4	3.2	0.0	0.0	1.0

gm=grams; mg=milligrams. Nutritional figures are approximate. Figures are based on findings of U.S. Department of Agriculture.

Apple-Glazed Zucchini

2 zucchini squash (³/₄ lb.)
6 oz. can unsweetened apple juice
¹/₂ tsp. arrowroot or cornstarch

1 tsp. instant dried onion
¹/₂ tsp. dried parsley flakes
salt
pepper

Slice the zucchini and combine it with the rest of the ingredients in a shallow saucepan. Simmer the mixture, uncovered, over moderate heat, stirring occasionally, until most of the liquid has evaporated, leaving a thick sauce.   *Makes 4 servings*

	Calories	Carbohydrate (gm)	Protein (gm)	Total Fat (gm)	Saturated Fat (gm)	Cholesterol (mg)
Total	145.1	35.4	3.3	0.0	0.0	0.0
Per Serving	36.3	8.9	0.8	0.0	0.0	0.0

Zucchini Italienne

6 medium zucchini
2 tbsp. diet margarine
¹/₄ tsp. butter-flavored salt

¹/₂ tsp. oregano
¹/₂ cup grated Parmesan cheese

Before cooking: Scrub the zucchini well with a brush, but do not pare them. Cut them into ¹/₄-inch slices.

Melt the margarine in a heavy non-stick skillet and add the zucchini. Season them with salt and oregano, cover the pan tightly and cook them over low heat for about 5 minutes — just long enough to heat the slices through. Remove the pan from the heat and sprinkle the cheese over the zucchini. Serve immediately.   *Makes 12 servings*

	Calories	Carbohydrate (gm)	Protein (gm)	Total Fat (gm)	Saturated Fat (gm)	Cholesterol (mg)
Total	904.0	46.8	69.6	55.2	26.0	129.6
Per Serving	75.3	3.9	5.8	4.6	2.2	10.8

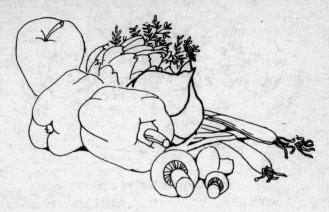

Ratatouille Provencale

3 onions
4 green peppers
1 medium eggplant
2 garlic cloves
4 small zucchini

4 tomatoes
1 tbsp. chopped
   black olives
1 tsp. salt
¼ tsp. freshly ground
   black pepper

Before cooking: Slice the onions and tomatoes. Slice the zucchini, but do not peel them. Seed the green peppers and cut them into eighths. Peel and cube the eggplant. Mince the garlic.

Arrange the vegetables in layers in a baking dish. Sprinkle the garlic, salt, pepper, and olives over each layer. Cover the baking dish and bake at 275° for about 40 minutes until the vegetables are soft. Then remove the cover, raise the heat to 500° and continue to cook for about 5 minutes longer — until the liquid is reduced. *Makes 6 servings*

	Calories	Carbo-hydrate (gm)	Protein (gm)	Total Fat (gm)	Saturated Fat (gm)	Choles-terol (mg)
Total	518.3	115.1	28.3	2.0	0.0	0.0
Per Serving	86.4	19.2	4.7	0.3	0.0	0.0

gm=grams; mg=milligrams. Nutritional figures are approximate. Figures are based on findings of U.S. Department of Agriculture.

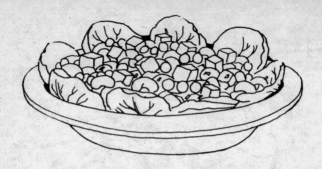

Romanian Ghivetch

1 potato
1 carrot
1 eggplant
17 oz. can Italian plum
    tomatoes
1 yellow squash
2 medium onions
1/2 cup fresh or frozen
    green peas

1/2 cup fresh or frozen
    cut green beans
2 ribs celery
1/2 tsp. hot pepper
    sauce
1 1/2 tsp. salt
10 1/2 oz. can condensed
    beef bouillon
1 clove garlic
1 tsp. dried dill weed

Before cooking: Pare and dice the potato and eggplant.
Pare the carrot and cut it into thin slices. Drain the can
of tomatoes. Thinly slice the squash, but don't pare it.
Slice the onions and celery. Crush the garlic in a garlic
press. Skim the fat from the bouillon by chilling it until
the fat rises to the top and can be whisked away.

Arrange the vegetables in layers in a 3- or 4-quart
casserole and sprinkle each layer with salt. In a
saucepan, heat together the hot pepper sauce,
bouillon, and garlic. Pour this over the vegetables and
sprinkle the dill over the top. Cover the casserole, and
bake it at 350° for 1 hour or longer until all the vegetables are tender.   *Makes 6 servings*

	Calories	Carbo-hydrate (gm)	Protein (gm)	Total Fat (gm)	Saturated Fat (gm)	Choles-terol (mg)
Total	516.4	104.5	34.0	2.5	0.0	62.9
Per Serving	86.1	17.4	5.7	0.4	0.0	10.5

*gm=grams; mg=milligrams. Nutritional figures are approximate. Figures
are based on findings of U.S. Department of Agriculture.*

Potatoes, Pasta, And Rice

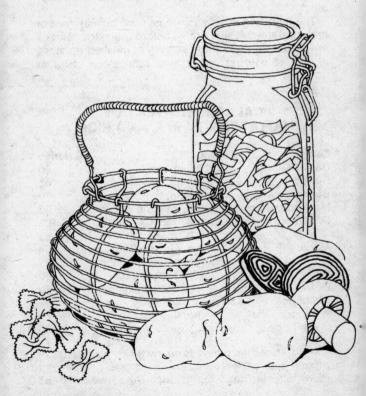

I f you pass up potatoes, skip spaghetti, or refuse rice — in favor of a second helping of steak — you are probably a victim of the carbohydrate myth. Low-Carb dieters seem to think some calories are more fattening than others and that somehow they can achieve slimness on limitless meat, cheese, cream, and other high-fat foods.

As a matter of fact, the so-called "starchy" potatoes, pasta, and rice are relatively low in calories. Most cost between 70 and 90 calories a serving, considerably less than the second helping of high-fat foods most low-carb dieters would replace them with. In fact, the only time these appetite-appeasers become fattening is when fat is added to them — in the form of butter, cream sauce, gravy, cheese, or other calorie-rich toppings.

The following chart shows just how low-cal most of these palate-pleasers are — before the extra calories are added on. A half-cup serving of mashed potatoes is only 63 calories, but a level tablespoon of butter adds 100 more.

CALORIE CONTENT OF POTATOES, PASTA, AND RICE

Item	Amount	Calories
Baked potato	1 medium, no fat	90
Boiled potato	1 medium, peeled	65
Boiled potato	1 medium, unpeeled	76
Mashed potato	$^1/_2$ cup, milk, no fat	63
Spaghetti	$^1/_2$ cup, cooked firm	108
	$^1/_2$ cup, cooked tender	83
Macaroni	$^1/_2$ cup, cooked firm	104
	$^1/_2$ cup, cooked tender	75
Egg noodles	$^1/_2$ cup, cooked	100
Brown rice	$^1/_2$ cup, cooked	89
White rice	$^1/_2$ cup, cooked	82
Long grain rice	$^1/_2$ cup, cooked	79
Instant rice	$^1/_2$ cup, prepared, no fat	80

A frozen stuffed potato is nearly triple the calories of a plain potato. Heat-and-serve fried rice is 40 percent more fattening than regular rice. And macaroni and cheese made from a convenience mix is double the calories of plain pasta.

But who wants plain potatoes or naked noodles? In this chapter we offer a variety of variations from standard fattening recipes — all aimed at keeping calorie counts low.

Recipes

Hi-Protein Cottage Potato Salad

- ¹/₄ cup plain yogurt
- 2 tbsp. diet Italian salad dressing
- 2 cups peeled, diced cooked potatoes
- 2 eggs
- 2 cups 99% fat-free cottage cheese
- ¹/₂ cup sliced celery
- ¹/₃ cup chopped ripe olives
- ¹/₃ cup sliced radishes
- ¹/₃ cup chopped green onions
- ¹/₂ tsp. salt

Before preparing: Hard-boil the eggs and then chop them.

Blend the yogurt and salad dressing together in a bowl. Add the potatoes and eggs and allow them to marinate at room temperature while you slice and chop the rest of the ingredients. Then add the rest of the ingredients to the bowl and mix everything well. Refrigerate the potato salad for several hours before serving.   *Makes 8 servings*

	Calories	Carbo-hydrate (gm)	Protein (gm)	Total Fat (gm)	Saturated Fat (gm)	Choles-terol (mg)
Total	834.4	59.0	78.7	29.7	6.9	547.8
Per Serving	104.3	7.4	9.8	3.7	0.9	68.5

gm=grams; mg=milligrams. Nutritional figures are approximate. Figures are based on findings of U.S. Department of Agriculture.

Red Onion Potato Salad

6 white potatoes
1 cup sliced celery
1 cup thinly-sliced red
  onion
1 cup cut-up parsley

4 tbsp. low-calorie
  Italian dressing
3 tbsp. wine vinegar
2 tsp. salt
dash of cayenne

Boil the potatoes, pare them, and cut them into slices. Toss them with the rest of the ingredients and chill the mixture before serving. *Makes 12 servings*

	Calories	Carbo-hydrate (gm)	Protein (gm)	Total Fat (gm)	Saturated Fat (gm)	Choles-terol (mg)
Total	586.0	127.0	14.0	4.0	0.0	0.0
Per Serving	48.8	10.6	1.2	0.3	0.0	0.0

Yogurt Potato Salad

8 cups boiled potatoes,
  pared and diced
1½ tbsp. vinegar
2 tbsp. corn or safflower
  oil
1½ tsp. garlic salt
1 tsp. dill weed
¼ tsp. pepper

¼ cup chopped
  pimiento-stuffed
  olives
1½ cups sliced celery
⅓ cup sliced green
  onion
8 oz. plain yogurt
1 tsp. prepared
  mustard
1 tsp. sugar

Mix the vinegar, oil, salt, dill weed, and pepper together. Pour this mixture over the potatoes and mix them gently. Chill the potato mixture for several hours. At serving time, add the olives, celery, and onion. Mix together the yogurt, mustard, and sugar, and fold this mixture into the potatoes gently but thoroughly.

Makes 16 servings

	Calories	Carbo-hydrate (gm)	Protein (gm)	Total Fat (gm)	Saturated Fat (gm)	Choles-terol (mg)
Total	1142.4	183.6	24.1	37.7	3.9	18.6
Per Serving	71.4	11.5	1.5	2.4	0.2	1.2

Basic Potato Salad

7 cups boiled potatoes,
    pared and diced
1½ cups diced celery
3 tbsp. finely chopped
    parsley
1 onion
1 cup diet mayonnaise

3 tbsp. vinegar
1 tsp. salt
    dash paprika
    dash pepper

Chop the onion and mix it with the rest of the ingredients. Cover the salad and chill it until ready to serve.
Makes 16 servings

	Calories	Carbo-hydrate (gm)	Protein (gm)	Total Fat (gm)	Saturated Fat (gm)	Choles-terol (mg)
Total	948.5	164.0	16.0	32.0	0.0	128.0
Per Serving	59.3	10.3	1.0	2.0	0.0	8.0

"Sweet Potato" Mock Pudding

2 packages frozen
    mashed squash
1 box (2 envelopes)
    low-calorie vanilla
    pudding mix
1 tsp. salt

2 tbsp. diet maple
    syrup
    pinch of pumpkin
    pie spice
1 egg white

Before cooking: Allow the squash to thaw.

Whip the squash, pudding mix, salt, syrup, and pumpkin pie spice together. Beat the egg white until it forms stiff peaks and fold it into the squash. Spoon the mixture into a non-stick baking dish and bake it in a preheated 350° oven for 30 minutes. *Makes 6 servings.*

	Calories	Carbo-hydrate (gm)	Protein (gm)	Total Fat (gm)	Saturated Fat (gm)	Choles-terol (mg)
Total	319.1	72.7	9.3	0.0	0.0	0.0
Per Serving	53.2	12.1	1.6	0.0	0.0	0.0

gm=grams; mg=milligrams. Nutritional figures are approximate. Figures are based on findings of U.S. Department of Agriculture.

Easy Au Gratin Potatoes

3 potatoes
1/2 cup celery chunks

10 3/4 oz. can cheddar
    cheese soup
1 tbsp. prepared
    mustard

Peel the potatoes and boil them until they are tender. Drain off the water and cut the potatoes into slices. Arrange the slices and the celery chunks in a non-stick baking dish. Mix the cheese soup and the mustard together in a bowl, and pour this mixture over the potatoes. Bake the potatoes at 375° for 30 minutes.

Makes 8 servings

	Calories	Carbo-hydrate (gm)	Protein (gm)	Total Fat (gm)	Saturated Fat (gm)	Choles-terol (mg)
Total	750.5	111.8	18.9	0.0	12.9	64.5
Per Serving	93.8	14.0	2.4	0.0	1.6	8.1

Potato Dumplings For Stew

2 large potatoes
1/4 cup skim milk
1 egg
4 tbsp. flour

1 tbsp. minced onion
1 tbsp. chopped
    parsley
1/2 tsp. salt
paprika

Peel the potatoes, cut them into chunks and boil them until they are tender. Drain off the water, and mash the potatoes, adding the skim milk a little at a time, until they are smooth. Then add all the rest of the ingredients, except the paprika. Scoop up rounded spoonfuls of the potato mixture and place them on top of the stew. Sprinkle them with paprika. Cover the pot and simmer the stew with the potatoes for 20 minutes.

Makes 12 dumplings
(6 servings)

	Calories	Carbo-hydrate (gm)	Protein (gm)	Total Fat (gm)	Saturated Fat (gm)	Choles-terol (mg)
Total	469.7	77.4	19.7	8.3	2.0	261.3
Per Serving	78.3	12.9	3.3	1.4	0.3	43.6

Protein Potato Patties

2 cups shredded raw
  potatoes
2 eggs, beaten
3 tbsp. grated onion

1 tbsp. flour
1/2 tsp. salt
2 tbsp. diet
  margarine

Combine the shredded potatoes with the eggs, onion, flour, and salt. Melt the margarine in a non-stick skillet. Drop the potato mixture from a tablespoon into the hot margarine and fry the patties on both sides until they are crisp. *Makes 10 servings*

	Calories	Carbo-hydrate (gm)	Protein (gm)	Total Fat (gm)	Saturated Fat (gm)	Choles-terol (mg)
Total	455.3	43.8	17.2	24.1	6.0	504.0
Per Serving	45.5	4.4	1.7	2.4	0.6	50.4

Cream Cheese Potato Casserole

3 potatoes
1/4 cup skim milk
4 oz. low-calorie
  cream cheese

1 tbsp. chopped
  chives
1 beaten egg
paprika

Peel the potatoes, cut them into cubes and boil them until they are tender. Drain the water and mash the potatoes. Add the skim milk, a little at a time, until the potatoes are smooth. Then add the diet cream cheese, and beat the mixture well. Stir in the egg and chives and spoon the mixture into a 1-quart casserole that has been sprayed with spray-on vegetable coating. Sprinkle paprika on the top and bake the potato casserole at 400° for 30 minutes. *Makes 8 servings*

	Calories	Carbo-hydrate (gm)	Protein (gm)	Total Fat (gm)	Saturated Fat (gm)	Choles-terol (mg)
Total	626.0	61.8	22.6	30.0	18.0	337.3
Per Serving	78.3	7.7	2.8	3.8	2.3	42.2

---

gm=grams; mg=milligrams. Nutritional figures are approximate. Figures are based on findings of U.S. Department of Agriculture.

Baked Potatoes Cottage Style

4 well-shaped baking
potatoes
1/2 cup plain yogurt
1 cup 99% fat-free
cottage cheese
1 tbsp. onion flakes

1/2 tsp. butter-flavored
salt
pinch of pepper
paprika
dried parsley
flakes

Scrub the potatoes and bake them in a preheated 400° oven for 50 to 60 minutes until they are tender. Remove them from the oven; carefully slice the potatoes in half. Scoop out the potato pulp and place it in a bowl. Mash together the potato pulp, yogurt, cottage cheese, onion flakes, salt, and pepper; or whip the mixture on the high speed of your electric mixer. Pile the potato mixture back into the baked potato skins and sprinkle the top with paprika and parsley. Return the potatoes to a 425° oven and bake them until they are lightly browned. *Makes 8 servings*

	Calories	Carbo-hydrate (gm)	Protein (gm)	Total Fat (gm)	Saturated Fat (gm)	Choles-terol (mg)
Total	613.0	99.0	46.3	4.0	2.2	29.4
Per Serving	76.6	12.4	5.8	0.5	0.3	3.7

Tangy Potatoes

6 potatoes (2 lbs. total)
4 tbsp. chopped fresh
parsley
2 tbsp. minced green
onion

4 tbsp. lemon juice
1 tsp. grated lemon
peel
1 tsp. butter-flavored
salt

Peel the potatoes and cube them. Toss them with the rest of the ingredients and place the mixture in a non-stick baking dish. Cover the dish, and bake the potatoes at 425° for 45 minutes. *Makes 12 servings*

	Calories	Carbo-hydrate (gm)	Protein (gm)	Total Fat (gm)	Saturated Fat (gm)	Choles-terol (mg)
Total	505.3	114.6	12.6	0.0	0.0	0.0
Per Serving	42.1	9.6	1.1	0.0	0.0	0.0

Creamed Potatoes with Bacon Bits

3 pared potatoes (1 lb. total)
10³/₄ oz. can condensed cream of celery soup

4 tbsp. water
4 tbsp. minced onion
pinch of pepper
1 tbsp. bacon-flavored bits

Boil the potatoes, drain them, and cut them into chunks. In a saucepan, combine the soup, water, onion, and pepper. Cook this mixture over low heat for 5 to 10 minutes, stirring occasionally. Then add the potatoes and continue to heat thoroughly. Serve the potatoes garnished with the bacon-flavored bits.

Makes 8 servings

	Calories	Carbo-hydrate (gm)	Protein (gm)	Total Fat (gm)	Saturated Fat (gm)	Choles-terol (mg)
Total	475.3	80.1	11.7	13.1	0.0	18.3
Per Serving	59.4	10.0	1.5	1.6	0.0	2.3

Scalloped Potatoes

2 cups thinly-sliced potatoes
¹/₂ cup sliced mushrooms
¹/₂ cup sliced onions
4 beef bouillon cubes

1¹/₂ cups boiling water
1 tsp. butter-flavored salt
pinch of pepper
pinch of nutmeg

Mix the potatoes, mushrooms, and onions in a non-stick baking dish. Dissolve the bouillon cubes in the water; blend in the salt, pepper and nutmeg, and pour this mixture over the vegetables. Cover the baking pan, and bake the potatoes for 45 minutes at 350°. Then uncover the pan and bake it for 20 minutes longer.

Makes 6 servings

	Calories	Carbo-hydrate (gm)	Protein (gm)	Total Fat (gm)	Saturated Fat (gm)	Choles-terol (mg)
Total	254.0	52.5	14.5	0.5	0.0	12.0
Per Serving	42.3	8.8	2.4	0.1	0.0	2.0

gm=grams; mg=milligrams. Nutritional figures are approximate. Figures are based on findings of U.S. Department of Agriculture.

Stuffed Potatoes

4 baking potatoes
2 egg whites
1 tsp. butter-flavored
  salt
pinch of cream of
  tartar
pinch of pepper

1 tsp. freeze-dried
  chives
$^1/_2$ to $^3/_4$ cup skim milk
3 tbsp. grated extra-
  sharp cheddar
  cheese
paprika

Scrub the potatoes, pierce them with a fork and bake them at 400° for about 1 hour until the potato is soft. Remove the potatoes from the oven and carefully slice them in half, lengthwise. Combine the salt, egg whites, and cream of tartar in a bowl. Using an electric mixer, whip the egg whites until stiff peaks form. Carefully scoop out the pulp of the potatoes and place them in another bowl. Add the pepper and chives and whip them with the electric mixer, adding a little milk at a time until they are fluffy. Fold the egg white mixture into the potatoes and pile the mixture back into the potato skins. Sprinkle the top of each potato with grated cheese and paprika and return the potatoes to the oven. Bake them at 425° until the cheese is melted and the potatoes are hot. *Makes 8 servings*

	Calories	Carbo-hydrate (gm)	Protein (gm)	Total Fat (gm)	Saturated Fat (gm)	Choles-terol (mg)
Total	686.6	94.8	40.8	18.0	10.0	59.8
Per Serving	85.8	11.9	5.1	2.3	1.3	7.5

Macaroni Salad

8 oz. elbow macaroni
$^1/_2$ cup diet mayonnaise
1 cup chopped celery
$^1/_2$ cup plain yogurt

2 tbsp. chopped
  onion
$1^1/_2$ tsp. salt
$^1/_4$ tsp. pepper
paprika

Cook the macaroni according to the directions on the package, drain it, and rinse it with cold water. Add the rest of the ingredients to the macaroni, mixing thoroughly, and chill the mixture for several hours.

Makes 8 servings

	Calories	Carbo-hydrate (gm)	Protein (gm)	Total Fat (gm)	Saturated Fat (gm)	Choles-terol (mg)
Total	490.8	73.0	12.2	19.6	1.0	74.0
Per Serving	61.4	9.1	1.5	2.5	0.1	9.3

Shell Salad

4½ tsp. dried onion flakes
2 tbsp. vinegar
1 cup diet mayonnaise
1¾ tsp. salt
¼ tsp. pepper
2 tsp. paprika

8 oz. small shell macaroni
3 medium tomatoes
½ cup chopped green pepper
2 tbsp. sliced black olives
3 eggs
2 tbsp. snipped parsley

Before preparing: Hard-boil the eggs and cut them into slices. Cook the macaroni according to the directions on the package and drain it. Cut the tomatoes into wedges.

Combine the onion and vinegar and let it stand for a few minutes. Then add the mayonnaise, salt, pepper, and paprika and mix well. Mix the macaroni, tomatoes, green pepper, and olives in a large salad bowl; and pour the mayonnaise mixture over all. Toss lightly. Chill the salad for several hours before serving. When serving, garnish with the egg slices and parsley.

Makes 8 servings

	Calories	Carbo-hydrate (gm)	Protein (gm)	Total Fat (gm)	Saturated Fat (gm)	Choles-terol (mg)
Total	985.0	102.3	33.0	55.7	6.0	884.0
Per Serving	164.2	17.1	5.5	9.3	1.0	147.3

---

gm=grams; mg=milligrams. Nutritional figures are approximate. Figures are based on findings of U.S. Department of Agriculture.

Macaroni and Cottage Cheese Salad

3 cups cooked elbow
 macaroni
1 1/2 cups 99% fat-free
 cottage cheese
1 onion
1/2 cup minced green
 pepper

1 carrot
salt
pepper
chili powder

Mince the onion and grate the carrot. Toss the vegetables lightly with the remaining ingredients. Chill the salad before serving. *Makes 10 servings*

	Calories	Carbo-hydrate (gm)	Protein (gm)	Total Fat (gm)	Saturated Fat (gm)	Choles-terol (mg)
Total	802.5	122.0	63.5	6.0	1.8	29.1
Per Serving	80.3	12.0	6.4	0.6	0.2	2.9

Italian Macaroni and Cheese

1 tbsp. diet margarine
1/2 cup chopped onion
1/2 cup chopped celery
1 garlic clove, crushed
3 1/2 cups water
6 oz. can tomato paste

1/2 lb. large #4
 macaroni
2 tsp. salt
1 tsp. oregano
1/2 cup chopped
 parsley
2 cups 99% fat-free
 cottage cheese
5 tbsp. grated extra
 sharp Romano

Melt the margarine in a large non-stick skillet. Sauté the onion, celery, and garlic until they are tender. Then stir in the water, tomato paste, macaroni, salt, and oregano. Cover the pan and simmer the mixture, stirring occasionally, until the macaroni is tender. Stir in parsley. Turn half the mixture into a baking dish and top it with 1 cup of cottage cheese, and sprinkle it with Romano cheese. Repeat the layers, ending with

Romano cheese. Bake the macaroni at 350° for about
15 minutes or until it is bubbly.   *Makes 6 servings*

	Calories	Carbo-hydrate (gm)	Protein (gm)	Total Fat (gm)	Saturated Fat (gm)	Choles-terol (mg)
Total	1530.5	664.7	119.9	40.6	18.4	119.8
Per Serving	255.1	110.8	20.0	6.8	3.1	20.0

Spaghetti and Meatballs

³/₄ lb. extra-lean round
   steak, ground
¹/₂ tsp. oregano
1 tsp. basil
¹/₂ tsp. salt
   pepper to taste
1 cup water
1 lb., 3 oz. can Italian
   tomatoes

6 oz. can tomato
   paste
1 cup chopped
   onion
1 green pepper
1 tbsp. oregano or
   mixed herbs
1 minced garlic
   clove
¹/₂ cup chopped
   celery
6 cups tender
   cooked
   spaghetti

Combine the meat with the oregano, basil, salt, and
pepper. Shape the mixture into 18 small meatballs, and
brown them under the broiler, turning them once. Chop
the green pepper and combine it with the water and the
remaining ingredients in a large saucepan. Bring this
mixture to a boil. Add the meatballs; cover the pot and
simmer over low heat for 1 hour or longer. Pour sauce
over spaghetti.   *Makes 6 servings*

	Calories	Carbo-hydrate (gm)	Protein (gm)	Total Fat (gm)	Saturated Fat (gm)	Choles-terol (mg)
Total	1787.6	260.0	148.7	21.5	4.4	315.2
Per Serving	297.9	43.4	24.8	3.6	0.7	52.5

*gm=grams; mg=milligrams. Nutritional figures are approximate. Figures
are based on findings of U.S. Department of Agriculture.*

Pasta Soup

$^1/_2$ cup chopped onion
$^1/_2$ tsp. oregano
2 cans chicken broth

1 cup chopped canned tomatoes, undrained
1 tbsp. chopped parsley
$^1/_4$ cup uncooked elbow macaroni

Skim the fat from the broth by using a bulb-type baster. Place the broth in a large saucepan and add all of the ingredients, except the macaroni. Bring the mixture to a boil. Then add the macaroni. Cook over low heat until the macaroni is tender, stirring occasionally.

Makes 6 servings

	Calories	Carbo-hydrate (gm)	Protein (gm)	Total Fat (gm)	Saturated Fat (gm)	Choles-terol (mg)
Total	273.5	43.4	21.6	1.6	0.0	73.6
Per Serving	45.6	7.2	3.6	0.3	0.0	12.3

Wild Rice and Mushrooms

4 oz. can sliced mushrooms
10$^1/_2$ oz. can condensed beef broth or chicken broth
5$^1/_2$ oz. water

2 medium onions
$^1/_2$ cup wild rice
1 cup long-grain rice
2 tbsp. snipped parsley

Before cooking: Drain mushrooms, reserving the liquid. Chop the onions. Combine the broth with enough water to make 2 cups. Wash the wild rice.

Bring the broth mixture, mushroom liquid, and onions to boiling in a saucepan. Add the wild rice, reduce the heat, cover the pan, and simmer the contents for 20 minutes. Then add the long-grain rice and mushrooms. Return the mixture to boiling; then reduce the heat, cover the pan, and simmer for about 20 minutes longer until the rice is tender. Serve garnished with parsley. *Makes 10 servings*

	Calories	Carbo-hydrate (gm)	Protein (gm)	Total Fat (gm)	Saturated Fat (gm)	Choles-terol (mg)
Total	1179.1	249.2	44.9	1.5	0.0	55.7
Per Serving	117.9	24.9	4.5	0.2	0.0	5.6

Golden Mushroom Rice

1 cup chopped onions	4 oz. can sliced
1 garlic clove, minced	mushrooms,
1 tbsp. diet margarine	drained
1 cup uncooked rice	1 tsp. curry
2 cups chicken broth	1 tsp. salt
	1/4 tsp. pepper
	1 tbsp. lemon juice

Melt the margarine in a non-stick skillet. Sauté the onions and garlic until the onions are tender. Then add the rice, broth, mushrooms, seasonings, and lemon juice. Heat the mixture to boiling; then cover the pan, lower the heat, and simmer for about 15 minutes until the rice is tender. Before serving, fluff the rice lightly with a fork. *Makes 6 servings*

Special hint: If you don't have chicken broth, you may use 2 chicken bouillon cubes mixed with 2 cups of water.

	Calories	Carbo-hydrate (gm)	Protein (gm)	Total Fat (gm)	Saturated Fat (gm)	Choles-terol (mg)
Total	796.4	163.6	19.0	7.0	1.0	6.0
Per Serving	132.7	27.3	3.2	1.2	0.2	1.0

gm=grams; mg=milligrams. Nutritional figures are approximate. Figures are based on findings of U.S. Department of Agriculture.

Baked Celery and Rice

1 cup uncooked rice
3 cups celery, sliced ¹/₂ inch thick
¹/₂ cup finely-chopped onion
2¹/₂ cups boiling chicken broth

¹/₂ tsp. marjoram
¹/₈ tsp. salt
¹/₈ tsp. pepper

Before cooking: Skim the fat from the broth, using a bulb-type baster.

Combine all of the ingredients in a 2-quart casserole. Cover the casserole and bake it in a preheated 400° oven for about 30 minutes until the rice and celery are tender. Garnish with chopped celery leaves. *Makes 6 servings*

	Calories	Carbo-hydrate (gm)	Protein (gm)	Total Fat (gm)	Saturated Fat (gm)	Choles-terol (mg)
Total	790.0	177.0	20.5	1.0	0.0	35.0
Per Serving	131.7	29.5	3.4	0.2	0.0	5.8

Spanish Rice

1¹/₂ cups chopped onion
1 tbsp. diet margarine
1 cup uncooked converted white rice
1 cup chopped green pepper
1 cup chopped celery

1 tsp. chili powder
8 oz. can whole tomatoes
1 tsp. salt
2 cups water
3 tbsp. bacon bits

Melt the margarine in a heavy skillet, and sauté the onion. Stir in the rice, green pepper, celery, chili powder, canned tomatoes, and salt. Add the water. Bring the mixture to a boil; then reduce the heat and simmer, covered, for about 20 minutes until the liquid is absorbed and the rice is cooked. Then garnish with the bacon bits. *Makes 8 servings*

	Calories	Carbo-hydrate (gm)	Protein (gm)	Total Fat (gm)	Saturated Fat (gm)	Choles-terol (mg)
Total	928.5	186.8	24.2	11.5	1.0	0.0
Per Serving	116.1	23.4	3.0	1.4	0.1	0.0

Clam Rice

1 cup sliced green onions	1 cup water
1 cup uncooked rice	1 tsp. salt
1 tbsp. diet margarine	dash of pepper
7½ oz. bottle clam juice	

Melt the margarine in a non-stick skillet. Using low heat, cook the onions and rice in the diet margarine until the rice is golden. Then add the remaining ingredients. Heat the mixture to boiling. Stir once, cover the pan, reduce the heat and simmer for 15 minutes. Toss the mixture lightly before serving. *Makes 6 servings*

	Calories	Carbo-hydrate (gm)	Protein (gm)	Total Fat (gm)	Saturated Fat (gm)	Choles-terol (mg)
Total	800.7	163.3	18.3	7.0	1.0	19.3
Per Serving	133.5	27.2	3.1	1.2	0.2	3.2

Skinny Rice

1 cup quick or instant rice	¼ cup finely-minced onion
1 cup water	½ tsp. salt or butter-flavored salt
1 cup finely-minced celery	⅛ tsp. pepper

Before cooking: The celery and onion should be chopped as fine as the grains of rice.

Combine all of the ingredients in a covered saucepan and simmer the mixture for 2 minutes. Remove the pan from the heat, and set it aside for 5 minutes or more, until serving time. *Makes 6 servings*

	Calories	Carbo-hydrate (gm)	Protein (gm)	Total Fat (gm)	Saturated Fat (gm)	Choles-terol (mg)
Total	205.0	48.5	4.5	0.0	0.0	0.0
Per Serving	34.2	8.1	0.8	0.0	0.0	0.0

---

gm=grams; mg=milligrams. Nutritional figures are approximate. Figures are based on findings of U.S. Department of Agriculture.

Unforbidden Sweets

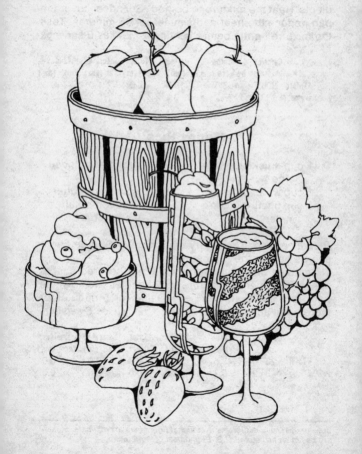

The trouble with sweets is sugar. Sugar is a "nutritional neuter" — empty calories with no redeeming nutritional value. "Raw" sugar, honey, molasses, maple syrup, and other "natural" sweets are equally high in calories. Despite the praise heaped on them by some health-food fans, the nutritional value of "natural" sweets is very small in comparison to their high calorie counts. As a waistline-watcher who must make every calorie carry its weight in nutritional value, you have very few calories to spend on sugar, be it natural or processed.

The dieter's best source of sweets is fresh fruit. This is sugar as nature intended it — a balanced "package" of vitamins, minerals, and appetite-appeasing roughage. A candy bar is gone in a minute, leaving you little but a sticky film to ruin your teeth while the calories ruin your waistline. An orange perfumes the air, fills your mouth with tangy sweetness, and makes vitamin C delicious. A cool, juicy peach provides generous quantities of vitamin A. So make fresh fruit your everyday dessert. Enjoy Mother Nature's bounty by picking the best of each season to cap your meals. Use fruit imaginatively in preparing homemade sweets and treats to take the place of empty-caloried snacks.

American sugar consumption approaches 115 pounds per person a year — or 200,000 calories' worth. Divided by 365 days a year, that is an average in excess of 500 calories a day.

Desirable as it might be to eliminate sugar altogether, most people would find it impossible, because much of our sugar intake is hidden in packaged and processed foods, canned vegetables, condiments, salad dressings, and other items not considered as "sweets." However, even cutting sugar consumption in half is a considerable savings — 100,000 calories a year. Since it takes a decrease of 3,500 calories to lose a pound, you could lose 28 pounds in a year, just by slicing sugar intake in half.

A taste for sweets is something that develops gradually. Critics of the American diet maintain that sugar-rich infant formulas and sweetened baby foods are the start of our national sweet tooth, followed later by sugared cereals and TV-touted snacks, sodas, and junk food. By the time we are adults, our sweet tooth may well be the only tooth left. But the taste for excessive sweetness can be reversed, simply by using diminishing amounts of sweetener in the dishes and desserts we prepare ourselves. Sugar-laden commercial cakes and pastries should be avoided altogether.

A Guide to Sugar Substitutes

One of the most painless ways to cut sugar calories without sacrificing sweetness is the use of modern sugar substitutes. Of course, it is better to learn to do without either — sugar or substitutes — but few overweights have the will power to swear off sweets entirely.

CYCLAMATE. Much concern has been elicited about the safety of sugar substitutes since the cyclamate scandal of the late 1960's, when massive doses of the then-most-popular sugar substitute was linked to tumors in test animals. Just which aspect of the episode constitutes the "scandal" depends on your point of view: opponents of sugar substitutes and supporters of the sugar industry interpret the findings to mean that the cyclamate sweeteners could cause cancer in humans, even though no human could match the test animals' intake. The other view is that cyclamate was a perfectly safe and beneficial substitute sweetener and that its removal from the market was totally unwarranted.

Cyclamate continues to be available in many European countries that did not follow the U.S. lead. The sweetener has been the subject of numerous scientific studies which fail to duplicate the cancer link that brought about the American ban. Abbott Laboratories, the drug firm which developed cyclamate, is continuing its fight with the Food and Drug Administration, hoping eventually to vindicate its product and resume marketing in this country.

After the demise of cyclamate, the only remaining non-nutritive sugar substitute was saccharin, which is the basic ingredient in most low-calorie sweeteners and diet products currently on the market. In the interim years, however, several other sugar substitutes have been developed.

Here is an update on present and future substitutes:

Saccharin. This no-calorie sweetener has been in use in the United States for more than 60 years. Saccharin is sold in a variety of forms — tablets, concentrated powders, packets, liquids, and granulated types which can be used spoon-for-spoon in place of sugar. Sodium saccharin is the most widely available type, although some manufacturers base their sweetener on calcium saccharin for those on low-sodium diets.

Modern saccharin-based sweeteners have eliminated much of the "bitter aftertaste" and heat instability that old forms had. Nevertheless, diet-conscious cooks are wise to avoid oversweetening food with too much saccharin. Once a certain limit is reached, additional artificial sweetener will produce bitterness instead of the desired sweetness. Unless you are on a totally sugar-free diet, you will be more satisfied with desserts that combine sugar substitute with sugar. You can cook with today's saccharin-based substitutes, but desserts that need only a minimum of heat are the most successful.

Sorbitol is a sweetener widely used in sugar-free diabetic products, but it's not available in this country as a table sweetener. Although it's useful for those with sugar intolerance, Sorbitol has no value to low-calorie dieters. Ounce-for-ounce, it has the same calories as sugar. But Sorbitol is less sweet than the same amount of sugar, so it takes more Sorbitol — and thus, more calories — to sweeten a product. That is why "dietetic" candies which are meant for diabetics may have the same (or more) calories than ordinary candy. Always check the label for the calorie count before buying and using "dietetic" products.

"Miracle Fruit." Some promise for the future is held by a natural extract from the berries of the "Miracle Fruit Tree," a tropical plant whose Latin name is Synsepalum dulcificum. The tree produces a small red cherrylike berry which contains a protein that has the unique ability to make sour foods taste sweet. It performs this function by coating the tongue with a substance that changes the way taste buds perceive flavors. After chewing a tablet containing the protein, sour foods — like lemon or grapefruit — taste as if they had been sprinkled with sugar. The problem is that all other acid-base foods also taste sweet, whether you want them to or not — salad dressing or dry wine, for example. Scientists are working on ways to combine this sweetening agent with foods to make it more useful. The fruit drops are currently marketed — mainly through mail order — under the trade name *Miralin*.

Fruit Sugar. Fructose, the natural sugar found in fruit and honey is very sweet. In certain combinations, it is nearly double the sweetness of sucrose (table sugar). Food technologists have developed new ways to produce fruit sugar more cheaply, and eventually hope to make it widely available as a low-calorie natural sweetener. Although fruit sugar still contains the same calories as sucrose — and little else in the way of nutrition — you can use less of it.

The exact sweetness level depends on other ingredients and temperature. Fruit sugar is at its most intense level when combined with fruit or other acid ingredients, especially when served chilled or frozen. Non-acid ingredients and hot temperatures minimize its sweetness to approximately the same level as ordinary sugar — in hot coffee, for example. A major marketer of fruit sugar had to pull its products from the shelves last year because of a label pitching it to diabetics. When available, fruit sugar will most likely be found first in health food stores.

Aspartame. In late 1974, the Food and Drug Administration gave approval to a new sweetener developed by G. D. Searle. Of all the sweeteners developed thus far, this is the most sugarlike in taste and texture.

Aspartame is composed of two naturally-occurring amino acids (the building blocks of protein). It has the same calories as sugar, but it has many times the sweetness of sugar. Therefore, only a tiny amount is needed — so little that the calories do not count.

The FDA approval limits Aspartame to table sweeteners: sugar substitute tablets for sweetening hot beverages, cold breakfast cereals; and for dry dessert mix bases such as instant coffee, tea and other beverages, gelatins, puddings, pie fillings, and whipped toppings. Aspartame is not approved for mixes that require long cooking because the sweetener is not stable when exposed to prolonged high heat. Prolonged cooking or high heat can cause loss of sweetness.

Until certain technological problems are worked out, it appears that Aspartame will have limited use in diet sodas and canned goods. Aspartame will also be off-limits to a small percentage of the population suffering from an inborn metabolic defect known as *phenylketonuria*. The defect requires such people to remain on a strict diet which is low in the amino acid, *phenylalanine*. And Aspartame is comprised partly of *phenylalanine*.

Calorie-Cutting Tricks with Sugar Substitutes

• For a minimum of tip-off aftertaste with saccharin-based substitutes, use them as a sweetness-booster instead of a total sweetness replacement. Combine both sugar and sugar substitutes in the same recipe. For example: if a recipe calls for 1 cup sugar, reduce the quantity to 1/2 cup, and replace the other half with its equivalent in sugar substitute.

• For even better results, combine sugar substitute with honey, brown sugar or maple syrup instead of white sugar.

• Most sweeteners include a table of equivalents on the label. Always check the label for information on how much to use. Remember: 3 teaspoons equals 1 tablespoon, and 16 tablespoons (48 teaspoons) equals one cup. Therefore, if you want to replace 2 tablespoons of sugar in a recipe, you would need sugar substitute equal to 6 teaspoons worth. To replace a 1/2 cup of sugar, you would need sugar substitute equal to 24 teaspoons worth.

• Tablet-type sweeteners should be dissolved in a little hot water before adding them to a recipe mixture.

• If possible, add sweeteners after cooking. Sprinkle sweeteners on a baked apple after it comes from the oven. Stir sweetener into pudding or gelatin desserts after you remove the pot from the heat.

• Desserts which need no cooking are especially

suitable for sugar replacement: refrigerator pies, puddings, gelatin molds, frozen desserts, layered parfaits.

• Check your supermarket diet shelf for sugar-free products which can be used as low-cal stand-ins for fattening ingredients. Low-calorie gelatin and pudding mixes can replace the fattening variety in many quick dessert recipes calling for these mixes. Sugar-free whipped topping mix can take the place of heavy whipped cream. Besides saving sugar calories, you will save fat calories, too!

More Calorie Saving Tricks to Make Sweets Less Fattening

• When a cake or pie comes from the oven, immediately mark the surface with a knife to divide it into eight or twelve equal-size servings. This helps eliminate the temptation to cut oversize helpings . . . or slice yourself an extra "sliver" of dessert.

• In most cake recipes, you can replace one egg with two egg whites — 30 calories instead of 80, and no cholesterol!

• To make a cake higher (and therefore offer more servings at fewer calories) separate the eggs and whip the egg whites stiff before folding them into the remaining batter. This works with packaged cake mixes as well.

• Cocoa powder can be used in place of chocolate, saving cocoa-fat calories. To replace one ounce of solid chocolate, use 3 level tbsp. of plain unsweetened cocoa. Do not add any additional fat.

• Chocolate extract, available on supermarket spice shelves, can supply chocolate flavor with a minimum of calories.

• Spices and extracts combine well with substitute-sweetened desserts. Avoid namby-pamby, bland-flavored desserts like plain puddings or simple custards. Well-spiced, strongly flavored blends with lots of fruit for flavor and texture are more interesting choices.

• If diet products taste bland, add a pinch of salt. Salt is often missing from these products in an effort to appeal to the low-sodium dieter as well.

- Boost the illusion of sweetness by adding or increasing vanilla.
- When a recipe calls for canned or frozen fruit, avoid unneeded sugar calories by choosing the fruits canned in juice instead of syrup, or the loose-pack frozen fruits without sugar. Or, freeze your own fresh fruit in season so you will have a handy supply in the freezer.
- Minimize the need for sugar or sweetener by cutting down on the amount of sour or bitter ingredients called for. Use less lemon juice, rind, coffee, or chocolate.
- Some sugar is needed for bulk in most cakes, cookies, and baked goods. However, you can often cut the amount called for in half and still get good results. Do not be afraid to experiment, but be prepared for some failures.

Sugar is not the only calorie-adder in desserts. Fat is also a culprit, in the form of butter, margarine, shortening, cream. Thus:

- When a recipe calls for cream, substitute evaporated skim milk.
- When a recipe calls for sour cream, substitute plain yogurt or buttermilk.
- Decrease or eliminate the butter called for in a dessert recipe, and add several drops of butter flavoring — available on the spice shelf in your supermarket. Or replace the salt called for with butter-flavored salt.
- Diet margarine can replace butter or margarine in many recipes, but other liquid will have to be reduced accordingly. For each 1/2 cup of diet margarine you use, delete 1/4 cup of other liquid.
- Low calorie "imitation" cream cheese or part-skim Neufchatel cheese can replace regular cream cheese in dessert recipes, thereby saving butterfat calories. Farmers cheese or low-fat cottage cheese, whipped smooth in your blender with a little skim milk, can serve as a stand-in for Ricotta cheese in Italian dessert recipes.
- Non-stick cake tins or pie pans, sprayed with vegetable coating for non-stick baking, completely eliminate the need for "greasing" pans with extra calories.

Recipes

Cream Puffs

¹/₂ cup diet margarine
¹/₂ cup water
¹/₂ tsp. salt

1 cup sifted all-
purpose flour
4 eggs

Heat the margarine with the water in a medium saucepan over high heat, stirring occasionally until the margarine is melted and the mixture is boiling. Turn the heat down to low. Add the salt and flour all at once, stirring vigorously until the mixture leaves the sides of the pan in a smooth compact ball. Remove the pan from the heat. Quickly add the eggs — one at a time — beating well after each addition until the mixture is smooth and shiny. Drop the mixture by spoonfuls, 3 inches apart, on an ungreased cookie sheet, shaping each into a mound. Bake the puffs in a 400° oven for 50 minutes. Remove them from the cookie sheet and cool them on a wire rack. To serve, slice the top off each cream puff and fill it with "Orange Filling." Then replace the tops.   *Makes 18 servings*

	Calories	Carbo-hydrate (gm)	Protein (gm)	Total Fat (gm)	Saturated Fat (gm)	Choles-terol (mg)
Total	1175.0	95.0	37.0	73.0	16.0	1008.0
Per Serving	65.3	5.3	2.1	4.1	0.9	56.0

Apple Kuchen

1 package flaky-style
biscuit dough (10
biscuits)
21 oz. can unsweetened
pie-sliced apples
sugar substitute to
equal 3 tbsp.

¹/₂ tsp. apple pie
spice
1 cup vanilla yogurt
1 beaten egg

Lay the biscuits out in a 9-inch pie pan and flatten them, sealing the edges together. Press the biscuit dough around the edges of the pie pan. Bake the dough in a preheated 350° oven for 5 minutes. Combine the apple slices, sugar substitute, and apple pie spice in a bowl, tossing the ingredients together, and spoon the mixture over the baked biscuit dough. Combine beaten egg with the yogurt and pour this over the fruit. Bake the kuchen at 350° for 20 minutes.

Makes 10 servings

	Calories	Carbo-hydrate (gm)	Protein (gm)	Total Fat (gm)	Saturated Fat (gm)	Choles-terol (mg)
Total	999.0	86.9	31.4	20.0	4.0	292.0
Per Serving	99.0	8.7	3.1	2.0	0.4	29.2

Cinnamon Coffee Cake

2 cups all-purpose flour
sugar substitute to
equal 1/4 cup
4 tsp. baking powder
1/2 tsp. salt
1 egg, well beaten

1 1/4 cups skim milk
1/2 cup water
2 tbsp. corn or
safflower oil
2 tsp. cinnamon
1/4 cup brown sugar

Stir the flour, sugar, baking powder and salt together. Mix the egg, skim milk, water and oil. Add them to the flour mixture and stir until moistened. Pour the batter into a greased 9-inch non-stick square pan. Combine the cinnamon and brown sugar and swirl them into the batter. Bake in a preheated 425° oven for 25 minutes or until top springs back when lightly touched.

Makes 9 servings

	Calories	Carbo-hydrate (gm)	Protein (gm)	Total Fat (gm)	Saturated Fat (gm)	Choles-terol (mg)
Total	1578.2	263.0	43.3	36.0	4.0	258.3
Per Serving	175.4	29.2	4.8	4.0	0.4	28.7

gm=grams; mg=milligrams. Nutritional figures are approximate. Figures are based on findings of U.S. Department of Agriculture.

Sponge Cake for Fruit

3 egg yolks
1 cup confectioner's
    sugar
1/4 cup boiling water
1 1/2 tsp. vanilla extract
1/4 tsp. grated lemon peel

1 cup cake flour
1 1/2 tsp. baking powder
4 egg whites
1/4 tsp. salt

Beat the egg yolks until they are light. Add the sugar and beat the mixture smooth. Add the boiling water, vanilla, and lemon peel; beat well. Then stir the flour and baking powder together, beating the dry ingredients into the batter until it is smooth. In another bowl, beat the egg whites and salt until stiff peaks form. Fold the batter into the egg whites gently but thoroughly. Spoon the batter into two 8-inch cake pans that have been sprayed with vegetable coating and bake them in a preheated 325° oven for about 25 minutes. Cool the layers thoroughly before removing them from the pans.

Makes 16 servings

	Calories	Carbo-hydrate (gm)	Protein (gm)	Total Fat (gm)	Saturated Fat (gm)	Choles-terol (mg)
Total	1072.2	200.5	32.0	16.0	6.0	756.0
Per Serving	67.0	12.5	2.0	1.0	0.4	47.3

Cranberry Nut Loaf

2 cups flour
2 tsp. baking powder
1/2 cup brown sugar
1 egg
    sugar substitute to
    equal 1/2 cup

1/2 cup diet margarine
3/4 cup orange juice
1 cup uncooked
    cranberries,
    chopped
5 tbsp. chopped
    walnuts

Sift the flour and re-measure it so there are only 2 cups. Then sift the flour again into a bowl with the baking powder and brown sugar. Beat the egg slightly; then combine it with the sugar substitute, margarine, and orange juice. Pour this mixture into the dry ingredients and stir only until they are well mixed. Then stir in the cranberries and walnuts. Pour the batter into a loaf pan that has been sprayed with vegetable coating and bake it in a 350° oven for about 1 hour until it is golden brown. *Makes 22 servings*

	Calories	Carbo-hydrate (gm)	Protein (gm)	Total Fat (gm)	Saturated Fat (gm)	Choles-terol (mg)
Total	2184.0	334.9	41.6	81.2	11.2	252.0
Per Serving	99.3	15.2	1.9	3.7	0.5	11.5

Spice Cake

1 cup sifted cake flour	1 tbsp. cold water
4 tbsp. brown sugar	2 egg yolks
1½ tsp. baking powder	1 tsp. vanilla
½ tsp. salt	sugar substitute to
1 tsp. cinnamon	equal 6 tbsp.
1 tsp. ground cloves	4 egg whites
1 tsp. nutmeg	¼ tsp. cream of tartar
1 tbsp. corn or safflower	2 tbsp. granulated
oil	sugar

Combine sifted flour, brown sugar, baking powder, salt, cinnamon, ground cloves, and nutmeg together in a large mixing bowl. Add the oil, water, egg yolks, vanilla, and sugar substitute. Beat the mixture until it is smooth. In a separate bowl, beat the egg whites and cream of tartar until stiff peaks form. Sprinkle the granulated sugar over the surface of the egg whites, then beat it in thoroughly. Gently fold the egg whites into the batter. Pour the batter into an ungreased 8-inch square cake pan and bake it at 325° for 1 hour. Invert the pan while the cake is cooling. *Makes 12 servings*

	Calories	Carbo-hydrate (gm)	Protein (gm)	Total Fat (gm)	Saturated Fat (gm)	Choles-terol (mg)
Total	967.3	158.9	29.0	25.0	5.0	504.0
Per Serving	81.4	13.2	2.4	2.1	0.4	42.0

gm=grams; mg=milligrams. Nutritional figures are approximate. Figures are based on findings of U.S. Department of Agriculture.

White Cake

4 tbsp. diet margarine
5 tbsp. sugar and
  granulated sugar
  substitute to equal 5
  tbsp.
1 tsp. vanilla extract

1 cup sifted cake
  flour
1 tsp. baking powder
1/4 tsp. salt
4 tbsp. skim milk
2 egg whites

Beat the margarine, sugar, and sugar substitute in a bowl until they are fluffy. Add the vanilla and blend well. Sift together the sifted flour and baking powder. Add the dry ingredients and the milk alternately to the margarine-sugar mixture, beating smoothly after each addition. Begin with the dry ingredients and end with the dry ingredients. In a separate bowl, add the salt to the egg whites and beat them until they are stiff. Gently fold the egg whites into the cake batter. Pour the batter into an 8-inch non-stick square pan that has been sprayed with vegetable coating. Bake the cake in a preheated 375° oven for 20 to 25 minutes.

Makes 8 servings

	Calories	Carbo-hydrate (gm)	Protein (gm)	Total Fat (gm)	Saturated Fat (gm)	Choles-terol (mg)
Total	855.3	147.2	17.3	25.0	4.0	1.3
Per Serving	106.9	18.4	2.2	3.1	0.5	0.2

Chiffon Cake

9 tbsp. sugar and sugar
  substitute to equal
  2/3 cup
2 1/4 cups sifted cake flour
3 tsp. baking powder
1 tsp. salt

1 cup skim milk
1/4 cup corn or
  safflower oil
1 1/2 tsp. orange
  flavoring
2 egg yolks
4 egg whites

Sift two tablespoons of the sugar into a bowl with the sugar substitute, sifted cake flour, baking powder, and salt. Pour in the milk, oil, and flavoring, and beat the mixture for 1 minute. Add the egg yolks, and beat for 1 minute more. Beat the egg whites in another bowl until they are frothy. Gradually add the remaining sugar, beating until the egg whites are stiff. Fold the egg whites gently but thoroughly into the cake batter. Spoon the batter into two 8- or 9-inch cake pans that have been sprayed with vegetable coating. Bake the cake for 25 to 30 minutes at 350°. *Makes 16 servings*

	Calories	Carbo-hydrate (gm)	Protein (gm)	Total Fat (gm)	Saturated Fat (gm)	Choles-terol (mg)
Total	1996.0	296.2	46.8	68.3	8.0	509.0
Per Serving	124.8	18.5	2.9	4.3	0.5	31.8

Refrigerator Wafer Cake

1 envelope plain gelatin
2 tbsp. cold water
1/2 cup boiling water
1 cup skim milk

1 package instant chocolate pudding
2 egg whites
half of 12 oz. box of vanilla wafers

Combine the gelatin and cold water in a blender. Add the boiling water and continue to blend on high speed until all the gelatin granules are dissolved. Then add the milk and pudding mix, and blend the mixture until it is smooth. Beat the egg whites in a bowl until they are stiff. Pour the mixture into the beaten egg whites, and gently but thoroughly fold them together. Place a layer of vanilla wafers in the bottom of an 8-inch cake pan. Cover the wafers with 1/3 of the chocolate mixture. Repeat the layers two more times, ending with the chocolate mixture. Chill the cake for several hours before serving. *Makes 8 servings*

	Calories	Carbo-hydrate (gm)	Protein (gm)	Total Fat (gm)	Saturated Fat (gm)	Choles-terol (mg)
Total	1249.8	214.2	42.6	35.5	0.0	67.2
Per Serving	156.2	26.8	5.3	4.4	0.0	8.4

gm=grams; mg=milligrams. Nutritional figures are approximate. Figures are based on findings of U.S. Department of Agriculture.

Classic Angel Food Cake

1½ cups sugar	½ tsp. salt
1 cup cake flour	2 tsp. cream of tartar
1¾ cups egg whites (12 to 14 eggs)	1 tsp. vanilla

Sift ½ cup of the sugar with the flour 3 times. Using an electric mixer or a rotary egg beater, beat the egg whites until they are frothy. Add the cream of tartar and salt to the egg whites. Continue to beat them until they are just stiff enough to hold their shape. This will take about 1 to 1½ minutes at medium speed. At medium speed, add the remaining cup of sugar to the egg whites, beating it in gradually. It should take about 1 minute to add the sugar. Then add the vanilla and beat an additional 2 minutes. Using a flat wire egg whip or a large spoon, fold in the flour and sugar mixture by sprinkling a few tablespoons at a time over the surface, cutting and folding it in. This should take about 2 minutes. Then carefully fold the mixture for an additional 2 minutes. Pour the batter into a large, ungreased angel food cake pan, turning the pan as the mixture is put in. Cut through the batter several times, and give it several hard taps on the table to fill up any air pockets. Bake the cake in a 350° oven for about 40 to 45 minutes. Remove the cake from the oven and invert the pan to cool. *Makes 16 servings*

	Calories	Carbo-hydrate (gm)	Protein (gm)	Total Fat (gm)	Saturated Fat (gm)	Choles-terol (mg)
Total	1727.0	377.5	63.0	1.0	0.0	0.0
Per Serving	107.9	23.6	3.9	0.1	0.0	0.0

Fudge Frosting for Angel Cake

1 pkg. chocolate fudge instant pudding mix	1 tsp. powdered instant coffee
1 pkg. (2 envelopes) low-calorie whipped topping mix	1¼ cups cold water

Combine the pudding mix, topping mix, and instant coffee in a deep bowl and add the water. Beat the mixture on the high speed of your electric mixer, scraping the sides of the bowl often. Beat until the mixture is light and fluffy. This is enough to frost a large 16-serving angel cake ring. *Makes 16 servings*

	Calories	Carbo-hydrate (gm)	Protein (gm)	Total Fat (gm)	Saturated Fat (gm)	Choles-terol (mg)
Total	884.0	84.6	2.8	65.9	0.0	0.0
Per Serving	52.8	5.3	0.2	4.1	0.0	0.0

Chocolate Cake

¹/₂ cup diet margarine
¹/₄ cup brown sugar and sugar substitute to equal 5 tbsp.
1 egg
1¹/₂ tsp. vanilla

¹/₄ cup skim milk
1²/₃ cups all-purpose flour
3 tbsp. unsweetened cocoa
2 tsp. baking powder
¹/₂ tsp. baking soda

Combine the margarine, brown sugar, sugar substitute, egg, vanilla, and milk in a bowl. Beat the mixture for 2 minutes at high speed. Then add the remaining ingredients and beat for 2 minutes at low speed. Spread the batter in a non-stick 8-inch square or round cake pan that has been sprayed with vegetable coating. Bake the cake in a preheated 350° oven for about 30 minutes until a toothpick inserted in the center comes out clean. *Makes 8 servings*

	Calories	Carbo-hydrate (gm)	Protein (gm)	Total Fat (gm)	Saturated Fat (gm)	Choles-terol (mg)
Total	1367.7	197.4	28.0	56.3	10.5	253.3
Per Serving	171.0	24.7	3.5	7.0	1.3	31.7

---

gm=grams; mg=milligrams. Nutritional figures are approximate. Figures are based on findings of U.S. Department of Agriculture.

Easy Frosting

1 package instant
   pudding mix (any
   flavor)
1 package low-calorie
   topping mix

1½ cups cold water

Combine the ingredients in a mixing bowl, beat them until the mixture is fluffy and of spreading consistency. This makes enough frosting for 4 layers.

Makes 24 servings

	Calories	Carbo-hydrate (gm)	Protein (gm)	Total Fat (gm)	Saturated Fat (gm)	Choles-terol (mg)
Total	844.0	84.6	2.8	65.9	0.0	0.0
Per Serving	35.2	3.5	0.1	2.7	0.0	0.0

Orange Filling

6 oz. can frozen orange
   juice concentrate
1 box (2 envelopes)
   low-calorie
   whipped topping
   mix

½ cup cold water

Allow the juice to thaw, but do not dilute it. Add the topping mix and water and whip the mixture until it is stiff.

Makes 18 servings

	Calories	Carbo-hydrate (gm)	Protein (gm)	Total Fat (gm)	Saturated Fat (gm)	Choles-terol (mg)
Total	872.0	87.0	5.0	64.0	0.0	0.0
Per Serving	48.4	4.8	0.3	3.6	0.0	0.0

Grape Whip

1 envelope unflavored
   gelatin
½ cup cold water

1¼ cups bottled grape
   juice
⅛ tsp. salt

Sprinkle the gelatin over the water in a saucepan and let it stand until the gelatin softens. Place the pan over low heat for about 3 minutes, stirring constantly until the gelatin dissolves. Remove the pan from the heat and stir in the grape juice and salt. Chill the mixture, stirring occasionally, until it has slightly thickened. Then, pour it into a chilled bowl and beat it with your electric mixer or rotary beater until it is light and fluffy and double in volume. Spoon the whipped mixture into dessert dishes and chill until firm.   *Makes 4 servings*

	Calories	Carbohydrate (gm)	Protein (gm)	Total Fat (gm)	Saturated Fat (gm)	Cholesterol (mg)
Total	231.3	52.5	7.3	0.0	0.0	0.0
Per Serving	57.8	13.1	1.8	0.0	0.0	0.0

Orange Whip

1 envelope (4-serving)
   orange flavored diet
   gelatin
1 cup boiling water
¾ cup cold water
1 tsp. freshly grated
   orange peel

1 egg white
2 tbsp. sugar
1 medium orange,
   peeled, cut into
   small bite-size
   pieces

Thoroughly dissolve the gelatin in the boiling water; add the cold water and the grated peel. Chill until partially set and very thick. Beat the egg white to the soft peak stage; gradually add the sugar and continue beating until stiff. Beat the thickened gelatin at high speed in small, deep bowl until foamy and double in volume. Continue to beat, adding the beaten white in 2 or 3 portions. When well blended, fold in the orange pieces. Spoon into a 1-quart mold; chill until set before turning out onto a serving plate.   *Makes 8 servings*

	Calories	Carbohydrate (gm)	Protein (gm)	Total Fat (gm)	Saturated Fat (gm)	Cholesterol (mg)
Total	541.1	77.6	63.0	0.0	0.0	0.0
Per Serving	67.6	9.7	7.9	0.0	0.0	0.0

gm=grams; mg=milligrams. Nutritional figures are approximate. Figures are based on findings of U.S. Department of Agriculture.

Cheese Cake

2 tbsp. diet margarine
1/2 cup graham cracker
   crumbs
2 cups 99% fat-free
   cottage cheese
1/4 cup sugar and sugar
   substitute to equal
   1/4 cup
2 tbsp. flour

1/4 tsp. butter-flavored
   salt
4 eggs, separated
1 cup evaporated
   skim milk
2 tsp. vanilla
1 tbsp. fresh lemon
   juice

Coat the bottom of a 9-inch spring pan with the diet margarine. Sprinkle the cracker crumbs over the margarine. In a bowl, whip the cottage cheese, sugar, sugar substitute, flour, and butter-flavored salt until the mixture is smooth. Add the egg yolks one at a time, mixing well after each addition. Stir in the milk, vanilla, and lemon juice. In another bowl, beat the egg whites until they are stiff, and fold them into the cheese batter. Then pour the batter over the crumbs. Bake the cheese cake at 325° for 1 hour. Allow it to cool before removing the rim of the pan. Do not invert the cake.

Makes 12 servings

	Calories	Carbo-hydrate (gm)	Protein (gm)	Total Fat (gm)	Saturated Fat (gm)	Choles-terol (mg)
Total	1514.3	126.4	105.8	63.1	23.4	1124.8
Per Serving	126.2	10.5	8.8	5.3	2.0	93.7

Cheese Pie

"Graham Cracker
   Crust" (the recipe is
   in this section)
1 cup evaporated skim
   milk
5 tbsp. sugar and sugar
   substitute to equal 5
   tbsp.
4 eggs

1/4 tsp. butter-flavored
   salt
1 tbsp. fresh lemon
   juice
2 tsp. vanilla extract
2 tbsp. arrowroot or
   cornstarch
2 cups (1 lb.) low-fat
   cottage cheese

In your blender container, combine all the ingredients except the graham cracker crust. Blend the mixture until it is completely smooth and pour it into the crust. Bake the pie in a 250° oven for 1 hour. Turn the oven off and leave the pie in the oven 1 more hour. Then remove the pie from the oven and chill it. If you wish, prepare one of the fruit glazes that follow and spread it on top of the pie after it is cool. Chill for several hours before serving. *Makes 8 servings*

Special hint: This recipe calls for one cup of evaporated skim milk from a 12-ounce can. The remaining canned milk can be chilled and whipped and served as a low-fat "whipped cream" with the pie.

	Calories	Carbohydrate (gm)	Protein (gm)	Total Fat (gm)	Saturated Fat (gm)	Cholesterol (mg)
Total	1732.4	172.6	107.4	122.0	23.4	1124.8
Per Serving	216.6	21.6	13.2	15.3	2.9	140.6

Buttery Pastry Shell

1 cup flour
1½ tsp. butter-flavored salt

2 tbsp. diet margarine
2 tbsp. butter, softened

Sift the flour and butter-flavored salt into a bowl. Cut in the margarine and butter. Knead the mixture just long enough for the dough to form a ball. Roll the dough out thinly on a well-floured board. This makes enough for an 8-inch double-crust pie.

Makes 8 servings

	Calories	Carbohydrate (gm)	Protein (gm)	Total Fat (gm)	Saturated Fat (gm)	Cholesterol (mg)
Total	757.5	95.3	13.3	36.0	14.8	70.8
Per Serving	94.7	11.9	1.7	4.5	1.9	8.9

gm=grams; mg=milligrams. Nutritional figures are approximate. Figures are based on findings of U.S. Department of Agriculture.

Apple Pie

"Buttery Pastry Shell"
(the recipe is in this
section)
sugar substitute to
equal 1/2 cup
1 tbsp. cornstarch
1 tsp. ground cinnamon

1/2 tsp. ground
nutmeg
1/4 tsp. butter-flavored
salt
6 cups cooking
apples, pared,
cored, and
sliced

Roll out half the pastry and place it in an 8-inch pie plate. In a bowl combine the sugar substitute, cornstarch, cinnamon, nutmeg, butter-flavored salt, and apple slices. Spoon this mixture into the pastry-lined pie plate. Roll out the remaining pastry and place it on top for the top crust. Press the edges of the top and bottom crust together and flute them. Cut vents in the top crust to allow steam to escape. Bake the pie for 40 minutes at 425° until it is golden brown.

Makes 8 servings

	Calories	Carbo-hydrate (gm)	Protein (gm)	Total Fat (gm)	Saturated Fat (gm)	Choles-terol (mg)
Total	1062.8	173.5	13.3	36.0	14.8	70.8
Per Serving	132.9	21.7	1.7	4.5	1.9	8.9

Single Crust Pie Pastry

1/2 cup all-purpose flour
pinch of salt

2 tbsp. salad oil
1 tbsp. ice water

Stir all of the ingredients together in a bowl with a fork. Then knead the mixture lightly until the pastry forms a ball. Flatten out the dough; wrap it in waxed paper and chill thoroughly. Roll the dough out on a lightly floured board. (For a two-crust pie, double the recipe.) *Makes 8 servings*

	Calories	Carbo-hydrate (gm)	Protein (gm)	Total Fat (gm)	Saturated Fat (gm)	Choles-terol (mg)
Total	477.5	47.5	6.5	28.5	2.0	0.0
Per Serving	59.7	5.9	0.8	3.6	0.3	0.0

Easy Yogurt Pie

"Single Crust Pie
Pastry" (the recipe
is in this section)
2 eggs, well beaten
1 tbsp. flour
½ tsp. cinnamon

1 cup sweetened
fruit yogurt, any
flavor
1 tsp. grated lemon
peel
pinch of butter-
flavored salt

Prepare the single crust pie pastry and line an 8-inch pie plate with it. Blend the filling ingredients thoroughly. Pour them into the pie shell. Bake the pie in a preheated 400° oven for 50 minutes until set. Chill before serving. (Garnish with fresh fruit, if desired.)

Makes 8 servings

	Calories	Carbo-hydrate (gm)	Protein (gm)	Total Fat (gm)	Saturated Fat (gm)	Choles-terol (mg)
Total	925.4	532.4	27.1	43.3	7.0	524.0
Per Serving	115.7	66.6	3.4	5.4	0.9	65.5

Graham Cracker Crust

⅔ cup graham cracker
crumbs

2 tbsp. diet
margarine

Lightly combine the graham cracker crumbs and diet margarine. Press them firmly into the bottom of an 8- or 9-inch non-stick pie pan. This crust is quite tender. For a sturdier crust, quick-bake it in a pre-heated, hot 425° oven for 6 to 8 minutes. Watch the crust — it burns easily. Cool before filling. *Makes 8 servings*

	Calories	Carbo-hydrate (gm)	Protein (gm)	Total Fat (gm)	Saturated Fat (gm)	Choles-terol (mg)
Total	390.4	55.4	5.3	19.9	2.0	0.0
Per Serving	48.8	6.9	0.7	2.5	0.3	0.0

gm=grams; mg=milligrams. Nutritional figures are approximate. Figures are based on findings of U.S. Department of Agriculture.

Pumpkin Chiffon Pie

"Single Crust Pie
Pastry" (the recipe
is in this section)
1 envelope unflavored
gelatin
1/3 cup cold water
1 lb. can pumpkin

brown sugar
substitute to
equal 1/2 cup
1 1/2 tsp. pumpkin pie
spice
1/4 tsp. salt
2 egg whites
4 tbsp. sugar

Prepare the pastry; place it in an 8-inch pie plate and bake it at 350° until it is lightly browned. Sprinkle the gelatin over the water in a saucepan and stir the mixture over low heat until the gelatin has dissolved. Allow it to cool. Stir in the pumpkin, brown sugar substitute, pumpkin pie spice, and salt. Beat the egg whites in a bowl until they are foamy. Add the sugar gradually and continue beating until stiff peaks form. Fold the egg whites gently but thoroughly into the pumpkin mixture. Pour the mixture into the cool pastry shell and chill the pie for about 3 hours until it is firm.

Makes 8 servings

	Calories	Carbohydrate (gm)	Protein (gm)	Total Fat (gm)	Saturated Fat (gm)	Cholesterol (mg)
Total	876.0	133.5	24.5	30.5	2.0	0.0
Per Serving	109.5	16.7	3.1	3.8	0.3	0.0

Pumpkin Pie

"Single Crust Pie
Pastry" (the recipe
is in this section)
1 cup canned pumpkin
(not sweetened pie
filling)
2 eggs
1 1/4 cups skim milk

1/2 tbsp. cornstarch
1/4 cup firm-packed
brown sugar and
sugar substitute
to equal 1/4 cup
1/4 tsp. salt
2 tsp. pumpkin pie
spice

Prepare the pie crust and line an 8-inch pie plate with it. Combine the rest of the ingredients in a bowl and beat them thoroughly. Pour the mixture into the prepared pastry shell. Bake the pie for 1 hour at 350°.

Makes 8 servings

	Calories	Carbo-hydrate (gm)	Protein (gm)	Total Fat (gm)	Saturated Fat (gm)	Choles-terol (mg)
Total	1045.3	137.0	31.9	41.6	6.0	512.8
Per Serving	130.7	17.1	4.0	5.2	0.8	64.1

Strawberry Topping

8 oz. frozen, unsweetened strawberries
5 tbsp. sugar and sugar substitute to equal ½ cup

2 tbsp. arrowroot or cornstarch
1 cup water
2 tbsp. lemon juice

Allow the strawberries to thaw and combine them with the rest of the ingredients in a saucepan. Cook and stir the mixture over moderate heat until it simmers and thickens. Serve the topping warm or cold over slices of cake.

Makes 12 servings

	Calories	Carbo-hydrate (gm)	Protein (gm)	Total Fat (gm)	Saturated Fat (gm)	Choles-terol (mg)
Total	541.3	139.8	0.9	0.8	0.0	0.0
Per Serving	45.1	11.7	0.1	0.1	0.0	0.0

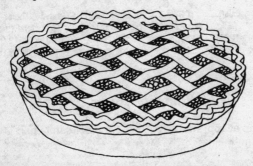

gm=grams; mg=milligrams. Nutritional figures are approximate. Figures are based on findings of U.S. Department of Agriculture.

Mile High Lime Pie

"Single Crust Pie
    Pastry" (the recipe
    is in this section)
6 eggs, separated
½ cup water
¼ tsp. salt
½ cup lime juice

1 envelope
    unflavored
    gelatin
1 tsp. grated lime
    peel
½ tsp. cream of tartar
5 tbsp. sugar and
    sugar substitute
    to equal 5 tbsp.

Prepare the pastry shell; place it in an 8-inch pie plate and bake it at 350° until it is lightly browned. In the top of a double boiler, beat the egg yolks with the water, salt, and lime juice. Stir in the gelatin. Place the double boiler over boiling water and stir constantly for about 6 minutes until the gelatin dissolves and the mixture thickens slightly. Then add the grated lime peel. Chill the mixture, stirring occasionally, until it mounds slightly when dropped from a spoon. Beat the egg whites with the cream of tartar in a bowl until they are stiff but not dry. Gradually add the sugar and sugar substitute and continue beating the egg whites until they are very stiff. Fold the gelatin mixture into the egg whites. Chill the mixture until it will pile up and stay mounded. Spoon it into the pastry shell, piling it high in the center. Chill the pie for several hours or overnight until it is firm. *Makes 8 servings*

	Calories	Carbo-hydrate (gm)	Protein (gm)	Total Fat (gm)	Saturated Fat (gm)	Choles-terol (mg)
Total	1253.7	120.2	49.0	64.5	14.0	1512.0
Per Serving	156.7	15.0	6.1	8.1	1.8	189.0

"Whipped Cream"

1 cup evaporated skim
    milk

2 tsp. fresh lemon
    juice

Chill the evaporated skim milk in your freezer until ice crystals begin to form. Also chill your bowl and the beaters of your electric mixer. Whip the milk on the high speed of your mixer until it triples in volume. If you add 1 or 2 teaspoons lemon juice for each cup of milk, it will speed the whipping.

	Calories	Carbo-hydrate (gm)	Protein (gm)	Total Fat (gm)	Saturated Fat (gm)	Choles-terol (mg)
Total	352.8	26.6	18.1	20.0	11.0	78.0

Frosty Pineapple Pie

"Single Crust Pie Pastry" (the recipe is in this section)
1½ cups 99% fat-free cottage cheese
sugar substitute to equal 4 tbsp.
1 tsp. vanilla

1 tsp. grated orange peel
½ tsp. salt
8¾ oz. can crushed unsweetened pineapple, undrained
1 envelope diet whipped topping mix, prepared

Prepare the pastry; place it in a 9-inch pie plate and bake it at 350° until it is lightly browned. Beat the cottage cheese in a small bowl or in a blender until it is smooth. Then beat in the sugar substitute, vanilla, orange peel and salt. Fold in the pineapple. Whip the topping mix in a separate bowl until it is stiff. Fold it into the cottage cheese mixture. Spoon the mixture into the pie shell and freeze it until it is firm. Remove the pie from the freezer and place it in the refrigerator for 4 to 6 hours before serving. *Makes 10 servings*

	Calories	Carbo-hydrate (gm)	Protein (gm)	Total Fat (gm)	Saturated Fat (gm)	Choles-terol (mg)
Total	1115.0	85.0	51.5	63.5	3.8	29.1
Per Serving	111.5	8.5	5.2	6.4	0.4	2.9

gm=grams; mg=milligrams. Nutritional figures are approximate. Figures are based on findings of U.S. Department of Agriculture.

Fresh Fruit Glaze

2 cups hulled fresh
strawberries or
fresh blueberries
1 tbsp. arrowroot or
cornstarch

1 cup unsweetened
white or red
grape juice
sugar substitute to
taste

If you are using strawberries, leave the small ones whole and slice the large ones in half lengthwise. Arrange the strawberries cut side down on top of the cooled cheese pie. If you are using blueberries, spread them in a single layer over the surface of the pie.

Stir the arrowroot and grape juice together in a saucepan over medium heat until the mixture clears and thickens. Set the pan aside for 10 minutes to cool. Sweeten the mixture to taste with sugar substitute. Using a spoon, drip the glaze over the fresh fruit. Use only as much as needed to completely coat the fruit. Discard the rest. *Makes 8 servings*

Special hint: If fresh fruit is not available, a 20 oz. can of unsweetened red pitted cherries may be used instead. Use the canned juice in place of the grape juice. If there is not enough juice to make one cup, add water.

	Calories	Carbo-hydrate (gm)	Protein (gm)	Total Fat (gm)	Saturated Fat (gm)	Choles-terol (mg)
Total	300.3	74.2	3.0	2.0	0.0	0.0
Per Serving	37.5	9.3	0.4	0.3	0.0	0.0

Pineapple Topping

16 oz. can unsweetened
crushed pineapple,
undrained
2 tbsp. sugar

2 tbsp. cornstarch
juice of 1/2 lemon
sugar substitute to
equal 5 tbsp.

Combine all of the ingredients, except the sugar substitute, in the top of the double boiler. Cook the mixture over hot water, stirring often until it has thickened. Remove the pan from the heat, and stir in

364

the sugar substitute. When the topping is cool, spread it on pound cake or angel food cake. *Makes 16 servings*

	Calories	Carbo- hydrate (gm)	Protein (gm)	Total Fat (gm)	Saturated Fat (gm)	Choles- terol (mg)
Total	433.3	129.0	182.1	0.0	0.0	0.0
Per Serving	26.5	8.1	11.4	0.0	0.0	0.0

Peach or Apricot Sauce

4 tsp. cornstarch
1 cup apricot or peach
   nectar

2 tsp. brandy extract

Combine all of the ingredients in a medium saucepan. Heat the mixture, stirring constantly, until it bubbles and thickens. Then remove it from the heat. Serve the sauce over pound cake, angel food cake, or over vanilla ice milk. *Makes 8 servings*

	Calories	Carbo- hydrate (gm)	Protein (gm)	Total Fat (gm)	Saturated Fat (gm)	Choles- terol (mg)
Total	211.3	52.1	0.0	0.0	0.0	0.0
Per Serving	26.4	6.5	0.0	0.0	0.0	0.0

Tangy Topper For Fruit

4 oz. low-calorie
   ("imitation") cream
   cheese, or
   Neufchatel cheese,
   softened

³/₄ cup vanilla
   flavored yogurt

Combine the ingredients and beat until fluffy. Chill before serving. *Makes 1¹/₄ cup, 20 tbsp.*

	Calories	Carbo- hydrate (gm)	Protein (gm)	Total Fat (gm)	Saturated Fat (gm)	Choles- terol (mg)
Total	373.8	13.8	14.0	27.0	17.5	99.0
Per Serving	18.7	0.7	0.7	1.4	0.9	5.0

gm=grams; mg=milligrams. Nutritional figures are approximate. Figures are based on findings of U.S. Department of Agriculture.

Sugar-free Oatmeal Drop Cookies

1 cup diet margarine
  sugar substitute to
  equal ³/₄ cup
1¹/₂ tsp. vanilla
1 egg
1 cup all-purpose flour

1 tsp. apple pie
  spice or
  cinnamon
¹/₂ tsp. soda
¹/₄ cup cold water
1 cup quick-cooking
  rolled oats
¹/₃ cup currants

Beat the diet margarine, sweetener, vanilla and egg with an electric mixer at high speed, scraping the bowl occasionally, until well blended. Add the flour, spice, soda and water. Beat about 2 minutes at low speed until the ingredients are well combined. Stir in the rolled oats and currants. Drop by teaspoon 2 inches apart on non-stick cookie sheets. Bake in a preheated 375° oven for 12 to 15 minutes until cookies are set.

Makes 3¹/₂ dozen

	Calories	Carbo-hydrate (gm)	Protein (gm)	Total Fat (gm)	Saturated Fat (gm)	Choles-terol (mg)
Total	1718.1	70.4	32.0	109.0	163.7	252.0
Per Serving	40.9	1.8	0.8	2.6	3.9	6.0

Chocolate Chip Cookies

¹/₂ cup margarine
²/₃ cup brown sugar and
  sugar substitute to
  equal ²/₃ cup
2 tsp. vanilla
2 eggs

2¹/₂ cups sifted all-
  purpose flour
1 tsp. baking powder
1 tsp. salt
¹/₂ cup semi-sweet
  chocolate chips

With the high speed of your electric mixer, cream the margarine, brown sugar, sugar substitute, vanilla, and eggs together until the mixture is light and fluffy. Stir the flour, baking powder and salt into the creamed mixture, blending well. Then stir in the chocolate chips. On a non-stick cookie sheet that has been sprayed with vegetable coating, drop the batter from a teaspoon, placing the drops 2 inches apart. Bake the cookies at 375° for 10 to 12 minutes. Remove the cookies from the cookie sheet immediately, and allow them to cool on a wire rack.   *Makes 100*

	Calories	Carbo-hydrate (gm)	Protein (gm)	Total Fat (gm)	Saturated Fat (gm)	Choles-terol (mg)
Total	3088.8	413.4	45.4	144.8	46.0	504.0
Per Serving	30.9	4.1	0.5	1.4	0.5	5.4

Lemon Cookies

1/2 cup butter
1/4 cup sugar and sugar substitute to equal 1/4 cup
1 egg
1 tbsp. water
1 tbsp. fresh lemon juice
1 tbsp. grated lemon peel
1 tsp. vanilla
1/2 cup shredded dry coconut
2 cups sifted flour
1 tsp. baking powder
1/2 tsp. salt

Cream the butter in a small mixing bowl with the high speed of your mixer. Add the sugar, sugar substitute, egg, water, lemon juice, lemon peel, and vanilla. Beat the mixture until thoroughly blended. Mix in the coconut. Sift the sifted flour with the baking powder and salt, and add this to the creamed mixture, mixing thoroughly. Form the dough into a roll 2 inches in diameter and wrap it in waxed paper. Chill the rolled dough until it is firm. Then cut it into thin slices. Place the slices on an ungreased cookie sheet and bake them at 400° for 10 to 15 minutes.   *Makes 4 1/2 dozen*

Diet hint: The cholesterol-conscious cook will want to use margarine instead of butter for a savings of 34 gm. saturated fat and 283 mg. cholesterol.

	Calories	Carbo-hydrate (gm)	Protein (gm)	Total Fat (gm)	Saturated Fat (gm)	Choles-terol (mg)
Total	2165.6	237.1	33.6	122.8	72.5	535.0
Per Serving	40.1	4.4	0.6	2.3	1.3	9.9

gm=grams; mg=milligrams. Nutritional figures are approximate. Figures are based on findings of U.S. Department of Agriculture.

Chocolate Kisses

3 egg whites
pinch of salt
1/2 tsp. cream of tartar

1 cup granulated
sugar
2 tbsp. cocoa

Beat the egg whites with the salt until they are foamy. Add the cream of tartar and continue beating until they form soft peaks. Then gradually beat in the sugar. Fold in the cocoa, 1 tablespoon at a time. Use a measuring teaspoon to drop level spoons of the mixture onto a non-stick cookie sheet. Bake them at 275° for 20 minutes. Let kisses cool before removing from sheet. Store in dry place. *Makes 9 dozen*

	Calories	Carbo-hydrate (gm)	Protein (gm)	Total Fat (gm)	Saturated Fat (gm)	Choles-terol (mg)
Total	830.0	203.6	13.6	0.6	0.3	0.0
Per Serving	7.7	1.9	0.1	0.0	0.0	0.0

Ginger Cookies

14 1/2 oz. package
gingerbread mix

1/3 cup skim milk

Blend the gingerbread mix with the milk. Form the dough into a firm ball, then flatten it slightly. Wrap the dough with foil or plastic wrap and chill it for at least 2 hours. Then roll the dough to 1/8-inch thick, and cut it with cookie cutters. Lift the cookies with a spatula and place them on a non-stick cookie sheet that has been sprayed with vegetable coating. Bake the cookies in a preheated 375° oven for 5 to 8 minutes. Immediately remove the cookies from the sheet to a wire rack to cool. *Makes 100*

	Calories	Carbo-hydrate (gm)	Protein (gm)	Total Fat (gm)	Saturated Fat (gm)	Choles-terol (mg)
Total	1789.2	326.9	23.7	41.4	12.4	1.7
Per Serving	17.9	3.3	0.2	0.4	0.1	0.0

---

gm=grams; mg=milligrams. Nutritional figures are approximate. Figures are based on findings of U.S. Department of Agriculture.

U.S. Recommended Daily Allowances

TWO CHARTS for Recommended Daily Allowances have been developed by the National Research Council. One chart, reprinted below, is used for
purposes of food labeling only. The figures represent
the *upper limit* of all figures on the full RDA chart. This
means that your food intake can fall somewhat below
these figures without endangering your health.

In this chart, the symbols are:

   g — gram   IU — International Unit
   mg — milligram   mcg — microgram.

When a manufacturer lists (for example) vitamin C as
80% of U.S.RDA on the package label of a food, you
will know that the vitamin C content is 80% of 60mg.

By checking the columns of the full RDA chart (printed on the following pages) you will discover the other
figures for vitamin C and all other nutrients. The recommended figures vary for age and sex, as would be
expected; what is most significant is the stability of the
figures from age eleven to the later years. Knowing
these figures are recommended for good health, you
can see how little your needs for certain types of foods,
and balanced nutritional composition of meals,
change as you age. At the age 50, your body requires
basically what it required in your teens (though calorie
requirements do drop noticeably and protein rises).

	Adults and Children		Adults and Children
Protein	65 g[a]	Vitamin B_6	2.0 mg
Vitamin A	5,000 IU	Folacin	0.4 mg
Vitamin C	60 mg	Vitamin B_{12}	6 mcg
Thiamin	1.5 mg	Phosphorus	1.0 g
Riboflavin	1.7 mg	Iodine	150 mcg
Niacin	20 mg	Magnesium	400 mg
Calcium	1.0 g	Zinc	15 mg
Iron	18 mg	Copper	2 mg
Vitamin D	400 IU	Biotin	0.3 mg
Vitamin E	30 IU	Pantothenic Acid	10 mg

[a] *If protein efficiency ratio of protein is equal to or better than that of
casein, U.S. RDA is 45 g.*

U.S. Recommended Daily Allowances

	(years) From Up to	Weight (kg)	Weight (lbs)	Height (cm)	Height (in)	Calories (kcal)[2]	Protein (g)	Vitamin A Activity (RE)[3]	Vitamin A Activity (IU)	Vitamin D (IU)	Vitamin E Activity[5] (IU)
Infants	0.0-0.5	6	14	60	24	kg × 117	kg × 2.2	420[4]	1,400	400	4
	0.5-1.0	9	20	71	28	kg × 108	kg × 2.0	400	2,000	400	5
Children	1-3	13	28	86	34	1300	23	400	2,000	400	7
	4-6	20	44	110	44	1800	30	500	2,500	400	9
	7-10	30	66	135	54	2400	36	700	3,300	400	10
Males	11-14	44	97	158	63	2800	44	1,000	5,000	400	12
	15-18	61	134	172	69	3000	54	1,000	5,000	400	15
	19-22	67	147	172	69	3000	54	1,000	5,000	400	15
	23-50	70	154	172	69	2700	56	1,000	5,000		15
	51+	70	154	172	69	2400	56	1,000	5,000		15
Females	11-14	44	97	155	62	2400	44	800	4,000	400	10
	15-18	54	119	162	65	2100	48	800	4,000	400	11
	19-22	58	128	162	65	2100	46	800	4,000	400	12
	23-50	58	128	162	65	2000	46	800	4,000		12
	51+	58	128	162	65	1800	46	800	4,000		12
Pregnant						+ 300	+ 30	1,000	5,000	400	15
Lactating						+ 500	+ 20	1,200	6,000	400	15

	Age (years) From Up to	Weight (kg)	Weight (lbs)	Height (cm)	Height (in)	Water-Soluble Vitamins Ascorbic Acid (mg)	Folacin[6] (µg)	Niacin[7] (mg)	Riboflavin (mg)	Thiamin (mg)	Vitamin B_6 (mg)	Vitamin B_{12} (µg)
Infants	0.0-0.5	6	14	60	24	35	50	5	0.4	0.3	0.3	0.3
	0.5-1.0	9	20	71	28	35	50	8	0.6	0.5	0.4	0.3
Children	1-3	13	28	86	34	40	100	9	0.8	0.7	0.6	1.0
	4-6	20	44	110	44	40	200	12	1.1	0.9	0.9	1.5
	7-10	30	66	135	54	40	300	16	1.2	1.2	1.2	2.0
Males	11-14	44	97	158	63	45	400	18	1.5	1.4	1.6	3.0
	15-18	61	134	172	69	45	400	20	1.8	1.5	1.8	3.0
	19-22	67	147	172	69	45	400	20	1.8	1.5	2.0	3.0
	23-50	70	154	172	69	45	400	18	1.6	1.4	2.0	3.0
	51+	70	154	172	69	45	400	16	1.5	1.2	2.0	3.0
Females	11-14	44	97	155	62	45	400	16	1.3	1.2	1.6	3.0
	15-18	54	119	162	65	45	400	14	1.4	1.1	2.0	3.0
	19-22	58	128	162	65	45	400	14	1.4	1.1	2.0	3.0
	23-50	58	128	162	65	45	400	13	1.2	1.0	2.0	3.0
	51+	58	128	162	65	45	400	12	1.1	1.0	2.0	3.0
Pregnant						60	800	+2	+0.3	+0.3	2.5	4.0
Lactating						60	600	+4	+0.5	+0.3	2.5	4.0

	(years)	Weight		Height		Minerals					
	From Up to	(kg)	(lbs)	(cm)	(in)	Calcium (mg)	Phosphorus (mg)	Iodine (µg)	Iron (mg)	Magnesium (mg)	Zinc (mg)
Infants	0.0-0.5	6	14	60	24	360	240	35	10	60	3
	0.5-1.0	9	20	71	28	540	400	45	15	70	5
Children	1-3	13	28	86	34	800	800	60	15	150	10
	4-6	20	44	110	44	800	800	80	10	200	10
	7-10	30	66	135	54	800	800	110	10	250	10
Males	11-14	44	97	158	63	1200	1200	130	18	350	15
	15-18	61	134	172	69	1200	1200	150	18	400	15
	19-22	67	147	172	69	800	800	140	10	350	15
	23-50	70	154	172	69	800	800	130	10	350	15
	51+	70	154	172	69	800	800	110	10	350	15
Females	11-14	44	97	155	62	1200	1200	115	18	300	15
	15-18	54	119	162	65	1200	1200	115	18	300	15
	19-22	58	128	162	65	800	800	100	18	300	15
	23-50	58	128	162	65	800	800	100	18	300	15
	51+	58	128	162	65	800	800	80	10	300	15
Pregnant						1200	1200	125	18+[8]	450	20
Lactating						1200	1200	150	18	450	25

[1] The allowances are intended to provide for individual variations among most normal persons as they live in the United States under usual environmental stresses. Diets should be based on a variety of common foods in order to provide other nutrients for which human requirements have been less well defined.

[2] Kilojoules (KJ) = 4.2 x kcal

[3] Retinol equivalents

[4] Assumed to be all as retinol in milk during the first six months of life. All subsequent intakes are assumed to be one-half as retinol and one-half as β-carotene when calculated from International Units. As retinol equivalents, three-fourths are as retinol and one-fourth as β-carotene.

[5] Total vitamin E activity, estimated to be 80 percent as α-tocopherol and 20 percent other tocopherols.

[6] The folacin allowances refer to dietary sources as determined by Lactobacillus casel assay. Pure forms of folacin may be effective in doses less than one fourth of the RDA.

[7] Although allowances are expressed as niacin, it is recognized that on the average 1 mg of niacin is derived from each 60 mg of dietary tryptophan.

[8] This increased requirement cannot be met by ordinary diets; therefore, the use of supplemental iron is recommended.

Index